THE MASTER ADAPTIVE LEARNER

THE MASTER ADAPTIVE LEARNER

The AMA MedEd Innovation Series: Innovations From the Accelerating Change in Medical Education Consortium

WILLIAM B. CUTRER, MD, MEd
Associate Dean for Undergraduate Medical Education
Vanderbilt University School of Medicine
Nashville, Tennessee

MARTIN V. PUSIC, MD, PhD
Director of the Division of Learning Analytics
Institution for Innovations in Medical Education
New York University School of Medicine
New York, New York

LARRY D. GRUPPEN, PhD
Professor of Learning Health Sciences
Director of the Master of Health Professions Education Program
University of Michigan Medical School
Ann Arbor, Michigan

MAYA M. HAMMOUD, MD, MBA
Professor, Obstetrics and Gynecology
University of Michigan Medical School
Ann Arbor, Michigan
Senior Advisor, Medical Education Innovation
American Medical Association
Chicago, Illinois

SALLY A. SANTEN, MD, PhD
Senior Associate Dean, Evaluation, Assessment and Scholarship
Virginia Commonwealth University School of Medicine
Richmond, Virginia

SERIES EDITORS
Susan E. Skochelak MD, MPH | Kimberly D. Lomis, MD | Maya M. Hammoud, MD, MBA

ELSEVIER

Elsevier
1600 John F. Kennedy Blvd.
Ste 1800
Philadelphia, PA 19103-2899

THE MASTER ADAPTIVE LEARNER   ISBN: 978-0-323-71111-1

Notice

Practitioners and researchers must always rely on their own experience and knowledge in evaluating and using any information, methods, compounds or experiments described herein. Because of rapid advances in the medical sciences, in particular, independent verification of diagnoses and drug dosages should be made. To the fullest extent of the law, no responsibility is assumed by Elsevier, authors, editors or contributors for any injury and/or damage to persons or property as a matter of products liability, negligence or otherwise, or from any use or operation of any methods, products, instructions, or ideas contained in the material herein.

Library of Congress Control Number: 2019949162

Publisher: Elyse O'Grady
Senior Content Development Specialist: Anne Snyder
Publishing Services Manager: Catherine Jackson
Senior Project Manager: Claire Kramer
Design Direction: Brian Salisbury

Printed in the United States of America

Last digit is the print number: 9   8   7   6   5

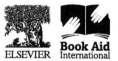 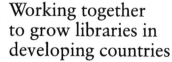

CONTRIBUTORS

Holly G. Atkinson, MD
Clinical Professor and Medical Student
Advisor
CUNY School of Medicine
New York, New York
*Chapter 4: What Are the Four Critical
Personal Characteristics That
Support the Master Adaptive
Learning Process?*

Kathy Boutis, MD, MSc
Professor of Pediatrics
University of Toronto
Toronto, Canada
*Chapter 16: How Does Master
Adaptive Learning Ensure
Optimal Pathways to Clinical
Expertise?*

Julie S. Byerley, MD, MPH
Executive Vice Dean for Education
and Chief Education Officer
University of North Carolina School
of Medicine
Chapel Hill, North Carolina
*Chapter 10: How Will the Master
Adaptive Learner Process Work
at the Bedside?*

Susan M. Cox, MD
Executive Vice Dean of Academics,
Dean's Office
Dell Medical School at the University
of Texas at Austin
Austin, Texas
*Chapter 14: How Can the Master
Adaptive Learner Model Advance
Leadership Development?*

William B. Cutrer, MD, MEd
Associate Dean for Undergraduate
Medical Education
Vanderbilt University School of
Medicine
Nashville, Tennessee
*Chapter 1: Who Is the Master Adaptive
Learner?*

*Chapter 2: How Does Master
Adaptive Learning Advance Expertise
Development?*
*Chapter 16: How Does Master Adaptive
Learning Ensure Optimal Pathways
to Clinical Expertise?*

Michelle M. Daniel, MD, MHPE
Assistant Dean for Curriculum
Clinical Associate Professor of
Emergency Medicine and Learning
Health Sciences
University of Michigan Medical School
Ann Arbor, Michigan
*Chapter 10: How Will the Master
Adaptive Learner Process Work at the
Bedside?*

Nicole M. Deiorio, MD
Associate Dean for Student Affairs
Virginia Commonwealth University
School of Medicine
Richmond, Virginia
*Chapter 12: How Can I Best Support Master
Adaptive Learners Using Coaching?*

Michael Dekhtyar, MEd
Research Associate
American Medical Association
Chicago, Illinois
*Chapter 11: How Does Master Adaptive
Learning Interact With the Learning
Environment?*
*Chapter 15: How Can the Master
Adaptive Learner Model and Health
Systems Science Collaborate to
Improve Health Care?*

Leslie H. Fall, MD
Executive Director and Chief Academic
Officer
Aquifer, Inc.
Geisel School of Medicine at Dartmouth
Hanover, New Hampshire
*Chapter 9: How Will the Master
Adaptive Learner Process Work in
the Classroom?*

Michael J. Fowler, MD
Associate Professor of Medicine
Vanderbilt University School of Medicine
Nashville, Tennessee
*Chapter 3: The Master Adaptive Learner: A
Conceptual Model*

Erica Friedman, MD
Interim Dean
CUNY School of Medicine
New York, New York
*Chapter 4: What Are the Four Critical
Personal Characteristics That Support
the Master Adaptive Learning Process?*

Jed D. Gonzalo, MD, MSc
Associate Professor of Medicine
Associate Dean, Health Systems
Education
Penn State University College of Medicine
Hershey, Pennsylvania
*Chapter 15: How Can the Master
Adaptive Learner Model and Health
Systems Science Collaborate to
Improve Health Care?*

Larry D. Gruppen, PhD
Professor of Learning Health Sciences
Director of the Master of Health
Professions Education Program
University of Michigan Medical School
Ann Arbor, Michigan
*Chapter 11: How Does Master Adaptive
Learning Interact With the Learning
Environment?*

Maya M. Hammoud, MD, MBA
Professor, Obstetrics and Gynecology
University of Michigan Medical School
Ann Arbor, Michigan
Senior Advisor, Medical Education
Innovation
American Medical Association
Chicago, Illinois
*Chapter 14: How Can the Master
Adaptive Learner Model Advance
Leadership Development?*

Vishesh Jain, MD
Medical Student
Vanderbilt University School of
    Medicine
Nashville, Tennessee
*Chapter 1: Who Is the Master Adaptive
    Learner?*

Rosa Lee, MD
Associate Dean of Curriculum and
    Assessment
CUNY School of Medicine
New York, New York
*Chapter 8: How and Where Do I Teach
    My Learners About the Master
    Adaptive Learner Model?*

Amy Miller Juve, MEd, EdD
Director of Education for the
    Department of Anesthesiology
    and Perioperative Medicine
Professional Development and
    Program Improvement
    Specialist, Graduate Medical
    Education
Oregon Health & Science University
    School of Medicine
Portland, Oregon
*Chapter 12: How Can I Best Support
    Master Adaptive Learners Using
    Coaching?*

Lynnea M. Mills, MD
Assistant Professor
University of California, San Francisco,
    School of Medicine
San Francisco, California
*Chapter 13: Can the Master Adaptive
    Learner Process Help the Struggling
    Learner?*

Donald E. Moore, Jr., PhD
Professor of Medical Education and
    Administration
Vanderbilt University School of
    Medicine
Director, Office for Continuing
    Professional Development
Vanderbilt University Medical
    Center
Nashville, Tennessee
*Chapter 3: The Master Adaptive Learner:
    A Conceptual Model*

Patricia S. O'Sullivan, EdD
Professor
University of California, San Francisco,
    School of Medicine
San Francisco, California
*Chapter 13: Can the Master Adaptive
    Learner Process Help the Struggling
    Learner?*

Klara K. Papp, PhD
Graber Term Professor of Health
    Learning
Director of the Center for the
    Advancement of Medical Learning
Case Western Reserve University
    School of Medicine
Cleveland, Ohio
*Chapter 5: Which Cognitive Processes
    Are Involved in the Master Adaptive
    Learner Process?*

Martin V. Pusic, MD, PhD
Director of the Division of Learning
    Analytics
Institution for Innovations in Medical
    Education
New York University School of Medicine
New York, New York
*Chapter 2: How Does Master
    Adaptive Learning Advance
    Expertise Development?*
*Chapter 16: How Does Master Adaptive
    Learning Ensure Optimal Pathways
    to Clinical Expertise?*

Nicole K. Roberts, PhD
Associate Dean, Medical Education and
    Faculty Development
CUNY School of Medicine
New York, New York
*Chapter 8: How and Where Do I Teach
    My Learners About the Master
    Adaptive Learner Model?*
*Chapter 11: How Does Master Adaptive
    Learning Interact With the Learning
    Environment?*

Sally A. Santen, MD, PhD
Senior Associate Dean, Evaluation,
    Assessment and Scholarship
Virginia Commonwealth University
    School of Medicine
Richmond, Virginia

*Chapter 2: How Does Master Adaptive
    Learning Advance Expertise
    Development?*
*Chapter 6: What Is the Role of Self-
    Assessment in the Master Adaptive
    Learner Model?*
*Chapter 7: How Do You Measure the
    Master Adaptive Learner?*
*Chapter 16: How Does Master Adaptive
    Learning Ensure Optimal Pathways
    to Clinical Expertise?*

Stephanie R. Starr, MD
Director, Science of Health Care
    Delivery Education
Associate Professor of Pediatrics
Mayo Clinic Alix School of
    Medicine
Rochester, Minnesota
*Chapter 15: How Can the Master
    Adaptive Learner Model and Health
    Systems Science Collaborate to
    Improve Health Care?*

JK Stringer, PhD
Postdoctoral Fellow
Virginia Commonwealth University
    School of Medicine
Richmond, Virginia
*Chapter 7: How Do You Measure the
    Master Adaptive Learner?*

Patricia A. Thomas, MD
Amasa B. Ford Professor of Medicine
Vice Dean of Medical Education
Case Western Reserve University
    School of Medicine
Cleveland, Ohio
*Chapter 5: Which Cognitive Processes
    Are Involved in the Master Adaptive
    Learner Process?*

Richard N. Van Eck, PhD
Associate Dean for Teaching and
    Learning
Monson Endowed Chair for Medical
    Education
University of North Dakota School of
    Medicine and Health Sciences
Grand Forks, North Dakota
*Chapter 8: How and Where Do I Teach
    My Learners About the Master
    Adaptive Learner Model?*

Alice Walz, MD
Assistant Professor
Medical University of South Carolina
Charleston, South Carolina
*Chapter 1: Who Is the Master Adaptive
    Learner?*

Amy L. Wilson-Delfosse, PhD
Professor of Pharmacology
Associate Dean for Curriculum
Case Western Reserve University
    School of Medicine
Cleveland, Ohio
*Chapter 9: How Will the Master Adaptive
    Learner Process Work in the Classroom?*

Margaret Wolff, MD, MHPE
Associate Professor
University of Michigan Medical School
Ann Arbor, Michigan
*Chapter 6: What Is the Role of Self-
    Assessment in the Master Adaptive
    Learner Model?*
*Chapter 7: How Do You Measure the
    Master Adaptive Learner?*

Katherine R. Zurales, MD, MBA
Resident, Obstetrics and Gynecology
University of Michigan Medical School
Ann Arbor, Michigan
*Chapter 14: How Can the Master
    Adaptive Learner Model Advance
    Leadership Development?*

FOREWORD

The American Medical Association (AMA) Accelerating Change in Medical Education Consortium is working to create new approaches to health professions training to ultimately improve patient outcomes. Our consortium has produced significant innovations in a number of areas that are being adopted at multiple schools. To assist in the dissemination of these innovations, we are pleased to introduce a series of books to aid the adoption of these ideas at additional health professions schools and training programs.

The AMA MedEd Innovation Series will provide practical guidance for local implementation of the education innovations tested and refined by the AMA consortium. This AMA *Master Adaptive Learner* book is the first in this series. Future subjects will include ways for students to add value to health systems, change management for faculty, the implementation of health systems science, and the incorporation of the electronic health record into curriculum.

The Master Adaptive Learner book presents a new model for self-directed learning designed to produce the habits of mind for lifelong learning in medicine. Important skills of curiosity, understanding gaps in knowledge and the need to change, researching and gaining new expertise, and obtaining feedback and self-monitoring are detailed. *The Master Adaptive Learner* framework integrates educational theories and methods of expertise development and provides a practical roadmap for faculty and students who wish to adopt this approach.

We are pleased to offer this first book in the AMA MedEd Innovation Series and look forward to learning about your experience in developing master adaptive learners.

Susan E. Skochelak, MD, MPH
Chief Academic Officer
AMA

We are pleased to present *The Master Adaptive Learner* book. We developed it based on the work of the Master Adaptive Learner special interest group of the American Medical Association's Accelerating Change in Medical Education Consortium. The interest group is comprised of a broad representation from the 32 consortium schools.

This new model details a metacognitive approach to self-regulated learning within health professions education. It builds on the work of Don Moore, Larry Gruppen, Casey White, Joseph Fantone, and many others. The goal is to create a shared mental model and language for the development of Master Adaptive Learners: trainees and clinicians who have mastered the art of learning and who can use that learning skill in optimal service to their patients.

The model emphasizes critical learning skills, including recognizing the need to change and the need to question current practices, planning for how to research and gain new expertise, feedback-seeking and self-monitoring, assessing the effect of the new learning, and finally, candidly assessing whether to advocate for a systematic change based on what was learned.

The Master Adaptive Learner framework is meant to integrate and summarize educational theories and methods of expertise development in ways that make them accessible to educators in the field. This book builds on the Master Adaptive Learner special interest group's work to date and seeks to offer practical tangible suggestions for the implementation and application of the Master Adaptive Learner framework to current undergraduate, graduate, and continuing medical education efforts.

You will note that each of the chapters is framed with a question. The ability to ask good questions is central to recognizing gaps in one's own knowledge, skills, and attitudes, as well as to planning for learning to be completed. Such framing illustrates how we have aspired to "walk the walk" as Master Adaptive Learners ourselves in creating this book. The book is not formatted to be read serially; instead, we encourage you to consider the first three chapters, which define the model, and then pick and choose according to your needs and interests.

We hope that you find this book helpful as you seek to improve the learning and adaptive expertise development of yourselves and your learners.

William B. Cutrer, MD, MEd
Martin V. Pusic, MD, PhD
Larry D. Gruppen, PhD
Maya M. Hammoud, MD, MBA
Sally A. Santen, MD, PhD

ACKNOWLEDGMENTS

The editors and authors of this book would like to thank Katie Pajak of the American Medical Association (AMA) for her project management. Without her, this book would not exist. We would like to thank Victoria Stagg Elliott, also of the AMA, for her copyediting and catching our misspellings and misused words. Kevin Heckman of the AMA and project manager of the AMA MedEd Innovation Series gets our gratitude for his support of this book. Thank you to the members of the Master Adaptive Learner working group of the AMA Accelerating Change in Medical Education Consortium.

In addition, we thank Paul Mazmanian, who provided input on Chapter 3, and Grace Huang, who provided input on Chapter 5.

And we would like to thank those who reviewed the chapters:

John Andrews
Katherine Fedder
Rachel Gottlieb-Smith
Sarah Hartley
Deborah Heath
Janet Lindsley

Kimberly Lomis
Kyriaki Marti
Anne Messman
Elizabeth Nelson
Robin Ohkagawa
Timothy Reeder

Nicole Roberts
LuAnn Wilkerson
Margaret Wolff
Mohammad Zaher

CONTENTS

THE MASTER ADAPTIVE LEARNER

Who Is the Master Adaptive Learner?

William B. Cutrer, MD, MEd; Vishesh Jain, MD; and Alice Walz, MD

LEARNING OBJECTIVES

1. Describe the characteristics of the ideal master adaptive learner.
2. Compare behaviors, skills, and attitudes used by a master adaptive learner with those of a less effective learner.
3. Identify characteristics within the learning environment that foster learning.
4. Discuss potential outcomes that demonstrate master adaptive learning.

CHAPTER OUTLINE

CHAPTER SUMMARY

Health care is provided in many different environments, including both inpatient and outpatient settings. Often the clinical teams are composed of members at various levels of training, which can provide both challenges and opportunities for effective care delivery and learning in the workplace. At its best, the clinical team can demonstrate that individuals across the undergraduate-graduate-continuing medical education spectrum can learn with and from each other, ultimately meeting the needs and improving the care of the patients they are serving. In this chapter, we describe the ideal master adaptive learner who utilizes a metacognitive approach to self-regulated learning that leads to the development and demonstration of adaptive expertise. The Master Adaptive Learner model offers a common language and shared mental model to facilitate conversation and learning among individuals across the training continuum.

INTRODUCTION

Before we explore the ideal master adaptive learner and supportive learning environment, let us first begin by considering a more typical scenario.

"Typical Day" Vignette

Lindsey Wong is a medical student who is (properly) excited to be on her pediatrics clerkship. She is working with attending physician Dr. Ludovico Smith and resident Dr. Nia Bloomberg on a general pediatrics inpatient ward team. In the morning, Lindsey joins Dr. Bloomberg in the workroom before rounds.

Lindsey: "Good morning! Were there any new patients overnight that I could pick up?"

Dr. Bloomberg: "Absolutely! We got slammed on top of our huge census. How many patients can you see?"

Lindsey: "I'm comfortable with my two patients, so let me pick up one today."

Dr. Bloomberg: "Why don't you see this 11-month-old with cough for 5 days that got worse yesterday. I'd love to go over the important factors of his case with you, but I'm already behind on prepping all my notes for rounds. I need time just to get my work done."

Lindsey reviews Simon's chart. She sees that his respiratory rate has progressively gotten higher and wonders at what point he might need extra respiratory support. She starts to ask Dr. Bloomberg what criteria she should look for in impending respiratory failure but remembers Dr. Bloomberg is too busy to discuss the case. For her two current patients, Lindsey reviews notes since yesterday and prints their laboratory results and medications. She remembers one of her patients has copious data from her intensive care unit stay with diabetic ketoacidosis. Lindsey thinks to herself, "I hope Dr. Smith won't ask me about these electrolytes. I don't know why they were so off, and I won't have time to look it up." Avoiding that thought, she heads to Simon's room first. Looking at her notes, she reads that Simon's cough worsened yesterday along with a new fever. She hears him wheezing even before she enters the room. Looking up from the notes, she sees Simon's mom rising from a slumber.

Simon's mom: "Are you part of Simon's team?"

Lindsey: "Yes, I'm the medical student who will be helping care for him."

Simon's mom: "I'm exhausted after being in the ER all day, but I have some questions now. Simon's breathing pretty fast, and sometimes I hear him wheezing; does he have asthma? Why isn't he on antibiotics yet?"

As they talk through everything, Lindsey starts to get nervous that she is not sure of the answers and will not have time to see her other patients.

Lindsey: "Well, I really need to get to rounds, so I'll have to step out now."

Simon's mom: "I still have other questions. Will someone come back to talk with me?"

Lindsey (walking through the door): "The whole team will be back later this morning."

Lindsey looks at her watch and realizes she will not have time to see her other patients. She rushes back to the workroom to find Dr. Smith talking with Dr. Bloomberg.

Dr. Smith: "I hear you saw our new patient Simon? Just give me the high points now."

Lindsey feels flustered, but she pulls out her papers and prepares to give her presentation. She is not sure what to say or leave out, but she decides to start with her one-liner.

Lindsey: "Simon is an 11-month-old boy with no significant past medical history who presents with 5 days of cough, worsening yesterday with fever. He is now having trouble breathing and . . ."

Dr. Smith: "How high was the fever?"

Lindsey apologizes and starts looking through her papers. Dr. Smith looks at Dr. Bloomberg impatiently.

Dr. Bloomberg: "100.6, tachypneic at 65 bpm, satting at 92%. He has respiratory distress with nasal flaring and wheezing on exam. His older sister had a URI last week. Most likely severe bronchiolitis from RSV, though it could be . . ."

Dr. Smith: "Great. Give him oral dexamethasone, IV fluids, and some oxygen. Let's go see him."

Dr. Bloomberg thinks she remembers reading something about systemic glucocorticoids in bronchiolitis, but she focuses on writing down Dr. Smith's orders because they are in a rush.

Lindsey: "Simon's mom was wondering about antibiotics, in case it's bacterial?"

Dr. Smith: "No, don't even think about it. Antibiotic stewardship, Lindsey. Steroids, fluids, and oxygen. That's the way I've always done it, and I've been around long enough to know it works."

Many of us likely sympathize with the experiences of Lindsey, Dr. Bloomberg, and Dr. Smith as described in the vignette. Similar encounters are likely occurring in a variety of clinical settings. Many opportunities for learning were missed in the interest of "just getting the work done." When considering the student and team in the previous vignette, but also individuals at all levels within the health care system at large, the topic of learning is a critical one. Each person in this vignette has learning needs that were suboptimally addressed. The absence of a shared mental model for their workplace learning prevented both individual and collective growth. Despite frequent calls for physicians to be lifelong learners, evidence does not support the idea that physicians currently learn and practice in such a manner, or at least not optimally.[1] Physicians routinely continue to use existing solutions to problems they have previously solved rather than approaching patient care and health care system challenges in the context of new and ongoing learning. There is a gap between what is known in literature and the current practice of many physicians.[2] This gap must be addressed with more effective identification of knowledge and skill deficiencies and with targeted learning to address them.

Additionally, physicians face a second gap between their current knowledge and novel challenges presented in the health care environment. Clinicians need adaptive expertise to recognize when the routine approach will not work and to reframe the problem in a way that allows for the incorporation of new ideas and concepts (learning) and the creation of new solutions (innovation) when appropriate. We describe adaptive expertise more thoroughly in Chapter 2.

A different type of learner, a master adaptive learner—described as an "individual who utilizes the metacognitive approach to self-regulated learning that leads to adaptive expertise development"—is needed.[3] The Master Adaptive Learner (MAL) model brings together multiple strands from the general and medical education bodies of literature.[4] It provides a common language and framework to facilitate self-regulated learning in individuals throughout the spectrum from medical school through residency training and into clinical practice. Individuals of any level can develop the skills and process of master adaptive learning, and once they do, they can synergistically reinforce each other's learning and development.

The MAL model (Fig. 1.1) is described in far more detail throughout the subsequent chapters of the book, but we begin here with a high-level overview of its important components. The four gears of the MAL process form the center of the model representing the required phases of activity. The MAL model serves as a combination of staged physician learning and self-regulated learning.[5,6]

Planning is the first phase and includes three steps. The learner must first identify a gap in her practice, which could be one of knowledge, skill, or attitude. In the course of a given day in the clinical environment, learners ranging from students to practicing physicians likely encounter many such gaps.[7,8] Step 2 within the planning phase is prioritizing one of those gaps as an opportunity for learning. Step 3 then involves searching for appropriate resources necessary for learning. Junior learners often skip the planning phase in the interest of "just getting to the work of learning." The planning phase is important, however, in ensuring that the learning efforts are aligned with areas in need of practice change or improvement. The planning phase includes several critical skills (questioning, prioritizing, goal setting, and searching for resources).

Learning is the second phase in the MAL model. In this phase, individuals engage in the difficult process of meaningful learning. The learning phase includes the critical appraisal of learning resources to ensure time spent engaging in learning is appropriately focused. It has been said that, "Learning is deeper and more durable when it is effortful."[9,10] Learners in this phase are encouraged to use

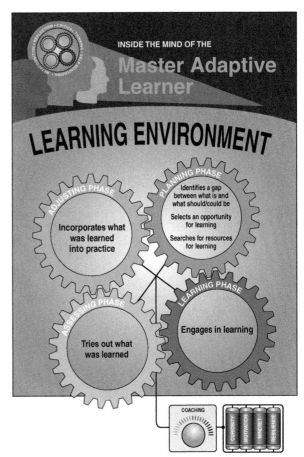

Fig. 1.1 Characteristics and contexts that allow the Master Adaptive Learner process. (From Cutrer WB, Atkinson HG, Friedman E, et al. Exploring the characteristics and context that allow Master Adaptive Learners to thrive. *Med Teach.* 2018; 40[8]:791-796.)

active learning strategies, as opposed to superficial approaches such as reading and rereading, highlighting and underlining, and cramming, all of which have repeatedly been shown to be ineffective in leading to long-term understanding and retention.[11] We make the claim throughout this book that if clinicians are to learn effectively, they must have explicitly mastered the scientific principles of learning (the "master" in master adaptive learning).

The third phase focuses on **assessing.** In this phase, learners try out what they have learned by comparing and contrasting their self-assessment with external feedback. This combination, termed *informed self-assessment* (see Chapter 6), supports learning by disciplining and aligning gut feelings and in-the-moment judgments with as much available data and evidence as possible. By pairing unguided self-assessment with external feedback, learners are able to continue to develop and calibrate their self-assessment skills while also benefiting directly from the external perspective.[12]

The final phase of the MAL model is **adjusting**. This phase involves making actual changes to one's practice based on the new learning that has occurred. For students, this can include incorporation of new ideas and understanding into their developing skill base, including clinical reasoning, approaches to given patient problems, and the creation and presentation of patient-specific assessments and plans. For practicing physicians, the adjusting phase involves changes to their own strategies for patient care. This can include everything from small changes, such as the selection of a different antibiotic for a given infection, to large changes, such as revising their approach to an entire category of patients. Skills necessary in this phase include the ability to differentiate how the new learning can and should be applied, as well as change management skills needed to implement change at the appropriate level of care provision (individual vs. health care system).

Readers familiar with the Plan-Do-Study-Act (PDSA) cycle from the field of quality improvement will recognize significant overlap with the MAL model.[13] This was intentional. Personal improvement by clinicians often goes hand-in-hand with health care system improvement. The original creators of the MAL model encourage learners to consider constant PDSA cycles of themselves as learners with their own practice gaps (i.e., cycles through the MAL process).

Learning does not happen in isolation. There are significant aspects of the learner's context that also impact the MAL process, as do other learner characteristics. Readers will note four batteries in the lower right corner of the MAL model in Fig. 1.1: curiosity, motivation, mindset, and resilience (see Chapter 4). These learner characteristics provide the power necessary for the learner to enter into and progress through the MAL process effectively. The concept of coaching is represented in the MAL model as a rheostat. While learning can and absolutely does occur without coaching, we firmly believe that learning will be more efficient and, importantly, more effective and coordinated with a coach's involvement (see Chapter 12).

Finally, it is vitally important to recognize that the clinical environment for learning is very different from the more controlled environment of the medical school classroom or the continuing medical education course. As evidenced by the initial "typical day" vignette in this chapter, as well as the revised vignette that follows, the learning environment can strongly impact the individual's learning in both positive and negative ways (see Chapter 11). Much has been written about the hidden curriculum within medical education, which can be both positive and negative for a given culture.[14] Certain learning environments will support and foster effective learning and improvement of patient care, while others unfortunately will impede learning and lead to bad habits.

WHO ARE OUR LEARNERS?

Within the vignette, there are three levels of medical learners: the medical student, the resident, and the attending physician. (The patients and families, such as the mother of Simon, are also learners-teachers but are not specifically addressed in this book.) While the MAL process applies to learners of every level, the focus of adaptive learning may be different for each of them. For example, the medical student still has to learn many aspects of basic care of a child with bronchiolitis. The resident is learning to supervise the medical student while consolidating and expanding her own learning. Finally, the attending physician must also adapt his learning to the trainees, while both maintaining current knowledge within his medical specialty and considering the overall system's impact on providing care for this type of patient. All three need to be master adaptive learners.

Using the previous vignette as an example and looking at the different phases of the MAL process, we could imagine how the learning of each member of this team could emphasize different stages of the MAL process. The medical student should be spending a significant amount of time in the planning and learning phases, developing clinical reasoning and illness scripts using evidence-based medicine. The resident in this scenario could be in the assessing phase, seeking direct feedback from her attending physician. Given that trainees and clinicians are historically poor at self-assessment (see Chapter 6), feedback within this phase is key to her development. The attending physician should be examining clinical practice guidelines from his specialty and, within the adjusting phase, changing his clinical practice. All four phases of the MAL process will apply to all levels of learners, though different learners may spend a larger proportion of time in a specific phase.

Now, we will examine a revised version of the "typical day" vignette to highlight how the MAL model and explicit consideration of the learning environment can improve learning for each member of the team.

Revised Vignette

Lindsey: "Good morning! Were there any new patients overnight that I could pick up?"

Dr. Bloomberg: "Absolutely! We got slammed on top of our huge census. How many patients can you see?"

Lindsey: "I'm comfortable with my two patients, so I could certainly pick up one patient."

Dr. Bloomberg: "Sounds good. I would like to get you to four patients by the end of this rotation. Why don't you pick up this 11-month-old—Simon? He's had a cough for 5 days that got worse yesterday with a fever. Before you go see him, what would be on your differential based on that information?"

[Note Dr. Bloomberg's explicit expectation and goal setting, reference to the patient by name rather than disease, and prompt question that can serve as an advance organizer to help prompt learner thinking.]

Lindsey names a few possibilities but struggles to think of more. She also tells Dr. Bloomberg that she is unsure what to look for when she examines Simon and worries that she will not be able to put the pieces together before rounds. Dr. Bloomberg quickly assesses Lindsey's knowledge base of the clinical presentation of bronchiolitis, and helps Lindsey expand her differential diagnosis and prioritize what to ask. Dr. Bloomberg would like to discuss the clinical features of severe respiratory distress in an infant, but she tells Lindsey that she is behind on prepping for rounds. She recommends that Lindsey read more about this complaint this afternoon, so they can discuss management together in more detail later.

[Note how Dr. Bloomberg's coaching helps Lindsey prioritize.]

After reviewing her three patients' charts, Lindsey prints their laboratory results and medications. One of her patients has copious data from her intensive care unit stay with diabetic ketoacidosis. Lindsey hopes to ask Dr. Smith about the strange electrolyte results, which she does not understand. She quickly sees the patients she knows and then heads to Simon's room. Before entering, she checks her watch to see how long she has. Simon's mom is sleeping, and Lindsey wonders whether to wake her because she will not have time to answer questions anyway. Starting her physical examination, she hears Simon wheezing. Looking up, she sees that Simon's mother is now awake.

[Note Lindsey's metacognition and consideration of communication skills.]

Simon's mother: "Are you part of Simon's team?"

Lindsey: "Yes, my name is Lindsey. I'm the medical student who will be caring for him. I sadly don't have much time now, but I'll be back with the rest of the primary team within 2 hours."

Lindsey encourages Simon's mom to write down her questions and takes her leave. She rushes back to the workroom to find Dr. Smith talking with Dr. Bloomberg.

Dr. Smith: "I hear you saw our new patient, Simon? I'll let you get situated while Dr. Bloomberg tells me about another patient, and then you can present. We're a little pressed for time, so just give me the high points: your one-liner, vitals, key symptoms and signs, and your assessment and plan. Does that sound all right to you? Any questions right now before you review your notes?"

[Note Dr. Smith's modeling of expectation setting and prioritization.]

Lindsey reveals her limited time in Simon's room and her uncertainty about the electrolyte results on her other patient. Dr. Smith asks Dr. Bloomberg if she could teach Lindsey about the latter as well as some tips for pre-rounding. As Dr. Bloomberg finishes up, Lindsey pulls out her papers and prepares to give her presentation.

Lindsey: "I never know exactly what to include, so your guidance was helpful. I would also love your feedback on whether I still included too much information or not enough. Simon is an 11-month-old boy with no significant past medical history who presents with 5 days of cough, worsening yesterday with fever. He was tachypneic at 65 bpm, satting at 92%, febrile to 100.6. On exam, he has nasal flaring and wheezing. It sounds like bronchiolitis, but it could be asthma or pneumonia . . . maybe we should get an x-ray? I feel good about the rest, but I'm not sure about the plan."

[Note Lindsey's feedback-seeking behavior and willingness to admit areas for growth.]

Dr. Smith: "Great, that was the right level of detail and a good differential. Dr. Bloomberg, anything to add?"

[Note Dr. Smith's specific feedback to Lindsey related to level of detail and differential diagnosis.]

Dr. Bloomberg: "Just that Simon's older sister had a URI last week. For the x-ray, what would you look for, Lindsey?"

Lindsey: "An opacity, like a pneumonia?"

Dr. Smith: "Not a bad thought, but a chest x-ray is pretty low-yield if bronchiolitis is the most likely diagnosis. How much do you know about bronchiolitis?"

[Note Dr. Smith's use of questioning to identify gaps and diagnose the learner.]

Lindsey outlines what she remembers from talking with Dr. Bloomberg and asks if it is accurate. In return, Dr. Smith makes a few clarifications and suggests that Lindsey read specifically about diagnostic evaluation for bronchiolitis. He then gives a 1-minute mini-lecture on management for bronchiolitis.

Dr. Smith: "Anyway, I usually treat a patient like this with oral dexamethasone, IV fluids, and some oxygen. Does that sound all right to both of you?"

[Note Dr. Smith's use of informed self-assessment and feedback seeking.]

Dr. Bloomberg: "I think the most recent guidelines suggest that systemic glucocorticoids don't improve outcomes in bronchiolitis. Sometimes a trial of inhaled bronchodilators can help, though."

Dr. Smith: "Interesting. I don't recall hearing that, but I may have missed it. Why don't you send us those guidelines for bronchiolitis management, and I'll do a quick literature search on the effectiveness of bronchodilator therapy. Then we can all meet this afternoon to discuss together. For now, we should get moving, so let's plan on at least starting with the IV fluids and respiratory support."

[Note Dr. Smith's growth mindset, willingness to learn, and critical appraisal of learning resources.]

On their way to Simon's room, Lindsey expresses her concern to Dr. Bloomberg that she has too many topics to look up, from diabetic ketoacidosis to a differential for cough. Dr. Bloomberg helps her prioritize based on where Lindsey feels weakest and what would be most helpful for her to know soon.

[Note Dr. Bloomberg's use of coaching to help with the prioritization step of the planning phase.]

As you might have noticed, the characteristics of the learners and the context for learning were significantly different in this second vignette (Table 1.1). We aimed to highlight the potentially very positive aspects of certain learner characteristics and the learning environment and their subsequent impact on the individuals' function as master adaptive learners. Let us now consider how the MAL process can differ across developmental levels.

Medical Students

Medical students hold a peculiar/wondrous/awkward/legitimate/sometimes peripheral position within the clinical workplace. Their primary objective is to learn and develop their skills, yet they must also contribute to the team's work. Medical students are expected to have knowledge and skill gaps because they lack knowledge and skill compared with other clinical learners, but they are also being assessed on those very domains. Furthermore, these expectations vary dramatically over the course of their clinical training but may not match their performance trajectory.[15] These conflicting pressures combined with students'

vulnerable status in the team make their motivation crucial. Students may be motivated extrinsically by attainment of positive assessments and would in that case be more reluctant to display their deficiencies. Conversely, curiosity can be a powerful driver for learning independently of the environment and learning culture. While in the "typical day" vignette, Lindsey is afraid to discuss a patient's electrolyte results; in the revised version her strong curiosity and intrinsic motivation drive her to ask Dr. Smith about them. Overlaid on this student's curiosity and motivation is her mindset regarding her intelligence and capacity for learning.

Because medical students will always have knowledge and skill gaps, depending on the motivation and resiliency of the student, these gaps may be framed by the student as failure. Without strong resilience and intrinsic motivation, a failure may be more likely to shut a student's mind down and induce avoidance of future learning opportunities. Support from supervisors, especially residents who spend the most time with students, can help them move forward through the MAL process rather than getting stuck. In the revised vignette, Dr. Bloomberg helps Lindsey on multiple occasions, such as setting goals for the number of patients to follow and prioritizing knowledge gaps to address.

Reviewing the learning and knowledge gained on the part of the student is another method of support. For example, Dr. Bloomberg confirmed the accuracy of Lindsey's understanding of bronchiolitis, as well as her recognition that Simon was in mild respiratory distress. In contrast to the missed opportunities in the first vignette, Lindsey is empowered by the team's shared mental model for her learning and its inclusion in the clinical workflow. Furthermore, her self-inculcation of curiosity and growth mindset enables her to gain more knowledge via concrete learning goals.

Residents

For residents, several issues that can affect their learning and performance, as well as that of their medical students, are important to highlight. Patient encounters form the foundation of clinical learning in residency, representing a formalized shift in the learning environment to be fully workplace based, rather than largely classroom based. This change opens up multiple external factors that can influence a resident's motivation and learning. Conflicting pressures exist because residents are both the central consumers of medical education in a patient interaction as they build their illness scripts and expertise and the individuals responsible for the actual delivery of medical care to patients. This is a key piece of a resident's ongoing professional identity formation and requires that the resident balance the needs of patients with his own learning.

TABLE 1.1 Vignette Comparison.

Behavior	"Typical Day" Vignette	Revised Vignette
Medical Student		
Planning	Hopes to hide knowledge gaps	Explicitly tracks knowledge gaps and seeks help
Learning	Passive approaches (e.g., unstructured reading)	Emphasizes active learning
Assessing	Avoids feedback opportunities	Seeks feedback and calibration
Adjusting	Slow to adapt studying habits away from test-oriented studying	Deliberate practice of clinical skills
Resident		
Planning	Reactive to clinical learning environment	Intentionally proactive
Learning	Prioritizes work over learning	Looks for opportunities to synergize work with learning (e.g., teaching)
Assessing	Sees quality improvement as separate from self-improvement	Demonstrates feedback-seeking behavior
Adjusting	Low levels of patient advocacy or self-advocacy	Change agent; uses high/intimate/detailed system knowledge to enact change
Attending		
Planning	Knowledge/skill gaps identified through self-assessment alone.	Growth/open mindset; informed self-assessment for identifying gaps
Learning	CME siloed structure	Active approaches
Assessing	Rare, episodic	Continuous feedback-seeking behavior
Adjusting	Accepts system as it is; emphasizes routinized practice; adversarial	Health care system aware; collaborative; interdisciplinary; innovative

CME, Continuing medical education.

Practicing in his chosen clinical medical specialty should foster curiosity to learn all aspects of the field. However, this deep dive into a single specialty has a difficult learning curve, which can be disorienting when coupled with a potentially unfamiliar hospital system or city, or both.

Residents are additionally responsible for extensive documentation in the electronic health record for each patient encounter. This administrative burden has been associated with higher rates of burnout and may erode some of the inquisitiveness a resident possessed during earlier medical training.[16] Without strong resilience, while working long hours with high documentation demands, residents may begin to view subsequent clinical encounters as taxing units of work, rather than focusing on the unique aspects of a patient's narrative. This change in attitude can be costly to their development and impede their role in medical student learning.

In the "typical day" vignette, Dr. Bloomberg feels overwhelmed with her necessary documentation for rounds and subsequently is unable to help Lindsey with her identified knowledge gap. This results in a missed opportunity for Lindsey to learn, as well as for Dr. Bloomberg to further develop herself as an educator. In the revised narrative, Dr. Bloomberg does a better job by conveying short learning points, preparing for rounds, and setting up a plan for future learning opportunities. Efforts should be made to balance documentation and bedside clinical care responsibilities to maximize learning opportunities for residents. This type of effort could produce changes resulting from an effective adjusting phase in the resident's own development as a clinician.

Residents may be hesitant to view themselves as teachers for medical students, feeling that they may not have sufficient experience or knowledge to pass along to someone more junior in her medical training. While some level of discomfort with uncertainty among trainees is expected, residents can capitalize on the opportunity to model for medical students the importance of recognizing and acknowledging one's own knowledge gaps, seeking answers to clinical questions, and asking for feedback from more senior members of the team.[17,18]

As shown in the revised vignette, Dr. Bloomberg could first start the conversation by assessing Lindsey's level of knowledge, perhaps by asking, "What have you learned thus far about bronchiolitis?" or "Describe for me how you would tell the patient's mother about bronchiolitis and our expectations for the patient's care." This would allow the resident to better plan targeted teaching efforts. Moreover, teaching medical students will consolidate the resident's knowledge and identify her own knowledge gaps.

Practicing Physicians and Faculty

For the faculty member, Dr. Smith, several important aspects could be examined. In the "typical day" vignette, it is obvious that Dr. Smith grounds his practice patterns in experience rather than adjusting his practice based on up-to-date clinical practice recommendations. He displays his rigidity by stating "That's the way I've always done it" when discussing treatment care plans, which closes the door for any additional conversation and learning. Conversely, in the revised vignette Dr. Smith is open to discussing treatment regimens different from his own, which allows all the learners on the team, himself included, to examine the primary literature and updated guidelines. If this vignette were to continue, we would likely see Dr. Smith adjusting his practice pattern after further discussion with his team regarding the evidence surrounding the lack of efficacy of steroids for bronchiolitis. As the field of medicine continues to evolve, it is imperative that practicing physicians keep up with the latest advances in medical care. The effective faculty member should emphasize that learning is a lifelong habit by fostering inquisitiveness and modeling adjustment to practice when new evidence comes forth (see Chapter 2).

Finally, Dr. Smith may not realize how his attitude in this encounter may inhibit learning. By saying he wants to hear "just the high points," Lindsey and the other team members may perceive that he is rushed and uninvested in their work and learning. Lindsey, who already feels flustered and who had already identified a gap in her knowledge, may be more hesitant to ask questions. In the revised vignette, Dr. Smith is a more effective educational leader. By setting shared expectations and listening attentively without interruption, he opens the door for additional learning opportunities for the medical student, the resident, and himself.

CONCLUSION

Adaptive expertise is needed in health care today to allow for the effective delivery of high-quality health care. The MAL model provides common language and a shared mental model to help learners at all stages of training develop the habits and approaches to learning that will lead to the development and demonstration of this adaptive expertise. The ideal master adaptive learners are those individuals who embody this process to continually improve themselves as learners and clinicians.

TAKE-HOME POINTS

1. Clinical teams are composed of learners at many different levels.
2. The Master Adaptive Learner model is a learner-centered metacognitive framework.
3. Learners at different levels of training have different practice gaps but can address them with effective learning.
4. The learning environment impacts the ability of those involved to learn effectively.

QUESTIONS FOR FURTHER THOUGHT

1. What attributes of the practice of medicine today would benefit from clinicians becoming master adaptive learners?
2. Do current medical students, residents, and clinical faculty typically learn like master adaptive learners? Why or why not?
3. How might a student learner adapt to function differently in various learning environments? How might a master adaptive learner interact with a suboptimal learning environment?

ANNOTATED BIBLIOGRAPHY

1. Cutrer WB, Miller B, Pusic MV, et al. Fostering the development of Master Adaptive Learners: a conceptual model to guide skill acquisition in medical education. *Acad Med.* 2017;92(1):70-75.
   The authors provide the original description of the Master Adaptive Learner model.
2. Regehr G, Mylopoulos M. Maintaining competence in the field: learning about practice, through practice, in practice. *J Contin Educ Health Prof.* 2008;28(suppl 1):S19-S23.
   The authors examine problematic assumptions about clinical self-directed lifelong learning behaviors.
3. McGlynn EA, Asch SM, Adams J, et al. The quality of health care delivered to adults in the United States. *N Engl J Med.* 2003;348(26):2635-2645.
   McGlynn and colleagues demonstrate substantial gaps between national guidelines of recommended care and actual clinical practice, indicating a need for continued learning and adjustment far beyond residency.
4. Cutrer WB, Atkinson HG, Friedman E, et al. Exploring the characteristics and context that allow Master Adaptive Learners to thrive. *Med Teach.* 2018;40(8):791-796.
   The authors examine factors within learners and in their learning environment that shape their learning process.

REFERENCES

1. Regehr G, Mylopoulos M. Maintaining competence in the field: learning about practice, through practice, in practice. *J Contin Educ Health Prof.* 2008;28(suppl 1):S19-S23.
2. Mylopoulos M, Brydges R, Woods NN, Manzone J, Schwartz DL. Preparation for future learning: a missing competency in health professions education? *Med Educ.* 2016;50(1):115-123.
3. McGlynn EA, Asch SM, Adams J, et al. The quality of health care delivered to adults in the United States. *N Engl J Med.* 2003;348(26):2635-2645.
4. Cutrer WB, Atkinson HG, Friedman E, et al. Exploring the characteristics and context that allow Master Adaptive Learners to thrive. *Med Teach.* 2018;40(8):791-796.
5. Cutrer WB, Miller B, Pusic MV, et al. Fostering the development of Master Adaptive Learners: a conceptual model to guide skill acquisition in medical education. *Acad Med.* 2017;92(1):70-75.
6. Moore DE, Green JS, Gallis HA. Achieving desired results and improved outcomes: integrating planning and assessment throughout learning activities. *J Contin Educ Health Prof.* 2009;29(1):1-15.
7. White CB, Gruppen LD, Fantone JC. Self-regulated learning in medical education. In: Swanwick T, eds. *Understanding Medical Education: Evidence, Theory, and Practice.* 2nd ed. West Sussex, UK: Wiley-Blackwell; 2013:201-211.
8. Magrabi F, Coiera EW, Westbrook JI, Gosling AS, Vickland V. General practitioners' use of online evidence during consultations. *Int J Med Inform.* 2005;74(1):1-2.
9. Festinger L. *A Theory of Cognitive Dissonance.* Stanford, CA: Stanford University Press; 1957.
10. Brown PC, Roediger HL, McDaniel MA. *Make It Stick: The Science of Successful Learning.* Cambridge, MA: Belknap Press of Harvard University Press; 2014.
11. Schmidt RA, Bjork RA. New conceptualizations of practice: common principles in three paradigms suggest new concepts for training. *Psychol Sci.* 1992;3(4):207-218.
12. Rohrer D, Pashler H. Recent research on human learning challenges conventional instructional strategies. *Educ Res.* 2010;39(5):406-412.
13. Sargeant J, Armson H, Chesluk B, et al. The processes and dimensions of informed self-assessment: a conceptual model. *Acad Med.* 2010;85(7):1212-1220.
14. Taylor MJ, McNicholas C, Nicolay C, Darzi A, Bell D, Reed JE. Systematic review of the application of the plan-do-study-act method to improve quality in healthcare. *BMJ Qual Saf.* 2014;23(4):290-298.
15. Hafferty FW. Beyond curriculum reform: confronting medicine's hidden curriculum. *Acad Med.* 1998;73(4):403-407.
16. Hauer KE, Lucey CR. Core clerkship grading: the illusion of objectivity. *Acad Med.* 2019;94(4):469-472. doi:10.1097/ACM.0000000000002413.
17. Robertson SL, Robinson MD, Reid A. Electronic health record effects on work-life balance and burnout within the I^3 population collaborative. *J Grad Med Educ.* 2017;9(4):479-484.
18. Busari JO, Scherpbier AJ, Van der Vleuten C, Essed GE. Residents' perception of their role in teaching undergraduate students in the clinical setting. *Med Teach.* 2000;22(4):348-353.

2

How Does Master Adaptive Learning Advance Expertise Development?

Martin V. Pusic, MD, PhD; William B. Cutrer, MD, MEd; and Sally A. Santen, MD, PhD

LEARNING OBJECTIVES

1. Describe adaptive expertise and how we develop it.
2. Define preparation for future learning as a core conceptualization for master adaptive learning.
3. Describe the intersection of master adaptive learning as a process model, as traits of an individual, as a metacognitive schema, and as a philosophy.

CHAPTER OUTLINE

CHAPTER SUMMARY

In this chapter, we first describe adaptive expertise as a new orienting goal for clinical training. We then describe how instructional designs can be altered to foster the development of adaptive expertise, with a particular emphasis on preparation for future learning— in essence, learning to optimally learn. Finally, we argue that the combination of the advanced learning target (adaptive expertise) accomplished by an advanced learning process (master adaptive learning) can result in a clinician with a complement of ingrained beneficial learning predispositions: a master adaptive learner.

Vignette

Vig and Emily are medical students on their emergency medicine clerkship. They just got back their clerkship knowledge examination scores. Vig scored much higher than Emily.

Emily: "How did that work? We always score the same."

Vig: "It's my superior emergency mind."

Emily: "Right. Like at that simulation where you held the laryngoscope backwards."

Vig (after an awkward pause): "Hey, we agreed to never talk about that."

Emily (chagrined): "Sorry, you're right. I'm just frustrated by this score—I didn't get any time to study."

Vig: "All good. Study time might actually be the difference. My preceptor let me off early from my last two shifts so that I could study. It really paid off."

Emily: "Not mine! Dr. Exemplar kept me right to the end of each shift, even when it wasn't busy. Even that would have been fine except the stuff I learned was about 'adaptive expertise' and was useless for the test."

Vig: "What do you mean by adaptive expertise?"

Emily: "Do you have all day? But, it was really interesting—about how to become a master learner. But clearly the people writing the exam aren't impressed with my master learner knowledge."

Vig: "But aren't we already master learners? Give me a topic, and some time, and watch me nail the exams."

Emily: "This is different. It's like he wanted me to relearn how to learn. How to learn for my patients. It was interesting and all, but it sure feels like I'm a malaligned learner right now."

WE NEED TO TARGET A NEW TYPE OF EXPERTISE

In Fig. 2.1, we present a simplified version of the popular Dreyfus model of expertise development.[1] In the usual version of this model learners start as novices whose legitimate participation is peripheral. They are not allowed to carry out any of the acts characteristic of the expert. Within a cognitive apprenticeship, learners progress with supports (also termed *scaffolds*) from instructors and the learning environment until they can be entrusted to practice in an unsupervised, independent manner. But what exactly is the expertise we are after? This is a complex question that we can begin to approach by considering an important tension: efficient care compared with innovative care.

One type of target clinical expertise is highly efficient and reliable—the automatic expert shown in Fig. 2.1. This type of expert can carry out her tasks in a routinized manner. She assesses the case quickly, understands deeply, and comes to action rapidly because she has a wealth of experience in prior cases to draw on, including known solutions to previously encountered problems.[2-4] In this

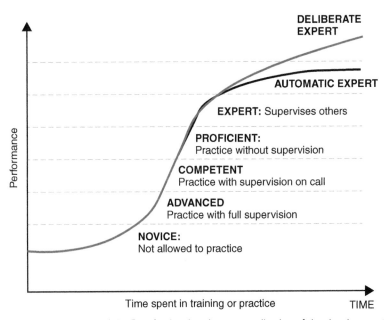

Fig. 2.1 A very simplified version of the Dreyfus brothers' conceptualization of the development of expertise in a learning environment.[1] We use this longitudinal representation to illustrate that the goal of the Master Adaptive Learner model is not only to develop a routinized, automatic expertise, but also to have the capacity to continue to improve and adapt to new situations and contexts. (From Kalet A, Pusic M. Defining and assessing competence. In: Kalet A, Chou CL, eds. *Remediation in Medical Education: A Mid-Course Correction.* New York, NY: Springer; 2014:3-15.)

type of expertise, further expertise gains take the form of greater efficiency and less cognitive effort. Bordage noted that the expert has "compiled" efficient knowledge; however, when encountering a novel problem, he reverts to reasoning that is "distributed" or novice-like.[5] The implied overall goal is to keep the expert in his routine wheelhouse and all will be fine.

While health professional experts can sometimes function in this automatic/routinized way in familiar structured environments, much of health care has changed. There are an increasing number of complex cases in increasingly complex care environments that require approaches outside the usual wheelhouse of any expert. Additionally, the diversification of health care teams to include a wide array of advanced practitioners can lead to a system in which the physician is selectively positioned to manage a panel of patients enriched for complexity. In other words, there is increasingly an imperative for the effective expert to innovate as part of her mandate.[3] This requires generating, for a complex patient, new specific solutions in the moment. This process of garnering cognitive resources and "figuring it out" is intensive and inefficient, but necessary. While the innovation imperative has long been the province of clinical researchers and entrepreneurs, what has changed is the increasing need for the active clinician to innovate as well, even if on a smaller scale.

However, this is not to say that efficiency has become irrelevant. Instead, while the modern practitioner is being asked to "slow down when he should," he still needs to maintain efficiency.[6,7] To negotiate this balance requires adaptive expertise, the ability to invoke the approach appropriate to the patients' and systems' needs for optimal health outcomes.[8] As we work with trainees, the goal is a curriculum and a culture that expect and nurture the development of adaptive expertise through master adaptive learning.

HOW DO WE DEVELOP ADAPTIVE EXPERTISE?

It may well be that developing adaptive expertise requires a different approach to learning from what has been emphasized in health professions education to date. *This is the key contention of this book: to become an adaptive expert, and to keep being one deep into the future, requires a new conceptualization—the clinician as expert learner.*

Consider the way clinicians typically learn to demonstrate clinical expertise. In the early stages, the material to be learned is *adapted* to the learner. Novices are heavily supervised. Simulations judiciously meter complexity to keep the learner in her zone of proximal development, such that cases are neither too easy nor too complex,

hitting the sweet spot for learning.[9] As the learner develops, supervision is gradually relaxed and complexity is layered in.[10] The environment and its representative problems are no longer novel. The learner no longer has to innovate to solve common problems. Her practice has become more routine. The less support required, the more we consider learners to be experts. The faster and more efficient they are, the more we consider them expert at what they are doing. Crucially, in this model, expertise can sometimes be regarded as no longer needing to learn, no longer needing to innovate. (We exaggerate for purposes of illustration.)

However, if we are to develop expertise by which the practitioner can innovate in the moment and can adapt, a pivot in instructional design is required. One cannot attain the expertise of a Tour de France cyclist, adapting to changing terrain and racing circumstances, by removing more and more training wheels. Where we have been adapting the environment to the learner before the pivot, we now must begin helping the learner-trainee learn adaptation and how to adjust to the full complexity of the clinical environment. This is not only a developmental process, but, ultimately, a way of becoming a different kind of clinician, one whose expertise is flexible and adaptive to a wide variety of contexts. This is an additional facet to clinical expertise, to which we would have a master adaptive learner aspire. Developing in the learner-clinician the skills of adaptation can itself result in ever-increasing expertise.

Thus learning for *adaptive expertise* is different from the way we usually think of learning. In Fig. 2.2, we illustrate one key method for learning this type of adaptive expertise, which is to situate learning whenever possible such that the learner has the opportunity to practice the balance between an innovation imperative and an efficiency one. This middle zone is termed the *Optimal Adaptability Corridor* (see Chapter 3). Examples of how a preceptor (such as Emily's) might arrange for this balanced learning include (Table 2.1):

- highlighting opportunities for innovation in routine cases
- highlighting opportunities for efficiency in complicated cases
- interrupting routinized care to probe for deeper, mechanistic understanding
- conversely, participating in quality improvement projects that look to make innovative care more routinized, more reliable
- practicing routine procedural skills in progressively more complex simulations
- pointing out the health care administrator's perspective on the way care is implemented

The Master Adaptive Learner (MAL) process specifically advantages transfer to new situations.

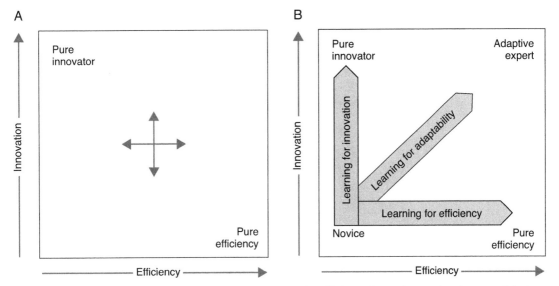

Fig. 2.2 Learning for Adaptive Expertise. (A) Negotiating the efficiency–innovation tension. In many clinical contexts, the clinician is asked to optimally balance innovation with efficiency. Routinized care, characterized by well-specified approaches, can emphasize efficiency *(bottom right)* while low-efficiency, high-innovation situations are typical of research and entrepreneurship *(top left)*. The adaptive expert is able to negotiate this space in a way that matches resources to the nature of the problem. (B) Learning the tension. With three channels for learning to become expert, situating the learner in the middle channel allows her to deliberately practice making the trade-off between efficient/routinized approaches and more innovative ones. This has been called the "Optimal Adaptability Corridor" because it allows the learner to continuously face the efficiency–innovation trade-off and to learn it well.[3,9] (From Schwartz D, Bransford J. Rethinking transfer: a simple proposal with multiple implications. *Rev Res Educ.* 2008;24[1999]:61-100 as adapted in Pusic MV, Santen SA, Dekhtyar M, et al. Learning to balance efficiency and innovation for optimal adaptive expertise. *Med Teach.* 2018;40[8]:820-827. https://doi.org/10.1080/0142159X.2018.1485887. Reprinted by permission of Taylor & Francis Ltd; retrieved from www.tandfonline.com.)

Instructional Parameter	Common Learning	Adaptive Expertise	Master Adaptive Learning
TABLE 2.1 How Learning for Adaptive Expertise Is Different.			
Emphasis	Efficient learning of well-known prototypes	Developing expertise that can match whatever situation is presented	Tripartite balance: efficiency, innovation, and blending them
Focus of adaptation	Adapt environment to learner	Adapt learner's approach to the environment	Increasing focus on the context and its richness/complexity
Scaffolding	Keep learner in zone of proximal development	Keep learner in the Optimal Adaptability Corridor (middle path in Fig. 2.2)	Less and less direct scaffolding and more at metacognitive level
Progression	Progressive withdrawal of scaffolds	Progressive challenges to encourage addition of adaptive behaviors	A progression of support from teaching/supervision to coaching
End point	Full withdrawal of scaffolds	No end point; coaching long-term for asymptotic improvement	Learning not a phase but part and parcel of being an adaptive expert

In the vignette, Emily felt disadvantaged in her learning, but was she, really? To develop adaptive expertise, we need a learning process that can be applied (transferred) to future, novel situations.[11] Consider the three levels of learning described in Fig. 2.3. They are common educational

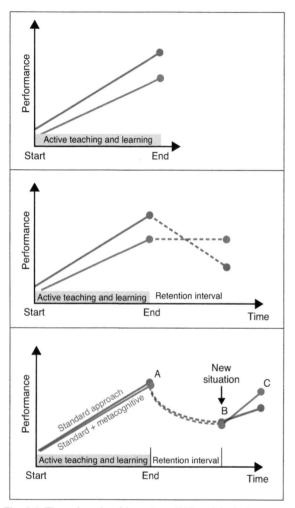

Fig. 2.3 Three Levels of Learning. (A) Level 1: A short-term focus on learning in which learning interventions are compared based on their ability to raise short-term outcomes *(blue line)*, with the assumption that the downstream transfer will also be improved. (B) Level 2: A desirable difficulties framework that advantages designs that produce durable learning even if immediate assessments are lower *(gray line)*. Durability is considered to have uncovered deeper learning. (C) Level 3: Even more ambitious, in preparation for future learning, material is learned with an additional consideration—that it be learned in such a fashion as to allow the rate of future learning to be improved (B→C). This is thought to be a combination of both deeper learning and, importantly, learning about learning: the Master Adaptive Learner process.

designs that differ in terms of their capacity to promote successful learning transfer to new contexts. The top pane (level 1) shows an education study in which two instructional designs are compared on their capacity to boost immediate posttest scores. How those higher posttest scores transfer to other contexts or over time is not within the scope of such a design. However, the worry is that this near target may advantage learning that is superficial and fragile, with considerable subsequent forgetting and poor transfer to new situations. In the middle pane (level 2), the desirable difficulties framework addresses some of these problems. It shows that some deeper learning contexts can make immediate posttest scores lower but the learning actually is shown to be more effective in the long run, resulting in better retention over time.[12] The learning is thought to be processed more deeply, taking more time and effort, with the reward of better retention and applicability.[12,13] While greater retention is associated with better later application, the middle framework does not explicitly address changing future contexts in which the retained knowledge becomes stale. Enter the third level (bottom pane), in which material is learned in a manner so as to advantage future learning ("preparation for future learning").[11,14] This requires careful attention to both the method of learning and advantaging deep approaches to learning that can be generalized to the variable context in which it will apply.[11,15,16] This specific attention to the nature of the learning sets up a virtuous cycle in which the clinician masters a set of flexible learning approaches that benefit both his clinical expertise and his future learning. This type of learning is difficult, as Emily experienced, and requires faith that it will pay off in the end. Engaging in the MAL process, at times, might look like level 2, where the students spend time goal setting, evaluating resources, and engaging in deep learning—as opposed to cramming facts that will subsequently be forgotten. As we work with learners, we might help them recognize that deep learning in the long run can actually be more effective and efficient.

What can we do today that prepares a learner for an uncertain future in which she is meant to function as an adaptive expert? We have highlighted one example, the concept of the Optimal Adaptability Corridor (see Fig. 2.2). Many of the chapters in this book provide perspectives on priming for future learning as it relates to master adaptive learning.

MASTER ADAPTIVE LEARNING IS AN INVESTMENT IN FUTURE LEARNING

So far we have described master adaptive learning from the perspective of aiming for a higher target, adaptive expertise, with which the clinician can adjust on the fly to the situation using the resources at hand. We have also

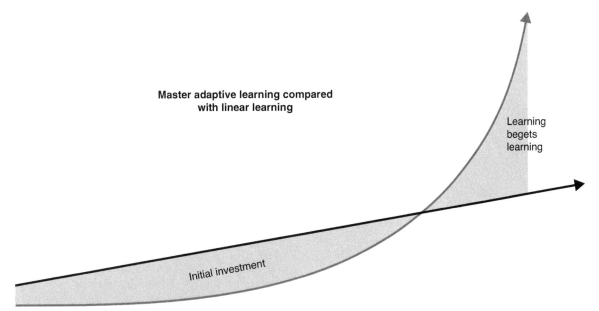

**Master adaptive learning compared
with linear learning**

Learning
begets
learning

Initial investment

Fig. 2.4 Learning Begets Learning in the Master Adaptive Learner Model. In many respects, investment in a master adaptive learner approach represents the difference between linear *(black line)* and exponential *(blue line)* learning. Exponential processes are those in which the innate process feeds off of itself in a manner that builds slowly initially but later explodes. It is within the nature of exponential processes that the early stages seem slower than those in linear ones.

described the idea that developing this type of expertise requires a different learning path, one with desirable difficulties that specifically advantage future learning.

In a time of overloaded curricula and training schedules, how do we convince a learner like Emily that this new approach will be worth it? Our claim is that, in specifically paying attention to mastery of learning early in the training of the adaptive clinician, we are *investing* in the optimal future clinician. Consider the two curves in Fig. 2.4.

One curve demonstrates linear learning. This can be a model for learning that is just a means to an end. When no specific attention is paid to how an individual learner learns, he develops idiosyncratic/individualized methods that are geared toward the next test or assessment, trusting that the assessments will guide the way to the expertise he wishes to develop. This can result in short-term thinking, learning only well enough for the moment. Think of cramming for a test as an extreme example. It accomplishes the short-term goal but does not serve the long-term one well. The result is steady improvement but at a fixed, limited rate. Each step results in the same amount of learning. It is steady, consistent, and satisfying, but it is mediocre. (Again, we exaggerate for purposes of illustration.)

Now consider the exponential curve. This is our aspiration for master adaptive learning. At first becoming a

master adaptive learner is frustrating. Not only does the master adaptive learner need to learn all the science or clinical content, just like the linear learner, but she also needs to learn how to learn. She needs to learn all the MAL processes. This is difficult because the assessment metrics, as currently constituted in a short-term linear fashion, will not show very much progress, especially when compared to the linear learner who steadily marches up the assessment ladder. However, as with compound interest where interest earnings eventually beget interest earnings so as to multiply the initial investment manyfold, knowing how to learn can beget ever more effective learning.[17] The learner for whom feedback seeking (see Chapter 6) is an ingrained habit from day 1 learns from every patient more and more efficiently in a way that compounds over time. The learner who systematically incorporates her learning into her clinical microsystem develops a platform with ever-higher performance standards that make the next improvement easier.

In the vignette, Emily and Vig live the difference between linear and potentially exponential learning. In many learning environments today, this is the difference between what is and what could be. In the succeeding chapters, we hope to convince you that the MAL framework can help develop in our learners and our systems a better way to learn.

WHAT IS MASTER ADAPTIVE LEARNING, REALLY?

We have laid down our first justification for the MAL approach: a new, more challenging target in the form of adaptive expertise and a new, more challenging way of learning. We have discussed development of expertise so as to provide a context for master adaptive learning and have discussed how routine and adaptive expertise differ. In subsequent chapters we will present in detail the elements necessary for developing adaptive expertise.

We now move on to an even broader consideration of master adaptive learning. In iteratively considering, testing, reflecting, and deepening their understanding of how clinicians develop expertise with the MAL model, the American Medical Association MAL interest group has come to appreciate the flexibility of Cutrer and Moore's original framework as it applies to a clinician's practice.[18]

Here we present four different perspectives on what master adaptive learning can be. The perspectives overlap and range from states to traits to behaviors. Combined, these perspectives outline a rich model that both creates a common language for what it means to be a learning clinician and is flexible enough to support the full range of learning endeavors. Master adaptive learning can be a process model. Master adaptive learning can define beneficial traits of an individual. Master adaptive learning can promote a metacognitive schema, and master adaptive learning might become a philosophy.

MAL: The Process

Engaging in master adaptive learning involves entering the MAL cycle at any of several points. Most classically, one enters at the top, in the planning stage where a gap is recognized (see Chapter 6), and generates an approach. What then follows is a step-by-step process that bears a considerable, intentional resemblance to the Plan-Do-Study-Act (PDSA) cycle that is central to quality improvement projects. The MAL process also resembles a number of learning models more directly from the field of education, such as Kolb's learning cycle (also four phases) and self-regulated learning.[19,20] Where the MAL process differs from these general conceptualizations is in contextualizing the learning process as not only learning for expertise but also learning as a core component of clinical expertise. In addition, the MAL process has the higher ambition of changing not only the individual but also the health care system with an explicitly stated adjusting phase (see Chapters 15 and 16). One phase of the process builds upon the next until the learning project has gone from recognizing in clinical practice that something could be better to an adjusted, improved health care system. The process is iterative and cyclical with a built-in acknowledgment that not all projects should or will succeed and, indeed, that learning can be difficult, requiring a great deal from the learner.

MAL: The Person

We speak of master adaptive learners as those who embody the predispositions and develop the skills necessary for optimal clinical practice; however, the full aspiration is for a master adaptive learner to be a superb clinician for whom intentional learning is not a separate activity but rather part and parcel of his professional identity. Consider the three words—master, adaptive, and learner—in reverse order. Being a master adaptive *learner* involves integrating a learning disposition into the core identity of the clinician. Learning is not a separate activity off to the side but is rather an intentional cultivated core skill and activity necessary for providing optimal care and maintaining an optimized health care system. In developing the capacity and volition to regularly invoke the MAL cycle, the clinician aspires to a higher level of expertise beyond routinized practice. The master *adaptive* learner is an adaptive expert who can shift between efficient routine approaches and slower, more reflective innovation-in-the-moment as required for optimal patient care (see Fig. 2.2). This requires more than just invoking the MAL cycle; the learner must also maintain a MAL disposition that includes curiosity, discernment, and openness to informed self-assessment, as well as the resilience necessary to confront the cognitive dissonance inherent in efforts to improve. Finally, being a *master* adaptive learner requires mastery of the theories and methods of individual learning and distributed cognition. These are skills to be engendered during professional school, refined in clinical training, and then continually adapted throughout a career in a rapidly changing health care system. One might not be able to predict what the health care system will look like 10 years from now, but one can certainly predict that intentional learning and adapting will be key components of successful approaches.

MAL: The Metacognition Lens

At a higher level, the MAL framework asks us to use a metacognitive perspective on the activities of a clinician; however, instead of asking a select few researchers, quality improvement officers, or educators to use metacognitive understanding for improvement, the MAL framework seeks to embed this way of seeing the world in every clinician. Historically, the evidence-based practice movement rightly sought to increase the degree to which critical thinking is used in applying research and experience to clinical care: "Am I using the best evidence?" Similarly, clinical reasoning cognitive models increase our understanding of biased decision making: "Am I making the best decision?" The MAL metacognitive framework seeks to increase and improve our awareness of *learning* in our processes and habits of mind: "Am I and the system learning the lessons that will help the next patient?" Learning for later application is more difficult than a routinized approach appropriate to the moment.

MAL: The Philosophy

Philosophy can be defined as the love of wisdom and the study of the basis of a particular branch of knowledge or experience. How perfect! In instituting the MAL model, we propose to create a better process for learning, to celebrate the characteristics of clinical learning for adaptive expertise, and to bring metacognition to bear within our everyday systems. However, the model itself has to walk the walk of continuing to evolve and improve. We point out one desirable attribute in this regard: the model is grounded in the clinical environment and not a separate educational environment (see Chapter 11). This is important because the model therefore will also be exposed to the evolutionary pressures that stress, mold, and infuriate us as clinicians. Perhaps it is an appropriate organizing myth that master adaptive learning is indeed a philosophy. A love of wisdom has to be the best preparation for future learning and the best predictor of future adaptive expertise.

TAKE-HOME POINTS

1. The MAL model establishes a new, higher goal for clinical expertise—that of the adaptive expert who can be both efficient and innovative in the measures required in a complex health care system.
2. The MAL model optimizes learning transfer, ensuring that what is learned today will still apply to new situations in the future.
3. The processes outlined in the MAL model, when encouraged over the longer term, can result in beneficial clinician traits such as adaptability, reflexivity, curiosity, and an ever-improving deep mechanistic understanding of medicine.

QUESTIONS FOR FURTHER THOUGHT

1. Who do you know who best exemplifies the beneficial characteristics of the master adaptive learner? How is that different from or the same as being a master clinician?
2. Name a time when you had to adapt to a change in your environment. To what extent was learning something new involved? Were you slow on the uptake, or were you among the first to recognize the need for the change? Why do you think this was the case?
3. You have an illness and are offered the choice to be cared for by one of two respected clinicians: an innovative, creative clinician-researcher or a highly efficient practitioner for whom you will be the umpteenth case that week. Under which circumstances would you choose one over the other?

ANNOTATED BIBLIOGRAPHY

1. Mylopoulos M, Brydges R, Woods NN, Manzone J, Schwartz DL. Preparation for future learning: a missing competency in health professions education? *Med Educ.* 2016;50(1):115-123.
   This paper is from a group that has promoted the Bransford and Schwartz "preparation for future learning" concept and has contextualized it for health professions education. They make the claim, as we do in this chapter, that attention to how we learn will be repaid downstream with a better clinician.
2. Pusic MV, Santen SA, Dekhtyar M, et al. Learning to balance efficiency and innovation for optimal adaptive expertise. *Med Teach.* 2018;40(8):820-827.
   This paper provides an exploration of how a master adaptive learner, in the adjusting phase, optimally and continually learns to balance routinization and innovation imperatives.
3. Bjork EL, Bjork RA. Making things hard on yourself, but in a good way: creating desirable difficulties to enhance learning. In: Gernsbacher MA, Pew RW, Hough LM, Pomerantz JR, eds. *Psychology and the Real World: Essays Illustrating Fundamental Contributions to Society.* New York, NY: Worth Publisher; 2011:56-64
   This chapter provides an overview of what a desirable difficulty is and why this can be a better way of learning.
4. Schwartz D, Bransford J. Rethinking transfer. A simple proposal with multiple implications. *Rev Res Educ.* 2008;24(1999):61-100.
   This seminal article lays out the logic for preparation for future learning, a better kind of learning transfer. It also describes how to create better instructional designs that promote preparation for future learning.

REFERENCES

1. Dreyfus S, Dreyfus H. *A Five-Stage Model of the Mental Activities Involved in Directed Skill Acquisition.* Berkeley, CA: United States Airforce Office of Scientific Research; 1980.
2. Mylopoulos M, Regehr G. How student models of expertise and innovation impact the development of adaptive expertise in medicine. *Med Educ.* 2009;43(2):127-132. doi:10.1111/j.1365-2923.2008.03254.x.
3. Pusic MV, Santen SA, Dekhtyar M, et al. Learning to balance efficiency and innovation for optimal adaptive expertise. *Med Teach.* 2018;40(8):820-827. doi:10.1080/0142159X.2018.1485887.
4. Hatano G, Inagaki K. Sharing cognition through collective comprehension activity. In: Resnick LB, Levine JM, Teasley SD, eds. *Perspectives on Socially Shared Cognition.* Washington, DC: American Psychological Association; 1991:331-348. Available at: http://dx.doi.org/10.1037/10096-014.
5. Bordage G. Elaborated knowledge: a key to successful diagnostic thinking. *Acad Med.* 1994;69(11):883-885. doi:10.1097/00001888-199411000-00004.
6. Berwick DM, Nolan TW, Whittington J. The triple aim: care, health, and cost. *Health Aff (Millwood).* 2008;27(3):759-769. doi:10.1377/hlthaff.27.3.759.
7. Moulton CA, Regehr G, Mylopoulos M, MacRae HM. Slowing down when you should: a new model of expert judgment. *Acad Med.* 2007;82(suppl 10):S109-S116. doi:10.1097/ACM.0b013e3181405a76.
8. Mylopoulos M, Woods NN. When I say … adaptive expertise. *Med Educ.* 2017;51(7):685-986. doi:10.1111/medu.13247.
9. Vygotsky L. *Mind in Society: The Development of Higher Psychological Processes.* Cambridge, MA: Harvard University Press; 1980.
10. Koens F, Mann KV, Custers EJ, Ten Cate OT. Analysing the concept of context in medical education. *Med Educ.* 2005;39(12):1243-1249. doi:10.1111/j.1365-2929.2005.02338.x.
11. Schwartz D, Bransford J. Rethinking transfer: a simple proposal with multiple implications. *Rev Res Educ.* 2008;24(1999):61-100.
12. Schmidt RA, Bjork RA. New conceptualizations of practice: common principles in three paradigms suggest new concepts for training. *Psychol Sci.* 1992;3(4):207-217. doi:10.1111/j.1467-9280.1992.tb00029.x.
13. Bjork EL, Bjork RA. Making things hard on yourself, but in a good way: creating desirable difficulties to enhance learning. In: Gernsbacher MA, Pew RW, Hough LM, Pomerantz JR, eds. *Psychology and the Real World: Essays Illustrating Fundamental Contributions to Society.* New York, NY: Worth Publishers; 2011:56-64.
14. Mylopoulos M, Brydges R, Woods NN, Manzone J, Schwartz DL. Preparation for future learning: a missing competency in health professions education? *Med Educ.* 2016;50(1):115-123.
15. Schwartz DL, Bransford JD, Sears D. Efficiency and innovation in transfer. In: Mestre JP, ed. *Transfer of Learning from a Modern Multidisciplinary Perspective.* Greenwich, CT: Information Age Publishing; 2005:1-51.
16. Woods NN, Brooks LR, Norman GR. The role of biomedical knowledge in diagnosis of difficult clinical cases. *Adv Health Sci Educ Theory Pract.* 2007;12(4):417-426. doi:10.1007/s10459-006-9054-y.
17. Bogle JC. *The Little Book of Common Sense Investing: The Only Way to Guarantee Your Fair Share of Stock Market Returns.* Hoboken, NJ: John Wiley & Sons; 2017.
18. Cutrer WB, Miller B, Pusic MV, et al. Fostering the development of master adaptive learners: a conceptual model to guide skill acquisition in medical education. *Acad Med.* 2017;92(1):70-75. doi:10.1097/ACM.0000000000001323.
19. Zimmerman BJ. Investigating self-regulation and motivation: historical background, methodological developments, and future prospects. *Am Educ Res J.* 2008;45(1):166-183. doi:10.3102/0002831207312909.
20. Zimmerman BJ, Kitsantas A. Self-regulated learning of a motoric skill: the role of goal setting and self-monitoring. *J Appl Sport Psychol.* 1996;8(1):60-75. doi:10.1080/10413209608406308.

The Master Adaptive Learner: A Conceptual Model

Donald E. Moore, Jr., PhD, and Michael J. Fowler, MD

LEARNING OBJECTIVES

1. Define the concept of adaptability in the context of the difference between routine and adaptive expertise.
2. Explain the importance of conceptual understanding in preparing master adaptive learners for future learning.
3. Be able to balance efficiency and innovation in evaluating patient presentations that are known and unfamiliar.
4. Describe the role of metacognition in adaptive expertise.
5. Explore how a master adaptive learner learns.

CHAPTER OUTLINE

CHAPTER SUMMARY

This chapter describes a model for a Master Adaptive Learner that medical educators could use as a guide to help medical students, residents, and fellows develop the skills associated with adaptive expertise in clinical reasoning. A master adaptive learner is characterized by his capability to recognize if a current approach to clinical reasoning is not working and by learning-in-practice a new approach that is more appropriate. The training of a master adaptive learner prepares her to learn in future practice settings by facilitating the integration of biomedical knowledge with clinical knowledge. The master adaptive learner follows a four-phase process to invent new approaches when older approaches do not seem to work.

INTRODUCTION

This chapter describes a model for a Master Adaptive Learner. Recent work has proposed that, to be successful in the increasingly complex challenges of the 21st century health care system, clinicians will have to develop the expertise of a master adaptive learner. A master adaptive learner's expertise will enable him to address the everyday tasks of a clinical practice but also to devise approaches to address the novel challenges that emerge in the clinical encounter.[1,2]

The Master Adaptive Learner model is a type of conceptual model, representing how complex things work the way they do. It draws on theories, evidence, assumptions, expectations, and beliefs and the presumed relationships among them to provide a representation that helps people know and understand a phenomenon.[3,4] The model outlined in this chapter describes a clinician in practice who has developed the expertise of a master adaptive learner, to complement and integrate with her expertise as a clinician. It is expected that this model would be used by curriculum planners in undergraduate and graduate medical education to guide the development of learning activities to help medical students, residents, and fellows develop the skills of a master adaptive learner.[5]

Vignette

Our model master adaptive learner is Dr. Ima Lerner. Dr. Lerner is a community-based primary care physician. She has been in practice for over 10 years in a medium-size multispecialty group. Researchers have suggested that many physicians reach expert status after 10 years in practice.[6] In the normal course of a day in her busy practice, Dr. Lerner sees a variety of patients. Because she has focused on diabetes, a significant proportion of her patients have type 2 diabetes. Most of her appointments for diabetes patients are return visits, and there are occasional visits from new patients.

WHAT IS THE EXPERTISE OF A MASTER ADAPTIVE LEARNER?

Ericsson suggested that there is a broad range of approaches to studying and conceptualizing expertise and expert performance.[7] In general, expertise refers to the combination of knowledge, skills, and dispositions that lead to expert performance; that is a consistently exceptional level of performance on a particular task or within a specific domain. Because clinical reasoning is the predominant activity of physicians in clinical practice, the particular task of concern for expert performance in this chapter is the clinical reasoning of a master adaptive learner.

Clinical Reasoning

Although a variety of conceptualizations of clinical reasoning exist, a consensus definition of clinical reasoning has not been established to guide efforts to develop medical student expertise in this important skill.[8] One group of researchers working on clinical reasoning has suggested that specifying boundary conditions when discussing clinical reasoning would clarify the conditions under which the discussion should be considered.[9]

The boundary for the term *clinical reasoning* in this chapter is influenced by a social constructivist perspective on learning.[10] The social constructivist perspective combines the perspectives of information processing, social cognition, and situated cognition learning theories. Such a boundary seems appropriate because clinical reasoning takes place in the clinical encounter, which is embedded in a dynamic health care environment,[11] and physicians engaged in clinical reasoning are learning as they interact with patients and the health care environment.[12]

In a clinical encounter, a physician engages in a dynamic contextual interaction with people, processes, technologies, artifacts, and sociocultural influences mediated by the physical setting and the physician's physical and mental condition.[12] Some have described the dynamic contextual interaction in terms of three levels—microsystem (clinical encounter), mesosystem (activities that support the care that the patient receives), and macrosystem (the health care system)—all embedded in a social system.[11] In the clinical reasoning process, a physician's formal learning and experience shape his perception of a patient's presenting information, and a mental representation of the patient's case will emerge. This mental representation will be used to guide further information acquisition, either from the patient or from resources afforded by the practice environment. A clinician will use the new learning obtained in this way to revise the mental representation until he is confident that it supports an actionable diagnosis or management plan or both.[8] The actionable diagnosis and the management plan usually draw on patterns that are stored in his long-term memory, but in some cases patterns do not exist or are incomplete. It is likely that this circumstance will be more common as novel patient presentations and more difficult patients increase and the number of therapeutic options multiplies.

Vignette Continued

On any given day, most of Dr. Lerner's patients are return patients whose needs are for reinforcement of current management strategies or minor adjustments that reflect improvements in health status. Other adjustments are needed for patients who are not following their management strategies as completely as they might. There is an occasional return patient with multiple comorbidities who is not doing well on a management strategy that has worked for other, similar patients. For the most part, new patients align with established management strategies, but an occasional new patient presents as a seemingly unsolvable puzzle.

Adaptability and Adaptive Expertise

As more difficult patients and novel patient presentations become more common and the number of therapeutic options multiplies, an important attribute of the expertise in clinical reasoning needed by a 21st-century physician is adaptability. Adaptability is the capability to be flexible and willing to change an approach to adjust to unfamiliar conditions.[13] Adaptability enables a physician to recognize that his usual approach to diagnosing and treating a patient may not always work in every situation and, as a result, he can modify his approach. The particular approach may be contingent on a variety of biologic/genomic, socioeconomic, cultural, and health care system forces that impact the physician and the patient.

Hatano and colleagues have provided a perspective of adaptability by drawing a distinction between expertise that is routine and expertise that is adaptive.[14] For example, an individual who demonstrates routine expertise has mastered procedures in her field to such an extent that she has become highly efficient and accurate in performing them, even appearing to perform the procedures automatically and without "thinking" about what she is doing. An individual who demonstrates adaptive expertise has developed a conceptual understanding about the procedures in her field in addition to routine expertise that enables her to innovate, creating new procedures that she can use to address unfamiliar circumstances effectively. She can balance efficiency and innovation to address problems that are routine or unfamiliar. To be able to do so successfully, she must have had training with two crucial characteristics. First, it must have prepared her for future learning. Second, it must have prepared her to balance efficiency and innovation.

Preparation for Future Learning

A clinician whose performance is characterized by adaptive expertise manages routine patients with known approaches and challenging patients with innovative approaches. This type of performance is the result of being "prepared for future learning." Essentially, preparation for future learning is a newer conception of transfer of learning. In clinical practice, transfer has traditionally been conceptualized as a clinician replicating or applying what he has learned in one setting to another setting. This kind of transfer works well for routine patients. When replicating or applying does not seem to work, a clinician who has developed adaptive expertise can reinterpret what he knows based on the available information and circumstances to create an innovative approach based on the patient's needs.[2,15-18] All clinicians adapt to novel situations to some extent, but with the Master Adaptive Learner conceptualization, we wish to highlight and promote this skill as an important educational objective.

Medical students, residents, and fellows can be prepared for future learning by providing them with opportunities to learn clinical knowledge and biomedical concepts concurrently during their continuum of training. In this way, basic science concepts become encapsulated with clinical facts in the mental representation of a disease. Knowledge encapsulation is one of the cognitive processes through which new knowledge is stored in neural networks in long-term memory and made available for retrieval. It is a learning mechanism in which the conceptual details of the biomedical sciences and their interrelations become associated in networks with representations of clinical experiences. When a clinical representation network is activated by a patient's presentation, an experienced clinician can diagnose and manage the patient by retrieving the representations stored in long-term memory without having to refer to the underlying biomedical concepts and principles. The integration of basic science concepts and principles with representation of clinical experiences is strengthened through increasingly challenging training and deliberate practice with both routine and challenging cases. With time, clinicians will be able to seamlessly recognize a group of clinical facts linked by underlying basic science concepts without needing to consciously consider the pathophysiology.[19-23] In this way encapsulation enables a clinician to use pattern recognition to diagnose and manage routine patient presentations with increasing automaticity.

In some cases, however, a patient's clinical presentation may activate a mental representation of a specific disease quickly, but the diagnosis, the management plan, or both pursued by the clinician were not effective. In other cases, a patient's clinical presentation might not activate a workable disease representation. In these and similar cases, a clinician would experience a surprise or cognitive dissonance, prompting reflection-in-action and a search for possible approaches to obtain an appropriate diagnosis.[24-27] Furthermore, reflection by a clinician who had developed adaptive expertise would raise to her consciousness the tacit biomedical concepts encapsulated with the clinical facts that had been activated by the patient's clinical presentation. The base biomedical concepts would serve as a platform for the generation/gap identification of need for new knowledge and the creation of an innovative approach to addressing the patient's needs.[2]

This capacity would be the result of clinical training that would have provided her with multiple opportunities to practice and receive feedback on unfamiliar or difficult clinical cases. The learning activities would have had to include opportunities to experiment with new ideas and to let go of (i.e., unlearn) old ones. Creating such a learning space for her would facilitate her being able to create a performance capacity that balances efficiency and innovation in her clinical work space.[28]

Balancing Efficiency and Innovation

People who are optimally adaptive can rearrange their thinking and reconceptualize their environments to reconstruct problems and to generate and use new knowledge based on the circumstances in which they are working. Schwartz and colleagues suggested that an adaptive expert reconstructs problems and generates and uses new knowledge by balancing efficiency and innovation within an Optimal Adaptability Corridor (Fig. 3.1).[1,28] Drawing on Pusic and colleagues[29] and Rebello,[30] however, it appears to be more likely that the adaptability that a clinician demonstrates can be represented more broadly by the intersection of two lines on a coordinate graph, one drawn from a point on the x-axis representing a clinician's efficient clinical reasoning capability and another line drawn from the y-axis representing the same clinician's innovative clinical

reasoning capability, each contingent on a patient's presentation and the sociocultural circumstances of the patient and the practice. A clinician demonstrating adaptive expertise in his work does not impose either an innovative or a routine solution on a patient but instead navigates a clinical encounter as necessary, drawing on capabilities that are characterized by either efficient clinical reasoning (horizontal axis) or innovative clinical reasoning (vertical axis) as needed. This judicious determination of the "as needed," matching approaches and resources to the patient, is the key expertise we wish to promote. In a routine clinical encounter in which a mental representation is retrieved efficiently based on a patient's presentation (routine expertise, located along the horizontal axis), the solution is known and is based on the training and experience of the clinician. In other cases when the mental representation is incompletely or not retrieved, a clinician would instead draw on his more resource-intensive innovative capability (creative exploration, located at a point on the vertical axis). His clinical

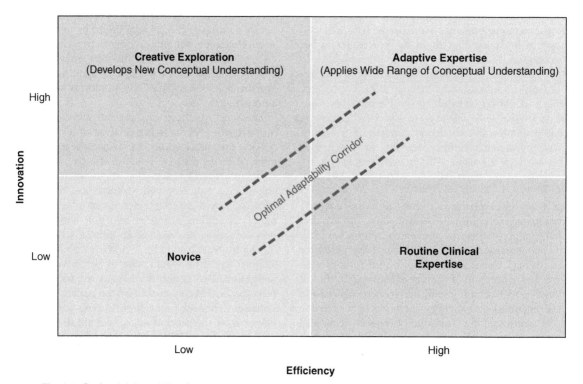

Fig. 3.1 Optimal Adaptability Corridor. Balancing routine and adaptive expertise in the Optimal Adaptability Corridor. (Adapted with permission from Bransford J, Barron B, Pea RD, et al. Foundations and opportunities for an interdisciplinary science of learning. In: Sawyer RK, ed. *The Cambridge Handbook of the Learning Sciences*. New York, NY: Cambridge University Press; 2006:27. Published in Cutrer WB, Miller B, Pusic MV, et al. Fostering the development of Master Adaptive Learners: a conceptual model to guide skill acquisition in medical education. *Acad Med.* 2017;92[1]:70-75.)

reasoning performance would be depicted as the optimal trade-off of efficient clinical reasoning capabilities and innovative clinical reasoning capabilities.

For a clinician to balance efficient with innovative clinical reasoning in performance, she needs to have been prepared for future learning by developing deep conceptual understanding of well-organized, fluently accessible sets of knowledge and skills that are represented on the efficiency dimension. In Fig. 3.2, four examples of adaptability are depicted. Examples 1 and 2 most closely represent what Schwartz and colleagues described as the Optimal Adaptability Corridor where a clinician has developed equal or close-to-equal capabilities in efficient and innovative clinical reasoning. This is an ideal situation in which the training a clinician would have received balanced the development of the two capabilities and, importantly, allowed the trainee the opportunity to practice balancing them. Example 1 could be a resident after ideal training; example 2 could be an experienced clinician who through ideal training and learning-in-practice would have developed ideal adaptive expertise. It is more likely, however, that the performance of most clinicians would reflect variants of examples 3 and 4. There are multiple intersection points between efficient and innovative clinical reasoning, all contingent on a clinician's capabilities and a patient's presentation and the sociocultural circumstances. Example 3 could be an experienced clinician who has developed significant routine expertise. Example 4 could be a clinician who is a pure innovator and spends most of her time in the research laboratory but has developed routine expertise in a very narrow area of patient care and sees patients one afternoon a week.

A Metacognitive Disposition

Central to the approach of a master adaptive learner to clinical reasoning and adaptability is a willingness and an

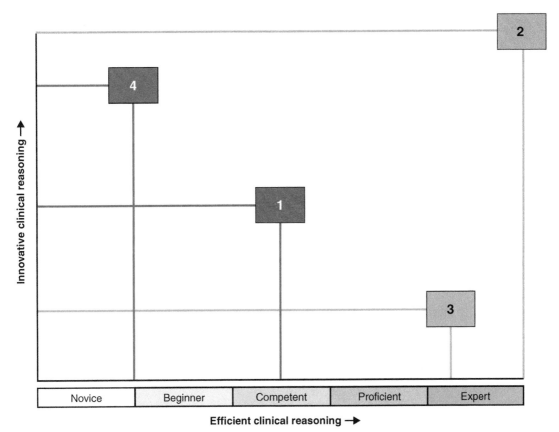

Fig. 3.2 Coordinate Graph. (Adapted from Pusic MV, Santen SA, Dekhtyar M, et al. Learning to balance efficiency and innovation for optimal adaptive expertise. *Med Teach.* 2018;40[8]:820-827; and Rebello NS. Can we assess efficiency and innovation in transfer? Paper presented at: Physics Education Research Conference; 2009; Ann Arbor, MI.)

intrinsic need to continuously review and analyze what she is doing and thinking and to make changes if the results of doing and thinking are not what is expected. This is called metacognition, a capability to rise above current thinking and activity to gain a better perspective. Metacognition has been described as higher-order thinking that enables understanding, analysis, and control of an individual's cognitive processes.[31]

Metacognition is important in the clinical encounter because it helps a clinician recognize what a patient needs and how to address those needs. As health care and the clinical encounter become increasingly complex, a clinician may more often become increasingly uncertain about what to do. Uncertainty varies from situations that are simple to those that are chaotic[32] (Fig. 3.3). Metacognition provides a clinician with three complementary approaches to thinking that address uncertainty: metacognitive monitoring, metacognitive control, and a predisposition to learn (growth mindset).[33]

For a clinician in a clinical encounter, metacognitive thinking generates awareness about the match between what a physician knows and can do and what is required for him to know and do in a particular situation.[31] Metacognitive monitoring, more commonly known as reflection, focuses on this. To address the health care needs of a patient, the abstract results of metacognitive monitoring stimulate a careful analysis of the evidence to generate an approach to the situation using a form of critical thinking termed *metacognitive control*.[31] If what a physician knows and can do match the requirements of the clinical encounter, the clinician can invoke a routine approach. If instead a match does not exist, cognitive dissonance results, which, especially if enabled by a growth mindset, will lead to learning an alternative approach or developing an innovation. Given the differentially greater demands of the latter, clinicians will naturally be predisposed to a tendency to judge situations as routine. The master adaptive learner approach promotes a cognitive disposition in the opposite direction.

Learning will take the form of self-regulated learning (SRL) or self-directed learning (SDL). SRL is defined as learning that is metacognitively guided, is at least partly intrinsically motivated, and follows a strategic plan.[34] SDL is often used interchangeably with SRL.[35] SDL is usually defined as a process in which individuals take the initiative to diagnose learning needs. They participate in learning and evaluate learning outcomes.[36] The two terms describe essentially the same process but differ because they are derived from different, though closely related disciplines: psychology (SRL) and adult education (SDL). SRL appears

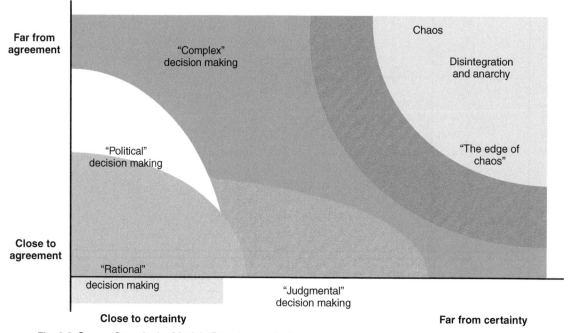

Fig. 3.3 Stacey Complexity Model. (From Innes AD, Campion PD, Griffiths FE. Complex consultations and the 'edge of chaos.' *Br J Gen Pract.* 2005;55[510]:47-52.)

to focus more on managing a project of learning while SDL appears to concentrate on the learning process.

In addition to SRL/SDL, the learning that a master adaptive learner would pursue requires yet another aspect of self.[37] Self-determination theory (SDT) describes a continuum of motivation that includes amotivation, external motivation, and internal motivation. Internal motivation, activated by cognitive dissonance, can be considered as the starting point of individual learning and change. Clinicians will learn only if the content (knowledge and skills) to be learned addresses what they consider to be their own problems in their own situations. Motivation is a hypothetical construct that describes the internal process whereby inner and outer forces produce the start, direction, intensity, and persistence of behavior, with a relevant example being engagement and persistence in learning projects. Motivation is not enough to achieve the desired results of demanding learning projects; a volitional dimension must come into play to sustain an agent's effort toward a personal goal. Self-regulation, as a dynamic combination of strategies and willpower (volition), is linked to success in academic and work performance in several research studies.[37] Self-direction represents the individual agency of a master adaptive learner to pursue learning in situations characterized by challenging uncertainty. Cutrer and his colleagues,[1] in their description of the Master Adaptive Learner model, used an SRL model derived by White and her colleagues.[38] We continue to use the Cutrer and colleagues choice of the SRL model but look forward to the time when researchers have combined SDT, SRL, and SDL into a comprehensive framework.[39]

A MASTER ADAPTIVE LEARNER IN PRACTICE

Vignette Continued

As mentioned previously, Dr. Lerner's return patients need reinforcement of or minor adjustments to current management strategies. She must also make adjustments for patients who are not completely following their management strategies or are not doing well on a management strategy that has worked for similar patients. Most of her new patients fall into established management strategies, but an occasional new patient presents management difficulties.

Over her 10 years in practice Dr. Lerner has developed routine approaches that address the needs of most of her patients. She has kept up to date with changes in diabetes care, regularly consulting the annual supplement in the journal *Diabetes Care* and articles in several other diabetes and internal

medicine journals. She is a frequent participant in grand rounds and patient care conferences at her hospital. Her hospital and practice are part of a clinically integrated network and the network's Quality Improvement and Patient Safety (QIPS) department conducts regular performance improvement studies as part of the network's goal to provide the best possible care.

We now describe how Dr. Lerner uses her skills as a master adaptive learner to address an unexpected outcome in her practice. We show how she follows the self-regulated learning model implicit to master adaptive learning to address an example case with an unexpected outcome. The model has four phases: planning, learning, assessing, and adjusting.[1] The divisions separating phases are not always straightforward. Activities in one phase occasionally overlap with activities in an adjacent phase (Table 3.1).

Planning Phase

The planning phase consists of recognizing a gap in practice, determining what needs to be learned, and creating a goal to guide learning activities. The planning phase began when Dr. Lerner sensed that something in her practice was not right.

TABLE 3.1 Metacognition and Master Adaptive Learning.

METACOGNITIVE DISPOSITION		
Metacognitive monitoring (Reflection)	Metacognitive control (Critical Thinking)	Predisposition to learn (Growth Mindset)
MASTER ADAPTIVE LEARNER MODEL PHASES		
Planning	Recognizing a gap Determining what needs to be learned Setting a goal	
Learning	Experimentation Activate encapsulated biomedical knowledge Formal learning activities Patient Care Conference	
Assessing	Informed self-assessment Coach	
Adapting	Microsystem (clinical encounter) Mesosystem (patient care support) Macrosystem (health care system)	

Vignette Continued

During a clinical encounter with John, a patient who has type 2 diabetes and is obese, Dr. Lerner reviewed his lab results and realized he was not improving. Among other indicators, his HbA_{1c} was considerably elevated. She wondered why he was not doing well on a management strategy that she was using routinely with other similar patients. The other patients seemed to be improving; their HbA_{1c} values were better than John's. She had made minor adjustments in John's medication and emphasized more strongly than usual the importance of exercise and diet. As she entered her notes in the network's electronic medical record, she wondered if there were other patients like John.

Like all physicians, Dr. Lerner wants to provide the very best possible care to her patients. After she saw John, she was uncomfortable because what she thought was the correct approach to managing his diabetes and obesity was not working the way she expected. She was confused about John's hemoglobin A_{1c} (HbA_{1c}) values because the approach that she was using was evidence based, having been developed with colleagues using the annual American Diabetes Association standards[40] and updated regularly. She wanted to find out if there were other patients like John. Several months ago, she had participated in a performance review in another clinical area conducted by the QIPS department and was impressed with the data that were used in the study and the approach of the QIPS staff. She asked the QIPS staff to generate a report that summarized the health status of patients like John. The report indicated that there were many patients like John who were on the same treatment approach and whose HbA_{1c} values were suboptimal.

The realization that there were more patients like John with suboptimal outcomes transformed the uncomfortable feeling that Dr. Lerner experienced after John's clinic visit into a stronger feeling that psychologists call cognitive dissonance. For Dr. Lerner, cognitive dissonance was a heightened discomfort that was the result of realizing that what she thought she was doing correctly to benefit a group of patients was contradicted by the less than optimal outcomes that she was seeing.[25] She began to recognize that there was a gap between what she was doing for patients like John and what she could or should be doing. Feedback from formal performance reviews can also highlight practice gaps for clinicians and cause cognitive dissonance. Developing a system for collecting this kind of external feedback is a kind of informed self-assessment, as discussed in Chapter 6.

Individuals who experience cognitive dissonance try to do something to reduce the discomfort. When Dr. Lerner realized that the dissonance she was experiencing was the result of the ineffectiveness of the approach she was using with John and patients like him, she wanted to know what approach she should use to produce more optimal outcomes. In this circumstance, Schön suggested that a clinician will experiment in practice to address the gap that created the cognitive dissonance or surprise.[24]

Dr. Lerner had managed her patients with routine problems using pattern recognition, a nonanalytic form of clinical reasoning that is largely automatic and unconscious.[41] When she interacted with these patients with routine problems, she recognized similarities between a patient's presentation and examples of similar presentations of previous patients (exemplars) stored in her long-term memory. Scripts of disease, exemplars of patients, and encapsulated knowledge play a significant role in nonanalytic reasoning, making it possible to reach a diagnosis without bringing a large amount of information into consciousness for processing. As a result of deliberate practice and encounters with patients as she developed from novice to expert, biomedical concepts became encapsulated under clinical knowledge, allowing Dr. Lerner to diagnose routine patient problems quickly and efficiently. Biomedical knowledge pertains to the (pathologic) processes underlying the manifestations of disease, and it incorporates knowledge about domains such as biochemistry, microbiology, and physiology. Clinical knowledge, on the other hand, concerns the ways in which a disease can manifest itself in patients.

However, the cognitive dissonance she felt due to the suboptimal results experienced by John and other patients with unexpectedly high HbA_{1c} values caused her to shift to a more reflective approach.[42] Although biomedical knowledge was not explicitly used by Dr. Lerner while diagnosing routine cases, it remained easily accessible when dealing with complicated or unfamiliar (complex) cases when nonanalytic reasoning failed to produce an adequate representation of a clinical case. If a match did not emerge between a patient's presentation and patterns that were stored in long-term memory, she would respond to the cognitive dissonance that she felt by shifting from the approach she used with routine patients to experiment with approaches with the goal of inventing an approach that will lead to more optimal outcomes for patients like John.[42] Therefore she begins to innovate, setting a goal to try out different approaches with patients like John for 6 months to determine if there is a better way to manage them.

Learning Phase

Learning for Dr. Lerner will emerge from her experimentation with patients like John. Reflecting-in-practice during clinical encounters with John and patients like him, she carefully considered the signs and symptoms in the patients' presentations.[43] When signs and symptoms were studied, biomedical concepts that had been encapsulated were activated. Information about signs and symptoms in a case point toward and activate specific, preexisting encapsulated concepts in long-term memory. Accessing the biomedical knowledge that was previously encapsulated, she looked for similarities that may not have been obvious initially in a patient's presentation. She spent a considerable amount of time using activated biomedical knowledge to make sense of signs and symptoms and inventing an approach to manage complex patients like John.[42]

Most clinicians learn by combining informal and formal approaches. While Dr. Lerner was learning informally through experimentation, she continued her typical formal learning activities but refocused her attention on what she was learning in her experiments with patients. She used PubMed searches to further investigate possibilities that her experimentation raised. She initiated conversations with endocrinologists and other colleagues in her practice and the network to solicit their ideas on her challenging patients. She continued to attend grand rounds and other hospital-based conferences but was more focused on attending activities that addressed some of the diabetes-related issues.

As she continued reflecting on John and her other challenging patients, Dr. Lerner considered the goals of care for them: glucose control and weight loss. She remembered that patients with untreated diabetes develop profound weight loss and wondered what the basic science mechanism was. Her reflections activated knowledge encapsulated around diabetes management, and as she researched the diabetes basic science literature, she realized that the subtype 2 sodium-glucose cotransporter (SGLT2) proteins were responsible for most of the renal glucose reabsorption. She wondered what the implications were for her patients. At a grand rounds presentation, she heard about a new class of diabetes drugs, SGLT2 inhibitors.[44] These drugs lower the threshold for the kidneys to excrete glucose into the urine such that whenever a patient's glucose is elevated, it is released into the urine. Dr. Lerner discussed the new drugs with her colleagues and learned that this new mechanism of lowering glucose levels also causes calories to be lost into the urine and could help with weight loss. Because the new drugs appeared to address the primary component of the goals of care for John and other similar patients, she decided to see if prescribing one of these new drugs would work for them. Because of the higher cost for the new drugs, she obtained prior approval from insurance companies and obtained copay discount cards to offset increased costs.

Assessing Phase

Informed self-assessment is the central activity during the assessing phase and overlaps with the learning phase. Research in several fields suggests that unguided self-assessment is not always accurate.[45-48] Informed self-assessment has been proposed as an alternative (see Chapter 6).[49,50] Informed self-assessment has been described as the process that an individual uses to assess his performance using an external standard, externally generated data, and external feedback.[51] As Dr. Lerner was conducting her experiments and was trying out what she was learning in practice, she was assessing the progress of her patients as well as her own capabilities with the new approaches. Because she recognized the importance of an additional, objective perspective on her work, she enlisted the help of the QIPS department and a senior colleague. The QIPS staff used data from her patient care experiences to compare her performance against institutional standards. Her senior colleague served as a coach to provide clear, timely, specific, and constructive external feedback.[49]

Initially Dr. Lerner was uncomfortable with the new approach. Adapting is resource intensive not only in terms of time but also psychologically, requiring of the learner a certain amount of resilience (see Chapter 4). However, as she learned more, made changes based on what she was learning, and received feedback that was positive, she became more confident and comfortable. After 6 months of informal learning, experimenting with patients, and participating in formal learning activities and consulting with colleagues, Dr. Lerner felt increasingly confident that while combining metformin and sulfonylurea was an acceptable approach for most patients with type 2 diabetes, incorporating a relatively new class of drugs into the regimen for John and patients like him was appropriate. She decided that it was important to get the approval of her colleagues and submitted the approach for review at a session of the Endocrinology Patient Care Conference (EPCC) at her hospital.

She attended the EPCC regularly and recalled that the community of practicing physicians who attend have helped other colleagues with their challenging cases. She reported at the EPCC session that after several months using the new approach, she was pleased to see improved glucose control and weight loss in John and other obese patients with type 2 diabetes. She explained the experiments she conducted with her challenging patients and how she used biomedical information to create the new approach to diagnose and manage them. She provided data that showed modest but sustained improvement in HbA_{1c} values. After a short discussion, her colleagues at the EPCC agreed that the new approach could be incorporated into routine practice. Although the new approach did not strictly follow the American Diabetes Association treatment algorithms, it was effective and was developed through a local consensus best practice process.

Adjusting Phase

During this final phase, Dr. Lerner integrated the new approach that she learned into her daily routines, and it became a part of what she did during clinical encounters with her obese patients who have type 2 diabetes. Adjustments were made in four areas:

- Clinical encounter (microsystem)—Nurses and practice staff were trained for the new approach; changes were made to the electronic medical record.
- Patient care support services (mesosystem)—The laboratory was notified that new tests were required; the physical therapy and nutrition departments were notified of a potential increase in consultations.
- Health care system (macrosystem)—The EPCC used Dr. Lerner's findings to modify the hospital-wide protocols for routine practice not only for Dr. Lerner but also her colleagues who see similar patients.
- Health care system (macrosystem)—Social services was notified that increased outreach was required to ensure that patients had access to nutritious food and exercise facilities.

CONCLUSION

This chapter describes a model for a Master Adaptive Learner that medical educators could use as a guide to help medical students, residents, and fellows develop the skills associated with adaptive expertise in clinical reasoning and management. Because we believe in the importance of starting with the end in mind, we based the model on the master adaptive learner target goal: an expert clinician who has developed adaptive expertise in clinical reasoning. Medical educators should use the model to create developmentally appropriate learning opportunities for medical students and residents using competencies and related milestones.

The essence of the skills of a master adaptive learner is adaptability: the capability to be flexible and willing to change. Adaptability can be developed by providing opportunities for medical students to be prepared for future learning by focusing in their training on the biomedical concepts that are the foundation of clinical knowledge and presenting them opportunities to practice shifting from routinized approaches to innovative ones. Biomedical concepts should be incorporated into clinical training so that they become encapsulated and yet still available. This will permit a clinician to both manage routine patients efficiently and accurately through pattern recognition and develop more innovative approaches for complex patients. Based on developmental level, medical students and residents should be provided increasingly challenging opportunities to learn in which they could develop the metacognitive capabilities to successfully pursue a four-phase master adaptive learning process to balance routine and innovative approaches to meet the needs of their complex patients.

TAKE-HOME POINTS

1. Physicians need both routine and adaptive expertise to successfully care for patients.
2. Case-based learning should begin early in the first years of medical education with explicit training in the integration of biomedical concepts and clinical knowledge.
3. Meaningful developmentally appropriate opportunities to develop metacognitive skills should be provided throughout medical school and residency training.

QUESTIONS FOR FURTHER THOUGHT

1. Would competencies and milestones for preparation for future learning facilitate the development of master adaptive learners?
2. Would qualitative research of how practicing physicians approach novel patient presentations contribute to our understanding of adaptive expertise?
3. Give an example from your own practice where you have had to take an encapsulated approach and consider each of its core components, in essence reasoning from first principles. What were the circumstances? What did you learn from the process of deconstruction and reflection?

ANNOTATED BIBLIOGRAPHY

1. Schmidt HG, Rikers RM. How expertise develops in medicine: knowledge encapsulation and illness script formation. *Med Educ.* 2007;41:1133-1139.

   This paper reviews research on the knowledge encapsulation and illness script hypotheses since their early formation. Findings in support of these views of expertise development are reported and conflicting data are discussed.

2. Mylopoulos M, Woods N. Preparing medical students for future learning using basic science instruction. *Med Educ.* 2014;48:667-673.

   Preparation for future learning has been proposed as a key competency supporting adaptive expertise. This study shows that the incorporation of basic science concepts in clinical instruction enables learning in practice when confronted with novel circumstances.

3. Mamede S, Schmidt HG, Rikers RM, Penaforte JC, Coelho-Filho JM. Breaking down automaticity: case ambiguity and the shift to reflective approaches in clinical reasoning. *Med Educ.* 2007;41:1185-1192.

   This study shows how case ambiguity caused clinicians to move from more automatic approaches to more analytic approaches.

REFERENCES

1. Cutrer WB, Miller B, Pusic MV, et al. Fostering the development of master adaptive learners: a conceptual model to guide skill acquisition in medical education. *Acad Med.* 2017; 92(1):70-75.
2. Mylopoulos M, Brydges R, Woods NN, Manzone J, Schwartz DL. Preparation for future learning: a missing competency in health professions education? *Med Educ.* 2016;50(1):115-123.
3. Bordage G. Conceptual frameworks to illuminate and magnify. *Med Educ.* 2009;43(4):312-319.
4. Earp JA, Ennett ST. Conceptual models for health education research and practice. *Health Educ Res.* 1991;6(2):163-171.
5. Dhaliwal G. Medical expertise: begin with the end in mind. *Med Educ.* 2009;43(2):105-107.
6. Ericsson KA, Kintsch W. Long-term working memory. *Psychol Rev.* 1995;102(2):211-245.
7. Ericsson KA. An introduction to Cambridge handbook of expertise and expert performance: its development, organization, and content. In: Ericsson KA, Charness N, Feltovich PJ, Hoffman RR, eds. *The Cambridge Handbook of Expertise and Expert Performance.* New York, NY: Cambridge University Press; 2006:1-19.
8. Gruppen LD. Clinical reasoning: defining it, teaching it, assessing it, studying it. *West J Emerg Med.* 2017;18(1):4-7.
9. Young M, Thomas A, Lubarsky S, et al. Drawing boundaries: the difficulty in defining clinical reasoning. *Acad Med.* 2018; 93(7):990-995.
10. Mann K, MacLeod A. Constructivism: learning theories and approaches to research. In: Cleland J, Durning SJ, eds. *Researching Medical Education.* Chichester, West Sussex, United Kingdom: Wiley Blackwell; 2015.
11. Nelson EC, Godfrey MM, Batalden PB, et al. Clinical microsystems, part 1: the building blocks of health systems. *Jt Comm J Qual Patient Saf.* 2008;34(7):367-378.
12. Moore Jr DE, Fleming GM, Miller BM. Learning in the practice setting: a synthesis of research and theory and suggestions for strengthening CPD. In: Rayburn WF, Turco MG, Davis DA, eds. *Continuing Professional Development in Medicine and Health Care.* Philadelphia, PA: Wolters Kluwer; 2017.
13. Nicolaides A, Marsick VJ. Understanding adult learning in the midst of complex social "liquid modernity". *New Dir Adult and Contin Educ.* 2016;2016(149):9-20.
14. Hatano G, Inagaki K, Stevenson H, Azuma J, Hakuta K. Two courses of expertise. In: *Child Development and Education in Japan.* New York, NY: W.H. Freeman and Company; 1986: 262-272.
15. Bransford JD, Schwartz DL. Rethinking transfer: a simple proposal with multiple implications. *Rev Res Educ.* 1999;24:61-100.
16. Mylopoulos M, Woods N. Preparing medical students for future learning using basic science instruction. *Med Educ.* 2014;48:667-673.
17. Mylopoulos M, Woods NN. When I say ... adaptive expertise. *Med Educ.* 2017;51(7):685-686.
18. Broudy HS. Types of knowledge and purpose of education. In: Anderson RC, Spiro RC, Montague WE, eds. *Schooling and the Acquisition of Knowledge.* Hillsdale, NJ: Lawrence Erlbaum; 1977:1-17.
19. Schmidt HG, Boshuizen HPA. On acquiring expertise in medicine. *Educ Psychol Rev.* 1993;5(3):205-221.
20. Schmidt HG, Rikers RM. How expertise develops in medicine: knowledge encapsulation and illness script formation. *Med Educ.* 2007;41:1133-1139.
21. Rikers RMJP, Schmidt HG, Moulaert VA. Biomedical knowledge: encapsulated or two worlds apart? *Appl Cogn Psychol.* 2005;19(2):223-231.
22. Rikers RM, Loyens SM, Schmidt HG. The role of encapsulated knowledge in clinical case representations of medical students and family doctors. *Med Educ.* 2004;38(10):1035-1043.
23. Schmidt HG, Boshuizen HPA. Encapsulation of biomedical knowledge. In: Evans DA, Patel VL, eds. *Advanced Models of Cognition for Medical Training and Practice.* New York, NY: Springer-Verlag; 1992:265-282.
24. Schön DA. Patterns and limits of reflection-in-action across the professions. In: *The Reflective Practitioner: How Professionals Think in Action.* New York, NY: Basic Books; 1983:21-73.
25. Festinger L. *A Theory of Cognitive Dissonance.* Stanford, CA: Stanford University Press; 1957.
26. Dewey J. *How We Think.* Boston, MA: Heath; 1933.
27. Mamede S, Schmidt HG. Reflection in diagnostic reasoning: what really matters? *Acad Med.* 2014;89(7):959-960.
28. Schwartz DL, Bransford JD, Sears D. Efficiency and innovation in transfer. In: Mestre J, ed. *Transfer of Learning from a Modern Multidisciplinary Perspective.* Greenwich, CT: Information Age Publishing; 2005:1-51.
29. Pusic MV, Santen SA, Dekhtyar M, et al. Learning to balance efficiency and innovation for optimal adaptive expertise. *Med Teach.* 2018;40(8):820-827.
30. Rebello NS. *Can we assess efficiency and innovation in transfer?* Paper presented at: Physics Education Research Conference, Ann Arbor, MI, 2009.
31. Winne PH, Azevedo R. Metacognition. In: Sawyer RK, ed. *The Cambridge Handbook of the Learning Sciences.* New York, NY: Cambridge University Press; 2014:63-87.
32. Stacey RD, Mowles C. *Strategic Management and Organizational Dynamics: The Challenge of Complexity.* 7th ed. Harlow, UK: Pearson Education; 2016.

33. Dweck CS. *Mindset; The New Psychology of Success.* New York, NY: Random House: Ballantine; 2006.

34. Winne PH, Perry NE. Measuring self-directed learning. In: Boekaerts M, Pintrich PR, Zeidner M, eds. *Handbook of Self-Regulation.* San Diego, CA: Academic Press; 2000:531-566.

35. Gandomkar R, Sandars J. Unravelling the challenge of using student learning goals in clinical education. *Med Educ.* 2017; 51(7):676-677.

36. Knowles MS. *Self-directed Learning: A Guide for Learners and Teachers.* New York, NY: Association Press; 1975.

37. Carre P. Heuristics of Adult Learning. In: Hiemstra R, Carre P, eds. *A Feast of Learning: International Perspectives on Adult Learning and Change.* Charlotte, NC: Information Age Publishing; 2013.

38. White CB, Gruppen LD, Fantone JC. Self-regulated learning in medical education. In: Swanwick T, ed. *Understanding Medical Education: Evidence, Theory, and Practice.* Chichester, West Sussex, UK: Wiley Blackwell; 2014:201-211.

39. Cosnefoy L, Carre P. Self-regulated and self-directed learning: why don't some neighbors communicate? *Int J Self Dir Learn.* 2014;11(2):1-12.

40. American Diabetes Association Professional Practice Committee. Standards of Medical Care in Diabetes 2019. *Diabetes Care.* 2019;42:S1-S204.

41. Norman G, Young M, Brooks L. Non-analytical models of clinical reasoning: the role of experience. *Med Educ.* 2007; 41(12):1140-1145.

42. Mamede S, Schmidt HG, Rikers RM, Penaforte JC, Coelho-Filho JM. Breaking down automaticity: case ambiguity and the shift to reflective approaches in clinical reasoning. *Med Educ.* 2007;41(12):1185-1192.

43. Mamede S, Schmidt HG. The structure of reflective practice in medicine. *Med Educ.* 2004;38(12):1302-1308.

44. Abdul-Ghani MA, Norton L, Defronzo RA. Role of sodium-glucose cotransporter 2 (SGLT 2) inhibitors in the treatment of type 2 diabetes. *Endocr Rev.* 2011;32(4):515-531.

45. Davis DA, Mazmanian PE, Fordis M, Van Harrison R, Thorpe KE, Perrier L. Accuracy of physician self-assessment compared with observed measures of competence: a systematic review. *JAMA.* 2006;296(9):1094-1102.

46. Friedman CP, Gatti GG, Franz TM, et al. Do physicians know when their diagnoses are correct? Implications for descision support and error reduction. *J Gen Intern Med.* 2005;20:334-339.

47. Eva KW, Cunnington JP, Reiter HI, Keane DR, Norman GR. How can I know what I don't know? Poor self assessment in a well-defined domain. *Adv Health Sci Educ Theory Pract.* 2004;9(3):211-224.

48. Eva KW, Regehr G. "I'll never play professional football" and other fallacies of self-assessment. *J Contin Educ Health Prof.* 2008;28(1):14-19.

49. Sargeant J, Armson H, Chesluk B, et al. The processes and dimensions of informed self-assessment: a conceptual model. *Acad Med.* 2010;85(7):1212-1220.

50. Mann K, van der Vleuten C, Eva K, et al. Tensions in informed self-assessment: how the desire for feedback and reticence to collect and use it can conflict. *Acad Med.* 2011;86(9): 1120-1127.

51. Epstein RM. Reflection, perception and the acquisition of wisdom. *Med Educ.* 2008;42(11):1048-1050.

4

What Are the Four Critical Personal Characteristics That Support the Master Adaptive Learning Process?

Erica Friedman, MD, and Holly G. Atkinson, MD

LEARNING OBJECTIVES

1. Describe the key internal characteristics of the master adaptive learner and understand how they function in supporting the master adaptive learning process.
2. Analyze a given learner's strengths and weaknesses in becoming a master adaptive learner.
3. Define interventions to enhance an individual learner's master adaptive learner characteristics.
4. Describe interventions to enrich the learning environment to foster the development of the master adaptive learner.

CHAPTER OUTLINE

CHAPTER SUMMARY

Four internal characteristics—curiosity, motivation, growth mindset, and resilience—drive the master adaptive learner process. They promote and sustain the learner's ability to engage in the learning cycle. Without curiosity, an individual does not have the drive to fill a gap in knowledge. Motivation puts curiosity into action.

A growth mindset sustains individuals' belief in their ability to acquire knowledge and develop talents and sustains their interest in learning. Resilience is key to weathering setbacks, overcoming obstacles, and surmounting failures. These critical master adaptive learner characteristics can be either promoted or stifled by individual factors, conditions in the learning environment, or both.

FOUR CRITICAL PERSONAL CHARACTERISTICS

Learning is influenced by both academic aptitude and noncognitive abilities or attributes. Academic aptitude is defined as the cognitive ability to acquire new academic knowledge and skills. Noncognitive personal abilities and attributes include "attention, will, and character."[1] Numerous studies have confirmed that such noncognitive abilities and attributes are powerful predictors of academic, social, economic, psychological, and physical well-being.[2-7] The term *noncognitive,* however, is inaccurate because it implies that attributes such as attention, will, and character are devoid of cognition, yet they often are modifiable by cognitive strategies. Nevertheless, the term is widely used to describe all characteristics other than academic ability/intelligence. Some educators prefer to use the term *social and emotional learning* to describe these characteristics.[8,9] Studies have shown that these characteristics can be modified by experiences[10-12] and by the learning environment.[13]

Challenges, personal beliefs, and cultural values all can alter the human mind in ways that affect both cognitive and noncognitive abilities.[14] In particular, the act of cognition is not an invariant system; rather, it is embedded in specific contexts and modified by individual characteristics and the learning environment. The ability to be self-aware while performing a task (metacognition) involves both cognition and affect and is critical for master adaptive learning. This self-regulation has profound consequences on intellectual functioning and development.

As described by Cutrer and colleagues, the Master Adaptive Learner (MAL) process is thought to be influenced by four personal noncognitive characteristics: curiosity, motivation, growth mindset, and resilience.[15] These characteristics act as batteries for the master adaptive learner (see Fig. 1.1); they provide the power to promote and sustain the learner's ability to engage in the MAL process. Without curiosity, an individual does not have the drive to identify and fill the gap in knowledge. Motivation puts curiosity into action. A growth mindset sustains the individual's belief in his ability to acquire knowledge and develop talents and sustains her interest in learning. Finally, resilience is key to weathering setbacks, overcoming obstacles, and surmounting failures that are all part of learning in challenging environments.

Although these four critical characteristics play a central role in the MAL process, there are, in addition, other characteristics thought to contribute to the development of the master adaptive learner, including tolerance of ambiguity[16-18] and a sense of belonging,[19,20] among others. These personal characteristics can be either promoted or stifled by conditions in the learning environment or in the individual. In this chapter, we concentrate on curiosity, motivation, growth mindset, and resilience—their definitions, tools for assessment (Table 4.1), research regarding their impact on learning, and their roles in medical education and the MAL process.

CURIOSITY

Curiosity, the first battery of the MAL process, is one of the intrinsic drivers of learning. Curiosity is basic to our nature and central to human development and adaptation. It confers survival benefit to individuals and species.[21,22] Intellectual curiosity has been described as individual preferences for engaging in mentally challenging tasks and the purposeful pursuit of knowledge.[5,23]

Curiosity in Higher Education

Curiosity has been divided into two individual-level attributes, called trait curiosity and state curiosity. Trait curiosity refers to an inherent and stable baseline trait, whereas state curiosity refers to a variable context-dependent state.[24-28] An individual demonstrates trait curiosity when

TABLE 4.1	Internal Characteristics of the Master Adaptive Learner	
Characteristic	**Definition**	**Selected Assessment Tools**
Curiosity	A desire for knowledge that leads to exploratory behavior.	• Melbourne Curiosity Inventory
Motivation	The general desire or willingness of an individual to engage in behavior to achieve a desired goal.	• Academic Motivation Scale • Reflection-in-Learning Scale
Growth mindset	The intrinsic belief that intelligence is malleable and improvable through effort and learning.	• The Mindset Assessment
Resilience	The ability to weather adversity and grow stronger in the face of challenges and failures.	• Academic Resilience Scale • Connor-Davidson Resilience Scale • Resilience Scale for Adults • Brief Resilience Scale

she pursues cognitively challenging or complex tasks and intellectual leisure time pursuits.[29] Both trait and state intellectual curiosity have been studied in higher education and measured using validated instruments.[26,28] They both are positively predictive of classroom and workplace learning and performance, suggesting that both types of intellectual curiosity may be beneficial for learning and can be promoted in adults through education.[30-32]

Using the Melbourne Curiosity Inventory, studies have shown that learner state curiosity can be stimulated.[21,27,28,33] This inventory is a validated, self-reported measure that employs distinct trait and state subscales. Forty items (20 per subscale) assess thoughts and feelings about learning, exploring, problem solving, and questioning. The trait subscale focuses on the individual in general, whereas the state subscale asks the respondent to focus on the current situation. Findings show that curiosity can be induced by a stimulus that is novel or attracts attention. Gaps in knowledge (an important part of the MAL process) can also stimulate curiosity, which then motivates the learner to find answers. The way information is presented can also influence curiosity and has implications for education and training. In addition, the perceived value of information and its personal relevance increase curiosity, which motivates the learner to learn more. Stimulating curiosity is central to education and learning.[34] The fact that teachers across the educational spectrum often prefer techniques of instruction that excite curiosity suggests that they believe it is instrumental to education, inquiry, and knowledge.[21]

Curiosity in Medical Education

Interest in the importance of curiosity has grown among medical educators, who have hypothesized that curiosity plays a critical role in intellectual discovery, problem solving, self-monitoring, and lifelong learning and caring.[35-43] In 1999, Faith Fitzgerald hypothesized that curiosity is key to the humanistic practice of medicine.[44] She believes that in order to empathize with patients, you must have curiosity to go beyond the science of their problems to learn about who they are—their fears, hopes, and spirituality and how they live their lives. In 2013, Richards and colleagues demonstrated that medical students with high trait curiosity used strategies that promoted understanding rather than memorization.[45] However, the learning environment plays an influential role. Fitzgerald and others[44] have expressed concern that current approaches to medical education can suppress curiosity through their use of passive learning techniques, focus on efficiency, and lack of acknowledgment of uncertainty.[35,38,40,46] Curiosity can also be suppressed by working hastily and driving for efficiency, which often requires immediate answers or responses.[47]

Sternzus and colleagues measured curiosity among medical students cross-sectionally across all 4 years of medical school using the Melbourne Curiosity Inventory.[48] They found that trait curiosity was significantly higher than state curiosity overall and for each year of training. They also found that trait curiosity was relatively stable across the 4 years, whereas there was more variability in state curiosity, which was consistently lower than trait curiosity. There are no published studies of how medical education itself influences trait or state curiosity and how it affects performance.

Promoting Curiosity

To maintain curiosity, the teacher and the environment should support connection of the new material to previously acquired knowledge through specific tasks.[27,49] Examples of these types of tasks include assigning problems or assessments, working in groups, and establishing personal or professional relevance. Educators can help learners sustain curiosity in challenging situations by providing direct encouragement of learners' abilities, providing feedback, creating opportunities for learners to ask questions, and providing resources that promote problem solving and strategy generation in order to promote autonomy and competence.[21,50] State curiosity can be sparked by environmental or content features such as incongruous, surprising information; character identification; and personal relevance and intensity. Environments that support this include group work, use of technology, presenting meaningful tasks, promoting personal involvement, project-based learning, and one-on-one tutoring/learning. Learners' curiosity is also enhanced when exposed to others' opinions.[51] Both team-based and problem-based learning capitalize on this aspect of curiosity and empower learners to educate their peers.

The environment must help learners shift from external support to internal support so that learners can generate questions to connect their present understanding with alternative perspectives.[51,52] Educational approaches that place an emphasis on learners identifying their own questions and investigation methods can enhance curiosity and, in turn, increase learning.[51] Medical educators should use approaches that stimulate learners' curiosity while assuring they are teaching knowledge and skills.

MOTIVATION

A second battery fueling master adaptive learning is the multidimensional concept of motivation. It is responsible for why a behavior is initiated, why it persists, and when it ends—the what, why, and where of goal-directed actions.[53] Motivation can be driven by the desire to solve a problem, rectify a knowledge or skill deficit, or gain a valued incentive. Motivation is key to learning in an academic setting and can improve trainee performance and well-being.[54-57]

In 1985, Deci and Ryan proposed two basic types of motivation: intrinsic motivation and extrinsic motivation. Intrinsic motivation drives an individual to pursue an activity because of a personal interest, whereas extrinsic motivation drives a person to seek a reward or avoid a punishment. Their self-determination theory (SDT) postulates that motivation is a continuum, ranging from amotivation (lack of motivation) to intrinsic motivation (pursuit of an activity for one's personal interest) self-generated by the individual. SDT hypothesizes that motivation can change during one's studies from extrinsic to intrinsic, depending on the learner's feelings of autonomy, competence, and relatedness experienced.[55] According to SDT, intrinsic motivation is associated with deeper learning.[56,57]

Maslow[58] proposed another theory about motivation involving self-efficacy, which was further elaborated by Bandura[59-61] and Zimmerman.[62,63] This theory states that individuals' beliefs about their abilities to achieve any given outcome are critical to their achievement motivation. Research has demonstrated that learners' goals, task value, and self-efficacy positively affect their efforts, the quality of their academic performances, and their willingness to take on challenging tasks.[61,63-68]

Investigation into motivation has been made even more complex by the introduction of the concept of "interest." Toward the end of the 20th century, research in interest as a motivational factor focused on the influence of interest on learning. One might intuit that the concept of interest would be more aligned with curiosity; however, "interest" has not been directly linked to "curiosity." Rather, interest is thought to play a role in motivation. It is a distinct concept that is important. Research on interest is positioned to make a significant contribution to understanding the functional relations among motivation, learning, and emotions.

Individual interest is considered the innate predisposition to attend to activities or objects with which one will reengage over time. Interest results in focused attention, engagement, or both. In contrast, situational interest is generated by a specific aspect of one's environment that engages attention and may be transient.[69] Three features of interest-based motivation set it apart from cognitively based motivation theories and call for the integration of the psychological aspects of interested engagement with findings of neuropsychological research.[70] Specifically, (1) interest is content specific, (2) it evolves in the interaction of the person and her environment, and (3) it is both a cognitive and an affective variable. Cognitive aspects of interest are associated with knowledge and value, and

affective aspects consist of emotions—most frequently positive emotions. Positive emotions create the development of interest and effort, resulting in focused, deep-learning behaviors.[51,70] Well-developed interest facilitates perseverance to continue working despite the extent of the challenge or frustration the work presents. Interest impacts learners' attention, memory for tasks,[71] and depth of processing.[72,73] It appears that interest has a significant impact on intellectual functioning. Furthermore, the ability to sustain and develop new interests has been associated with lifelong learning and suggests that interest should have a central role in pedagogical practice.[74-76]

Berninger and Richards have noted that emotions, motivation, and academic tasks are intricately linked with cognitive and executive functions in the neural circuitry spanning subcortical and cortical regions of the brain.[77] However, there is little information about ways to support the development of positive affect and motivation so that learners who do not have interest for particular content can become academically motivated individuals.[78-80] Work to support pedagogical use of situational interest as a scaffold to engagement is a step in this direction.[81,82] Case analyses of learners' interest in, for example, learning in Latin and history classes further suggest that teachers play a pivotal role in supporting learners' developing interest for specific content and a love of learning more generally.[70] In particular, teachers are in a position to adjust their instruction to meet learners' strengths, needs, and interests, and to structure the classroom environment so that learners can learn.[83] Interestingly, however, interventions to support the development of interest, or love of learning, have primarily targeted older learners and adults. Because of adults' metacognitive abilities, they are able to learn to self-regulate their learning if they have reason to undertake the necessary tasks to learn and will take steps themselves to make these tasks more interesting.[70]

Motivation in Medical Education

Most theories about the motivation to learn are predicated on a framework involving learners' thoughts and beliefs.[84] Theoretically, when a learner is considering future tasks required to learn content, she takes into consideration the value of learning (intrinsic, incentive, and utility value) and the cost. Relatively little research has been conducted to assess the motivation of health care professions learners to obtain the requisite knowledge and skills. In 1999, Williams and colleagues differentiated autonomous from controlled motivation. Autonomous (intrinsic) motivation indicates a person's interests and values, whereas controlled (extrinsic) motivation depends upon rewards or punishment or on an internalized belief of what is expected.[85] Williams and colleagues used the Academic Motivation Scale to assess the goal orientation of learners in colleges of medicine, nursing, and pharmacy. The majority of the learners were mastery oriented, with an internal locus of control, and had metacognitive learning strategies.

As is true in the general education literature, most studies of medical students have found that motivation is positively correlated with academic performance. Sobral used a series of rigorous scales to measure medical students' motivation in consecutive years.[86] He found that medical students had greater intrinsic motivation than extrinsic motivation and that increased intrinsic motivation correlated with increased persistence and effort in studies, academic achievement, reflective learning, and meaning orientation.

Kusurkar and colleagues reviewed the medical literature and identified 56 papers that assessed the role of motivation in predicting and understanding processes and outcomes in medical education.[87] They concluded that motivation affects learning and study behavior, academic performance, choice of medicine and the specialty within medicine, and the intention to continue to study medicine. Motivation is stimulated by medical students' need for autonomy, competence, and relatedness, supporting the validity of the self-determination theory. However, the studies had mixed results regarding the correlation between the amount and type of motivation (intrinsic versus extrinsic) and better academic performance. Kusurkar and colleagues and ten Cate and coworkers have suggested that autonomy-supportive teaching can enhance medical students' intrinsic motivation for medical education/studies.[88,89]

Promoting Motivation

Motivation is driven by numerous factors both internal and external. The environment, an individual's behavior, and internal characteristics (knowledge, emotions, and cognitive development) all influence one another and the motivation to learn. Extrinsic motivators include providing clear expectations and giving corrective feedback using scaffolding, providing rewards for achieving simple tasks, and allowing learners to engage in social learning activities in order to observe others doing things correctly.[51] Stimulators of intrinsic motivation include setting goals for learning; explaining or showing why the skill or knowledge is important and relating it to learners' needs; allowing learners to select their learning goals or tasks and helping them develop a plan of action; and creating or maintaining curiosity and providing a variety of activities and sensory stimulation, simulation, or both.[81,82]

Educators can influence environmental factors to enhance situational interest. Aspects of content that trigger situational interest include novelty, surprising information, intensity, concreteness, visual imagery, and value. In addition, prior knowledge, ease of comprehension, engagement, and emotional reactions are factors that create situational interest.[90] However, prior knowledge alone is insufficient to generate or increase situational interest. Situational interest is influenced by social aspects of the environment. A cooperative learning environment can elicit situational interest, as can providing scaffolding to help learners make connections.[81] Only meaningfulness of the task and personal involvement maintain interest.

Curricular design should recognize that incorporating teaching methods such as small group work and problem-based learning can increase learner motivation.[51] Also, environments that provide regular and constructive feedback, support autonomous behavior, and foster learner feelings of competence can enhance motivation.[51] Promoting learner relatedness through mentorship and positive role models can stimulate learners' autonomous motivation and lead to greater learner satisfaction.

Finally, it is important to note that extrinsic motivators only work while learners are under their direct influence, whereas intrinsic motivators are internalized and persist. Teachers should work to promote intrinsic motivators to assure persistence of the behavior.

GROWTH MINDSET

Implicit Theories of Self

The next MAL battery is growth mindset. Mindsets, or implicit theories of self, are defined as core assumptions individuals hold about the malleability of their personal traits, such as their intelligence or ability to learn.[91] Carol Dweck, a pioneer in mindset research, described the difference between "entity" and "incremental" self theories and their impact on learning as the "fixed mindset" and "growth mindset," respectively.[92,93] Individuals with fixed mindsets believe that basic qualities, such as intelligence or talents, are fixed traits. They believe talent alone creates success, without much effort, and are hesitant to take on challenges or obstacles for fear of not looking smart or for fear of failure. In contrast, individuals with growth mindsets believe they can develop their most basic abilities, including their intelligence, through dedication and hard work—brains and talent are just the starting point. Growth mindset individuals embrace challenges, accept critical feedback, and invest in learning. Dweck developed a diagnostic tool, composed of eight self-reported questions, drawn from research-validated measures to assess an individual's mindset for intelligence.[94]

Research has shown that learners' mindsets about their own intelligence predict their academic performance over

TABLE 4.2	Comparison of Common Traits for Individuals With Growth and Fixed Mindsets	
	Growth Mindset	**Fixed Mindset**
Attitudes about learning	• Pursue challenges • Value effort • Believe that mistakes and effort are critical to learning	• Feel smart when education comes easily • Avoid looking foolish or unlearned • Worry about making mistake • Sacrifice learning if it risks showing deficiencies
Responses to feedback	• Eagerly seek out formative feedback • Quickly implement feedback received	• Become discouraged and defensive about constructive feedback • Be more likely to cheat and lie about grades and performance
Responses to setbacks	• Demonstrate resilience to setbacks • Believe setbacks are a part of the learning process • Employ adaptive studying methods • Adapt to increasing challenges	• Give up easily • Believe setbacks are indictments of self • Assume that setbacks signal low ability and low intelligence • Make excuses and blame others • Avoid similar courses/situations in the future

Adapted from Cooley JH, Larson S. Promoting a growth mindset in pharmacy educators and students. *Curr Pharm Teach Learn.* 2018;10:675-679.

time, especially when they are challenged in their work and struggle to achieve their goals.[95] The two different mindsets appear to create different psychological worlds for learners (Table 4.2). The growth mindset promotes resilience in the face of challenges and setbacks, whereas the fixed mindset does not.[91,93] Several variables explain why learners who embrace a more incremental theory, or growth mindset, are more likely to succeed when confronted with a challenge:

> . . . an incremental [growth] versus entity [fixed] theory shapes students' *goals* (whether they are eager to learn or instead care mostly about looking smart and, perhaps even more important, not looking dumb), their *beliefs about effort* (whether effort is a key to success and growth or whether it is a signal that they lack natural talent), their *attributions* for their setbacks (whether a setback means that they need to work harder and alter their strategies or whether it means they might be "dumb"), and their *learning strategies* in the face of setbacks (whether they work harder or whether they give up, consider cheating, and/or become defensive).[96]

It is important to note that these two concepts—the fixed mindset and the growth mindset—represent two polarities, and that people do not always hold one or the other. They may have different mindsets toward various domains of their lives (i.e., professional vs. personal) or toward various qualities, such as their intelligence, ability for sports or music, or personality traits.[93,97] As Dweck explains,

> Everyone is a mixture of fixed and growth mindsets. You could have a predominant growth mindset in an area but

there can still be things that trigger you into a fixed mindset trait. Something really challenging and outside your comfort zone can trigger it, or, if you encounter someone who is much better than you at something you pride yourself on, you can think "Oh, that person has ability, not me." So I think we all, students and adults, have to look for our fixed-mindset triggers and understand when we are falling into that mindset.[98]

Ultimately, according to mindset theory, the beliefs that an individual holds about herself matter substantially. They influence motivation, goal setting, self-regulatory behavior, and responses to adversity in a number of facets in life, including academic pursuits, social relationships, the workplace, emotional health, and physical health.[99] Studies have documented the numerous ways in which a growth mindset contributes to behaviors that promote academic achievement in particular.[100-102] Especially when faced with challenges and setbacks, learners with a growth mindset tend to earn better grades than learners with a fixed mindset.[95,101,102] It is important to note that mindset matters most when learners encounter challenges.[103,104]

Importantly, extensive research among high school and college learners shows that fostering a growth mindset through targeted interventions and interactions with adults can improve learners' motivation, raise grades, and reduce social class, gender, and racial gaps.[95,105-107] For example, Aronson and colleagues[108] studied African-American and white learners in an effort to test a method to help learners resist responses to stereotype threat (being at risk of confirming, as a self-characteristic, a negative stereotype about one's social group).[109] Learners in the intervention group were encouraged to see intelligence as malleable rather than fixed. Over three sessions, they learned about the brain's capacity for neuroplasticity, imaged their brains growing denser connections between neurons when faced with academic challenges, and wrote a pen pal letter to teach the growth mindset message to a struggling middle-school learner. The investigators found that the African-American learners (and to some degree the white learners) who engaged with the growth mindset experienced an enduring and beneficial change in their own attitudes about intelligence. They reported greater enjoyment of the academic process and greater academic engagement, and obtained higher grade point averages than the control groups.

Because most field interventions have involved in-person trainings with small groups of learners, Paunesku and colleagues sought to determine if interventions to alter mindset could be scaled up to enhance academic achievement and close achievement gaps for a large number of learners.[110] They focused specifically on the poorly performing learners at risk of dropping out of high school (who comprised one-third of the sample). The researchers transformed in-person interventions into brief computer-based modules that presented two mindset interventions, one for growth mindset of intelligence and a second one for sense of purpose, designed to help learners persist in the face of academic difficulty. They delivered the online intervention to 1594 learners in 13 geographically diverse high schools. The 45-minute mindset intervention consisted of reading an article about the neurologic underpinnings for learners' ability to increase their intelligence through study and practice and performing two writing exercises. The first exercise asked learners to summarize the scientific findings in their own words, and the second asked learners to write a supportive letter to a struggling learner. The investigators found that the interventions raised grades and satisfactory completion rates in core academic subjects in a large and diverse group of underperforming learners over one academic semester. Among the learners at risk of dropping out, each intervention raised learners' semester grade point averages in core academic courses and increased the rate of satisfactory performance in core courses by 6.4 percentage points.

Yeager and Walton, in a review of the literature regarding the theoretical basis of several prominent social-psychological interventions, concluded that mindset interventions

> are not magic. They are not inputs that go into a black box and automatically yield positive results ... They do not teach students academic content or skills, restructure schools, or improve teacher training. Instead, they allow

students to take better advantage of learning opportunities that are present in schools and tap into existing recursive processes to general long-lasting effects.[7]

Mindset in Medical Education

Although there has been tremendous expansion of studies on mindset in the psychological and educational literature over the last two decades, primarily investigating high school and college learners, there have been surprisingly few studies to date exploring the role mindset plays or can play in training adult health professionals, including medical students and practicing physicians.

Feeley and Biggerstaff conducted a literature review to gauge the impact that two different aspects of learning—learning style and learning approaches—have on medical students' academic achievement.[111] The term *learning style* refers to the way in which learners prefer to receive information (e.g., visual, auditory, read-write, and kinesthetic modes). The term *learning approaches* refers to the motivations that drive their learning (e.g., deep, strategic, and surface). The researchers found that preferred learning styles do not correlate with examination performances, and that there was no evidence that designing curricula to explicitly match individual medical student's learning preferences had any effect on academic outcomes. In contrast, medical students' learning approaches did correlate with achievement; medical students with "strategic" and "deep" (less consistently) approaches to learning performed consistently better on medical school examinations than medical students with "surface" approaches. This was true across various medical student groups in different countries and cultures worldwide. Feeley and Biggerstaff's findings also revealed that medical students' learning approaches can change, and learners can learn more adaptive approaches to their studying. Feeley and Biggerstaff concluded,

> the evidence is that helping learners adopt a growth mindset, valuing effort, and emphasizing the utility of continuous development rather than fearing failure, is achievable. This approach may help learners adopt the strategic (and deep) learning approaches that have been shown to consistently correlate with medical school exam success.[111]

Jegathesan and colleagues sought to determine if pediatricians are of the fixed or growth mindset and whether individual mindsets affect perception of medical error reporting.[112] They hypothesized that physicians with different mindsets might react differently to the making of and admitting to a medical error, which could have educational implications for promoting enhanced clinical practice. They surveyed residents and attendings at a tertiary care pediatric hospital to determine their mindset and collected data on respondents' recall of medical errors by themselves or others. The researchers found that pediatricians did not have a dominant mindset, and that the distribution of fixed and growth mindsets was similar to that seen in the general population. Furthermore, there was no difference in the number of errors reported between fixed and growth mindset physicians, whether reporting their own errors or those of others. Although Jegathesan and colleagues found no correlation between mindset and the reporting of medical errors on a survey, they surmised,

> This finding is far from conclusive. Future research may still be able to delve further into evaluating whether variability in mindset affects a clinician's response to error or other feedback. . . . Future studies can elucidate how mindset interacts with a physician's response, when a physician is confronted with threats to self-perception of intelligence and worth and whether these responses have implications for future clinical decision-making and practice-based performance in medicine.[112]

Indeed, the occurrence of a medical error prompts individual physicians and provider teams to learn, improve systems, and enhance the quality of care if, in the aftermath of an adverse patient event, providers are motivated to reflect and engage in constructive ways.[113] Klein and colleagues argued that growth mindset instruction could help clinicians develop a more resilient response to medical errors, "allowing students and trainees—as well as more experienced doctors—to cope and even flourish in the wake of an error."[114]

As part of the proliferation of research on growth mindset, researchers in neuroscience are beginning to uncover the connections between growth mindset, intrinsic motivation, and learning processes. Ng reviewed the small body of existing growth mindset studies using neuroscience methods, primarily electroencephalography and functional magnetic resonance imaging, that reveal neural mechanisms of growth mindset.[115] For example, Moser and coworkers found that individuals with a growth mindset exhibit a higher error positivity waveform response, which is correlated with a heightened awareness of and attention to mistakes, supporting the notion that growth mindset learners are receptive to corrective feedback.[116] Myers and colleagues found that growth mindset was related to both ventral and dorsal striatal connectivity with the dorsal anterior cingulate cortex and the dorsolateral prefrontal cortex, both of which are critical to error monitoring and behavioral adaptation.[117] The neuroscience of growth mindset is still in its infancy and promises to impact our understanding of the interplay between growth mindset and intrinsic motivation, and, ultimately, how to

maximize growth mindset interventions in order to assist learners to reach their full potentials.

Given the need for physicians to engage in learning at every stage of their careers in order to provide high-quality health care, the growth mindset likely has an important role to play in helping medical students, residents, and practicing clinicians become master adaptive learners. Growth mindset individuals are forward-looking, believe in their ability to grow, and focus on improvement, and thus, from the outset, have a willingness to engage with the MAL process to capitalize on a learning opportunity.

Promoting the Growth Mindset

Multiple studies have shown that a number of methods can be utilized to promote a growth mindset. Administrators can incorporate validated academic mindset programs and practices into existing school programming and invest in classroom learning materials that teach the growth mindset.[20] Educational interventions can include single sessions, presented as an orientation, a workshop, or grand rounds; once-a-week sessions; or online modules. One of the most successful method for assisting learners to adopt a growth mindset is to provide direct instruction about growth and fixed mindsets.[7,93,95-97,108,118] Although still evolving, Klein and colleagues noted that the

> key components of the training appear to be: 1) participants are first exposed to scientific information on neuroplasticity—that the brain is "like a muscle" and greater learning, experience and practice leads to the development of denser networks of neurons in the brains; 2) participants write about a personal example of learning and getting smarter; and 3) participants are asked to write a letter to a future student who might be struggling in school.[114]

Educators can also develop and incorporate validated programs to instruct faculty on how to effectively promote a growth mindset among learners.[20] As Blackburn has succinctly stated, it starts with oneself: "Reinforcing a growth mindset with your students requires that you have a growth mindset."[119] Faculty can act like positive role models in a number of ways, promoting the growth mindset in the language they use with their learners,[120] in how they perceive the abilities of their learners,[121] and in how they provide feedback.[122] "Feedback on performance in simulations or in actual clinical work should focus on process as much as possible, pointing out the efforts and behaviours that led to positive outcomes and those that did not, with specific recommendations for the actions that can be taken to make improvements."[114] Educators can label constructive or corrective feedback as coaching and mentoring and stress that making errors of judgment and receiving feedback on how to improve is a valuable and necessary aspect of learning.[114] Simulation exercises, as a newer method of teaching, can play an important role in revealing errors of judgment in a safe environment, allowing learners to gain knowledge and skills without exposing patients to provider misjudgments and mistakes.[123-125] In addition, faculty as role models can share their own stories of setbacks and failures and how they persevered in the face of challenges during their careers.

Finally, the institution at large can play a critical role in promoting a growth mindset by creating a culture that deeply values it and supports it in a number of ways.[20,114] These can include instituting educational programs and engaging in research[20] to advance our understanding of mindset and its effects on learners' motivation, faculty teaching, and overall academic achievement and clinical performance. Research into implicit theories of self in medical education and practice is at an early stage, and there are extensive opportunities to develop meaningful interventions and best practices to assist medical students, residents, faculty, and practicing clinicians to adopt and nurture a growth mindset.

RESILIENCE

Resilience as a Dynamic Capacity

The fourth MAL battery is resilience. For over half a century, resilience has been the intense focus of research in several fields, including psychology, trauma studies, education, and medicine. It has emerged as a concept that represents a critical capability believed to be necessary to thrive in the complex and stressful field of medicine.[126] Resilience—predictors of it and its effect on well-being—has been studied in a number of populations, including individuals struggling to overcome traumatic experiences; living with debilitating, chronic conditions; and coping in stressful work environments. Initially, resilience was viewed as a personal attribute or fixed trait ("trait-oriented approach"). However, with the passage of time and the ever-expanding body of research findings, experts in the field have come to view resilience as a dynamic process[127] that can be developed ("process-oriented approach") or an outcome[128,129] to be achieved ("outcome-oriented approach").

The American Psychological Association has defined resilience as "the process of adapting well in the face of adversity, trauma, tragedy, threats, or even significant sources of threat."[130] In its most shorthand definition, resilience is the ability "to bounce back." The definition of resilience, however, varies greatly among researchers and experts involved in resilience work. In a review of the literature, Chmitorz and colleagues critically evaluated the definition of resilience, how it was assessed, and technical design issues in 43 randomized controlled trials of resilience interventions published between 1979 and 2014.[131] Twenty-five of the 43 trials gave no explicit definition of resilience, whereas the remaining 18 used a variety of definitions, including trait-based ones, process-oriented ones, and one outcome-oriented definition. Sanderson and Brewer, in a scoping review of articles on resilience in health education literature, found the same. There was no commonly accepted definition of resilience within the 36 papers they reviewed.[126] They did find, however, that the majority of definitions referred to resilience as a process, utilizing terms such as "ability," "capacity," or "capability." The process definitions tend to embody three phases: "1) an adverse or trauma event, 2) a process of learning or problem solving, and 3) the individual's return to their previous state or to an altered state."[126] Adopting a socioecological perspective[132] and drawing on the earlier work of Tempski and coworkers[133] and Wood,[134] Sanderson and Brewer proposed the following definition: "Resilience is the dynamic capacity to overcome adversity, drawing on personal, social and organizational resources, to achieve personal growth and transformation."[126] Adversity, according to Lazarus' Transactional Model of Stress and Coping,[135] is commonplace: many events that one must typically confront in the course of a lifetime create adversity (e.g., losses in one's personal and professional life, job stresses, illness, traumatic experiences). Thus the value of personal resilience, according to the Lazarus model, "lies in its potential as an internal resource for mitigating the negative effects of stress and for maintaining mental health through adversity."[136]

The notion of resilience is thus a very complex, multidimensional construct, and individuals' capacity for resilience varies widely. One's ability to respond to adversity depends on numerous genetic, developmental, cognitive, psychological, and neurobiologic risk and protective factors.[137] Researchers have identified a number of internal resilience factors that help protect a person from the potential negative effects of adversity, including cognitive factors, emotion regulation, social factors, physical health, and neurobiology factors (Fig. 4.1). External and environmental protective factors, such as access to material resources, play a role as well.[138] Emerging theory supports the notion that resilience is not static. Rather, at any given point, an individual's overall capacity for resilience is influenced by the dynamic interaction of the internal and external components. This capacity can be enhanced or compromised.[139-141] Given the neuroplasticity of the human brain, experts in the field believe that many of the protective factors can be enhanced through interventions

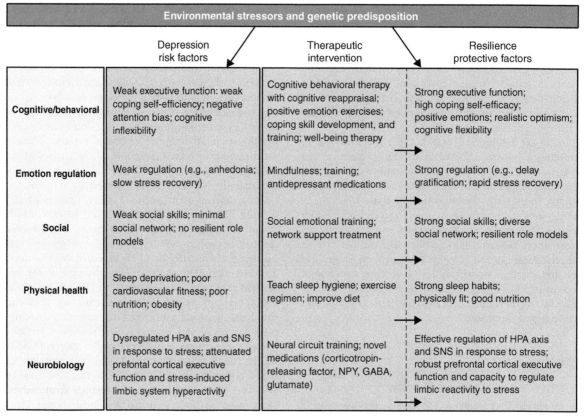

Fig. 4.1 Resilience as a multidimensional construct. *GABA,* Gamma-aminobutyric acid; *HPA,* hypothalamic-pituitary-adrenal; *NPY,* neuropeptide Y; *SNS,* sympathetic nervous system. (From Southwick SM, Charney DS. The science of resilience: implications for the prevention and treatment of depression. *Science.* 2012;338[6103]:79-82.)

and practice, although scientific investigations into this area are at an early stage.[137]

Resilience is typically assessed by using one of the numerous resiliency scales that have been developed for use in general and clinical populations. In 2011, Windle and colleagues conducted a systematic review[142] of the psychometric rigor of 15 resilience measurement scales and reported that the Connor-Davidson Resilience Scale,[143] the Resilience Scale for Adults,[144] and the Brief Resilience Scale[145] had the best psychometric ratings. They concluded, however, "We found no current 'gold standard' amongst 15 measures of resilience. A number of scales are in the early stages of development, and all require further validation work."[142]

In 2016, Cassidy reported the development of a reliable and valid 30-item instrument called the Academic Resilience Scale, which focuses on the process of resilience rather than attitudes about resilience.[146] The instrument provides a measure of academic resilience based on learners' specific adaptive cognitive-affective and behavioral responses to academic adversity. The concept of academic resilience is specifically concerned with the relevance of resilience in educational contexts and is defined as "a capacity to overcome acute and/or chronic adversity that is seen as a major threat to a student's educational development."[147] Cassidy concluded that the Academic Resilience Scale "has the potential to help identify limitations in existing student responses to academic adversity and to assist the development of interventions aimed at fostering adaptive responses, and to provide a measure of the efficacy of such interventions in terms of developing students' academic resilience."[146]

Although overall there is still a lack of clarity regarding the concept of resilience, a precise definition of the term, and an agreed upon method for measuring outcomes, resilience is believed to be a highly important human capability with which to master the vicissitudes of life and, importantly, is a capacity that can be enhanced through interventions that bolster the protective factors comprising a resilient response in the face of a challenge. For this reason, the medical field has taken great interest in resilience.

Resilience in Medical Education

Over the past two decades, medicine has witnessed an ever-increasing concern about the stress involved in medical education and clinical practice and about the level of burnout among medical students,[148,149] residents,[150,151] and practicing clinicians.[152-154] According to the extensive literature on burnout—defined as a work-related syndrome characterized by emotional exhaustion, depersonalization, and a sense of reduced accomplishment[155]—it now affects approximately one-half of all physicians in training and practicing physicians at some point in their careers. The consequences of burnout are well documented, ranging from a host of professional issues, including reduced productivity, increased medical errors, reduced quality of patient care, and decreased medical knowledge, to personal issues such as substance abuse problems, disrupted personal relationships, clinical depression, and suicide.[149,153,154] Medical students are known to struggle with high levels of depression, anxiety, and suicidal ideation.[148] Likewise, the literature documents high rates of depression and suicide among physicians.[152,156] The reality is that working in the health professions is stressful and presents the learner with numerous challenges at every stage of education and practice.

In the face of this reality, many educators and researchers have become interested in resilience, looking to develop it among medical students and practicing physicians as a way to mitigate burnout and, more importantly, enhance the learning process, maximize self-actualization, promote well-being, and, ultimately, improve patient care. In a 2009 review of the resilience literature in health disciplines, McAllister and McKinnon argued, in a way that supports the MAL process, that "resilience theory should be part of the educational content and taught in a way that promotes reflection and application in order to give students strength, focus, and endurance in the workplace."[157] The profession is now grappling with how to develop a culture that promotes and nurtures resilience starting in medical school and continuing throughout the education continuum. Studies have identified resilience as a central element of medical student and physician well-being.[158-160] Delany and colleagues recognized the importance of resilience especially in clinical learning environments.[161] Epstein and Krasner argued that resilience is "a key to enhancing quality of care, quality of caring, and sustainability of the health care workforce."[162]

Promoting Resilience

As noted previously, although many researchers and education experts called for resilience education as a solution to meeting challenges and mitigating burnout, initially there was little evidence that educational interventions could enhance resilience.[163] More recently, research is addressing the question of whether it can be enhanced and, if so, the best methods for doing so. Several recent systematic reviews have attempted to answer this question by analyzing the accumulated evidence.

In 2014, Leppin and coworkers conducted a systematic review and meta-analysis of 25 randomized trials assessing the efficacy of resiliency training programs to improve mental health and capacity in diverse adult populations and persons with chronic disease.[136] "Resiliency training programs" were loosely defined in the trials, with no single accepted theoretical framework or consensus statement guiding the development or application of the programs or a gold standard method of evaluating them. "There remains little clarity related to what is fundamentally required for a program to be considered resiliency training," the researchers wrote, "let alone for it to be considered effective."[136] Nonetheless, they reported that, after at least 3 months of follow-up, the findings supported a modest but consistent benefit of training programs in improving a number of mental health outcomes.

In a 2016 systematic review, Rogers analyzed the evidence from 16 papers on a variety of educational interventions aimed at enhancing resilience among health care workers.[163] The main interventions were resilience workshops, small group problem solving, sharing, reflection, cognitive behavioral interventions, mindfulness and relaxation techniques, and mentoring. Rogers found that, overall, education can improve health care workers' resilience and that there was reasonable evidence for resilience-enhancing workshops and cognitive behavioral interventions. There was also some evidence for small group problem solving. The strength of the evidence for reflection, mentoring, mindfulness, and relaxing techniques was mixed. One paper suggested that the effectiveness of an intervention might be influenced by the preexisting level of resilience, with those individuals with lower levels of resilience benefitting the most.[164] Rogers concluded that a combination of interventions might represent the best chance of success.[163]

In 2018, Fox and colleagues conducted a systematic review of 22 studies published between 2000 and 2016 (~73% since 2014) that assessed interventions to foster resilience in physicians.[165] Interventions included psychosocial skills training, mindfulness-based training, coaching interventions, and simulation-based interventions, with almost all focused on enhancing resilience at the individual level. The majority of interventions were delivered in group settings, and the majority (59%) were conducted in mixed groups of physicians along with other health care professionals and medical students. The remaining 41% were delivered exclusively to physicians. Fox and colleagues reported that the methodologic quality of the studies was low to moderate, and effect sizes were heterogeneous. Nevertheless, they concluded that initial data are promising and suggest that interventions can result in increases in resilience that may persist over time. Fox and colleagues called for more methodologic rigor in the research and a greater focus on a systems-wide approach to resilience building that targets both the individual and the organization.

It is important to underscore the role of the organization in either promoting resilience or driving burnout. Whereas interventions have traditionally focused on the individual, research suggests burnout is more the consequence of the organizational systems in place across many medical education and hospital settings.[165-167] Interventions that fail to address the underlying detrimental organizational factors that undermine well-being unduly place the burden of responsibility on the individual to resist burnout and to adapt through building resilience. Taking a systems approach may be significantly more impactful.[166,168] Increasingly, health care organizations are appointing senior personnel to serve in roles (e.g., chief wellness officer) focused on initiating or expanding strategies to improve physicians' and other team members' health and well-being.[169]

In summary, the literature suggests that resilience can be enhanced and has an important role to play in medical education. It is a complex phenomenon, and there is still much work to be done in terms of defining and measuring it, as well as determining best practices for enhancing and sustaining it. As part of our continuing investigation into resilience, it will be critical to ascertain its role in promoting and sustaining the master adaptive learner. The role of the organizational system—especially the learning environment—in promoting resilience and the other personal characteristics that drive the MAL process needs to be a central area of research and transformation.

THE FOUR PERSONAL CHARACTERISTICS AND THE MASTER ADAPTIVE LEARNER PROCESS

The MAL process is, at its core, a process of self-regulation of one's own intellectual functioning and development. This chapter has explored what we currently know from a number of different fields about the four critical personal characteristics that are believed to drive the MAL process, promoting and sustaining the learner's ability to engage in the learning cycle. Curiosity stimulates the learner's desire to gain information in order to understand and make sense of the world. Curiosity compels a learner to learn in order

to deeply understand a problem rather than to just complete a task, pass an assessment, or meet a minimal competency. Curiosity is critical for the MAL planning phase, which drives the learner to identify gaps between what she understands and what is actually occurring. It is also key to the learning phase because it helps ensure that a learner spends the time and effort to thoroughly understand the issue or question at a deep level. Learners who demonstrate curiosity are "less likely to accept what they are told uncritically. Instead, they enjoy asking questions, and are more willing to reveal their questions and uncertainties in public."[170] While curiosity makes the learner identify a gap in knowledge, motivation provides the impetus to identify how to fill the gap and the ability to ask the skillful questions (what, how, and why) in pursuit of the answers. Motivation also allows the learner to sustain the effort to continually seek out, engage in, enjoy, and pursue opportunities for effortful cognitive activity.

The attributes of a growth mindset can also assist in driving forward each of the four phrases of the MAL process. Positive attitudes about learning (pursuing challenges, valuing effort, and believing mistakes are critical to learning) trigger master adaptive learners to engage with the planning phase, especially stimulating their identification of a knowledge, skill, or attitude gap and setting a deep-learning–oriented goal. Adaptive responses to setbacks (believing setbacks are part of the learning process, demonstrating resilience to them, employing adaptive study methods, and adapting to increasing challenges) can assist in all four phases of the MAL process. These adaptive responses are particularly relevant in the learning phase, when the learner may be confronted with internal challenges, such as difficulties understanding the material, or with external challenges, such as a stressful learning environment. Responding positively to feedback (eagerly seeking out formative feedback and quickly implementing feedback received) is particularly useful in the assessing phase, because unguided self-assessment by medical trainees and clinicians is less accurate.[171] At each step of the way, the growth mindset is a critical foundation for learners to become master adaptive learners. The attributes of a growth mindset help drive each of the four phases of the MAL process.

Finally, resilience has an important role to play in supporting the trainee in becoming a master adaptive learner. Resilience is particularly important in the MAL process when the learner encounters inevitable challenges, setbacks, and failures. Resilient learners are individuals who cultivate specific attitudes, skills, and habits that enhance their capacity to achieve their goals with minimal psychological and physical cost and a healthy response to stress. This includes the capacity for self-awareness, mindfulness, self-monitoring, limit setting, and engaging with challenges at work in a constructive way. It also entails establishing practices and routines that incorporate leisure-time activity, cultivation of relationships with family and friends, limits on work hours, ritualized time-out periods, continuous professional development, physical exercise, spiritual nurturance and, ultimately, knowing and accepting one's personal boundaries and professional limits.[162]

These four critical personal characteristics interact in profoundly complex ways to power the MAL process. Much remains to be understood about how they actually drive the process, how they interact with one another and enrich the MAL process, and, importantly, how they each can be promoted within individuals and the learning environment. In addition, there are unquestionably other characteristics and factors critical to the MAL process that we have not discussed in this chapter. For example, what is the role that the tolerance of ambiguity plays in being able to engage with gaps in knowledge? How does an individual's sense of social belonging or lack thereof influence engagement with the MAL process? The prospects for research into defining and understanding all the personal characteristics and external factors that influence the MAL process are broad and deep and offer the health professions an array of exciting opportunities to support learners and enrich both the learning and workplace environments.

Health care continues to rapidly change in the 21st century due to multiple factors, including the expanding body of knowledge, technical advances, population dynamics, and issues of equity and inclusion. The knowledge and skills gap between what medical students and clinicians know and what they need to know to be successful in delivering the best possible care to patients and solve workplace challenges will only continue to expand.[172] Becoming a master adaptive learner, with the attendant curiosity, motivation, growth mindset, and resilience, is central to meeting the challenge of the ever-changing and demanding field of medicine.

TAKE-HOME POINTS

1. There are four critical personal characteristics—curiosity, motivation, growth mindset, and resilience—that drive the master adaptive learner process.
2. Medical students, residents, fellows, and practicing physicians can take steps to enhance these characteristics.
3. The learning environment can either promote or stifle MAL characteristics, and measures should be taken to assure that the environment fosters these characteristics.

QUESTIONS FOR FURTHER THOUGHT

1. How can we best alter the learning environment such that it promotes MAL characteristics?
2. What are the best ways to assess deficiencies and diagnose MAL challenges? Should we attempt to routinely assess these characteristics through testing?
3. What are the best ways to offer remediation for those learners who have significant issues related to MAL characteristics?
4. Should these characteristics be measured in medical school applicants and used as grounds for admission to medical school?
5. These characteristics do not function in isolation. How do other factors in the external environment impact the expression of MAL characteristics in learning situations?

ANNOTATED BIBLIOGRAPHY

1. Sternszus R, Saroyan A, Steinert Y. Describing medical student curiosity across a four year curriculum: an exploratory study. *Med Teach.* 2017;39(4):377-382.
   This study is the first to describe state and trait intellectual curiosity in undergraduate medical education. Findings suggest medical students' state curiosity may not be optimally supported. This paper also highlights avenues for further research.
2. Dyche L, Epstein RM. Curiosity and medical education. *Med Educ.* 2011;45:663-668.
   This paper discusses how curiosity, inquisitiveness, and related habits of mind can be supported in medical education through specific, evidence-based instructional approaches.
3. Kusurkar RA, Ten Cate TJ, van Asperen M, Croiset G. Motivation as an independent and a dependent variable in medical education: a review of the literature. *Med Teach.* 2011;33(5):e242-e262.
   This systematic review of the medical literature shows that motivation is an independent variable in medical education, influencing important outcomes. Motivation is also a dependent variable influenced by autonomy, competence, and relatedness.
4. Kusurkar RA, Croiset G, Ten Cate TJ. Twelve tips to stimulate intrinsic motivation in students through autonomy-supportive classroom teaching derived from self-determination theory. *Med Teach.* 2011;33(12):978-982.
   Grounded in the self-determination theory (SDT) of motivation, this article presents 12 practical tips for teachers in

health professions on how to engage in autonomy-supportive teaching behaviors in order to stimulate intrinsic motivation in medical students.

5. Rattan A, Savani K, Chugh D, Dweck CS. Leveraging Mindsets to Promote Academic Achievement: Policy Recommendations. *Perspect Psychol Sci.* 2015;10(6):721-726.

This article addresses how policy at all levels (federal, state, and local) can leverage mindsets—the growth mindset and the belonging mindset—to improve educational outcomes.

6. Dunn LB, Iglewicz A, Moutier C. A conceptual model of medical student well-being: promoting resilience and preventing burnout. *Acad Psychiatry.* 2008;32(1):44-53.

This review of the literature on medical student stress, coping, and well-being proposes a model of medical student coping termed the *coping reservoir,* with the goal of enhancing resilience, improving mental health, and mitigating distress and burnout.

7. Epstein RM, Krasner MS. Physician resilience: what is means, why it matters, and how to promote it. *Acad Med.* 2013;88(3):301-303.

This commentary by experts in the field proposes methods for enhancing individuals' resilience while building community, as well as articulating directions for future interventions, research, and institutional involvement.

REFERENCES

1. Binet A, Simon T. *The Development of Intelligence in Children (the Binet-Simon Scale).* Baltimore, MD: Williams & Wilkins; 1916.
2. Borghans L, Duckworth AL, Heckman JJ, ter Weel B. The economics and psychology of personality traits. *J Hum Resour.* 2008;43(4):972-1059.
3. Farrington CA, Roderick M, Allensworth E, et al. *Teaching Adolescents to Become Learners. The Role of Noncognitive Factors in Shaping School Performance: A Critical Literature Review.* Chicago, IL: University of Chicago Consortium on Chicago School Research; 2012.
4. Jackson JJ, Connolly JJ, Garrison SM, Leveille MM, Connolly SL. Your friends know how long you will live: a 75-year study of peer-rated personality traits. *Psychol Sci.* 2015;26(3):335-340.
5. Moffitt TE, Arseneault L, Belsky D, et al. A gradient of childhood self-control predicts health, wealth, and public safety. *Proc Natl Acad Sci U S A.* 2011;108(7):2693-2698.
6. Naemi B, Burrus J, Kyllonen PC, Roberts RD. *Building a Case to Develop Noncognitive Assessment Products and Services Targeting Workforce Readiness at ETS.* Princeton, NJ: Educational Testing Service; 2012.
7. Yeager DS, Walton GM. Social-psychological interventions in education: they're not magic. *Rev Educ Res.* 2011;81(2):267-301.
8. Elias MJ, ed. *Promoting Social and Emotional Learning: Guidelines for Educators.* Chicago, IL: Association for Supervision and Curriculum Development; 1997.
9. Durlak JA, Domitrovich CE, Weissberg RP, Gullotta TP. *Handbook of Social and Emotional Learning: Research and Practice.* New York, NY: Guilford; 2015.
10. Caspi A, Roberts BW, Shiner RL. Personality development: stability and change. *Annu Rev Psychol.* 2005;56:453-484.
11. Roberts BW, DelVecchio WF. The rank-order consistency of personality traits from childhood to old age: a quantitative review of longitudinal studies. *Psychol Bull.* 2000;126(1):3-25.
12. Roberts BW, Walton KE, Viechtbauer W. Patterns of mean-level change in personality traits across the life course: a meta-analysis of longitudinal studies. *Psychol Bull.* 2006;132(1):1-25.
13. Tough P. *How Children Succeed: Grit, Curiosity, and the Hidden Power of Character.* New York, NY: Houghton Mifflin Harcourt; 2013.
14. Kosslyn SM, Cacioppo JT, Davidson RJ, et al. Bridging psychology and biology. The analysis of individuals in groups. *Am Psychol.* 2002;57:341-351.
15. Cutrer WB, Miller B, Pusic MV, et al. Fostering the development of master adaptive learners: a conceptual model to guide skill acquisition in medical education. *Acad Med.* 2017;92:70-75.
16. Furnham A, Marks J. Tolerance of ambiguity: a review of the recent literature. *Psychology.* 2013;4:717-728.
17. Caulfield M, Andolsek K, Grbic D, Roskovensky L. Ambiguity tolerance of students matriculating to U.S. medical schools. *Acad Med.* 2014;89(11):1526-1532.
18. Simpkin AL, Schwartzstein RM. Tolerating Uncertainty - The Next Medical Revolution? *N Engl J Med.* 2016;375(18):1713-1715.
19. Walton GM, Cohen GL. A question of belonging: race, social fit, and achievement. *J Pers Soc Psychol.* 2007;92:82-96.
20. Rattan A, Savani K, Chugh D, Dweck CS. Leveraging mindsets to promote academic achievement: policy recommendations. *Perspect Psychol Sci.* 2015;10(6):721-726.
21. Loewenstein G. The psychology of curiosity: a review and reinterpretation. *Psychol Bull.* 1994;116:75-98.
22. Berlyne DE. Novelty and curiosity as determinants of exploratory behavior. *Br J Psychol.* 1950:41:68-60.
23. Goff M, Ackerman PL. Personality-intelligence relations: assessment of typical intellectual engagement. *J Educ Psychol.* 1992;84:537-552.
24. Berlyne DE. A theory of human curiosity. *Br J Psychol.* 1954;45:180-191.
25. Berlyne DE. *Conflict, Arousal, and Curiosity.* London, UK: McGraw-Hill; 1960.
26. Naylor FD. A state-trait curiosity inventory. *Aust Psychol.* 1981;16:172-183.
27. Pluck G, Johnson HL. Stimulating curiosity to enhance learning. *GESJ: Educ Sci Psychol.* 2011;2(19):24-31.
28. Reio Jr TG, Petrosko JM, Wiswell AK, Thongsukmag J. The measurement and conceptualization of curiosity. *J Genet Psychol.* 2006;167:117-135.
29. Mussel P. Intellect: a theoretical framework for personality traits related to intellectual achievements. *J Pers Soc Psychol.* 2013;104:885-906.
30. Chamorro-Premuzic T, Furnham A, Ackerman PL. Incremental validity of the typical intellectual engagement scale as predictor of different academic performance measures. *J Pers Assess.* 2006;87:261-268.

31. Arteche A, Chamorro-Premuzic T, Ackerman P, Furnham A. Typical intellectual engagement as a byproduct of openness, learning approaches, and self-assessed intelligence. *Educ Psychol.* 2009;29:357-367.

32. von Stumm S, Hell B, Chamorro-Premuzic T. The hungry mind: intellectual curiosity is the third pillar of academic performance. *Perspect Psychol Sci.* 2011;6:574-588.

33. Reio Jr TG, Callahan JL. Affect, curiosity, and socialization-related learning: a path analysis of antecedents to job performance. *J Bus Psychol.* 2004;19:3-22.

34. Gruber MJ, Gelman BD, Ranganath C. States of curiosity modulate hippocampus-dependent learning via the dopaminergic circuit. *Neuron.* 2014;84(2):486-496.

35. Kasman DL. Socialization in medical training: exploring "lifelong curiosity" and a "community of support". *Am J Bioeth.* 2004;4:52-55.

36. Epstein RM, Siegel DJ, Silberman J. Self-monitoring in clinical practice: a challenge for medical educators. *J Contin Educ Health Prof.* 2008;28:5-13.

37. Curry RH, Montgomery K. Toward a liberal education in medicine. *Acad Med.* 2010;85:283-287.

38. Dyche L, Epstein RM. Curiosity and medical education. *Med Educ.* 2011;45:663-668.

39. Roman B. Curiosity: a best practice in education. *Med Educ.* 2011;45:654-656.

40. Nanda A. Curiosity, compassion, and composure. *World Neurosurg.* 2012;78:14-17.

41. Kanter SL. Realizing full potential. *Acad Med.* 2012;87:1453.

42. Whitehead C, Kuper A. Beyond the biomedical feedlot. *Acad Med.* 2012;87:1485.

43. Ellaway RH. When I say ... epistemic curiosity. *Med Educ.* 2014;48:113-114.

44. Fitzgerald FT. Curiosity. *Ann Intern Med.* 1999;130:70-72.

45. Richards JB, Litman J, Roberts DH. Performance characteristics of measurement instruments of epistemic curiosity in third-year medical students. *Med Sci Educ.* 2013;23:355-363.

46. Norman G. On competence, curiosity and creativity. *Adv Health Sci Educ Theory Pract.* 2012;17:611-613.

47. Darley JM, Batson CD. From Jerusalem to Jericho: a study of situational and dispositional variables in helping behavior. *J Pers Soc Psychol.* 1973;27(1):100.

48. Sternszus R, Saroyan A, Steinert Y. Describing medical student curiosity across a four year curriculum: an exploratory study. *Med Teach.* 2017;39(4):377-382.

49. Crick RD. Learning how to learn: the dynamic assessment of learning power. *Curriculum J.* 2007;18(2):135-153.

50. Renninger KA, Hidi S. Student interest and achievement: developmental issues raised by a case study. In: Wigfield A, Eccles JS, eds. *Development of Achievement Motivation.* San Diego, CA: Academic Press; 2002:173-195.

51. Hidi S, Renninger AK. The four-phase model of interest development. *Educ Psychol.* 2006;41(2):111-127.

52. Renninger KA. Individual interest and its implications for understanding intrinsic motivation. In: Sansone C, Harackiewicz JM, eds. *Intrinsic and Extrinsic Motivation: The Search for Optimal Motivation and Performance.* San Diego, CA: Academic Press; 2000:375-407.

53. Petri HL. Introduction. In: Petri HL, eds. *Motivation: Theory, Research, and Applications.* 4th ed. Pacific Grove, CA: Brooks/Cole Publishing Co; 1996:3-21.

54. Bransford JD, Brown AL, Cocking RR. Learning and transfer. In: *How People Learn: Brain, Mind, Experience, and School.* Expanded ed. Washington, DC: National Academies Press; 2000:51-78.

55. Deci EL, Ryan RM. *Intrinsic Motivation and Self-Determination in Human Behavior.* New York, NY: Plenum; 1985.

56. Ryan RM, Deci EL. Intrinsic and extrinsic motivations: classic definitions and new directions. *Contemp Educ Psychol.* 2000;25:54-67.

57. Ryan RM, Deci EL. Self-determination theory and the facilitation of intrinsic motivation, social development, and well-being. *Am Psychol.* 2000;55:68-78.

58. Maslow AH. A theory of human motivation. *Psychol Rev.* 1943;50(4):370-396.

59. Bandura A. Self-efficacy: toward a unifying theory of behavioral change. *Psychol Rev.* 1977;84:191-215.

60. Bandura A. Self-efficacy mechanism in human agency. *Am Psychol.* 1982;37:122-147.

61. Bandura A. *Self-Efficacy: The Exercise of Control.* New York, NY: W.H. Freeman; 1997.

62. Zimmerman BJ. A social cognitive view of self-regulated academic learning. *J Educ Psychol.* 1989;81:329-339.

63. Zimmerman BJ. Self-efficacy: an essential motive to learn. *Contemp Educ Psychol.* 2000;25:82-91.

64. Ames C. Classrooms: goals, structures, and student motivation. *J Educ Psychol.* 1992;84:261-271.

65. Heckhausen H. *Motivation and Action.* Berlin, Germany: Springer; 1991.

66. Pajares F. Self-efficacy beliefs in academic settings. *Rev Educ Res.* 1996;66:543-578.

67. Pintrich PR, de Groot EV. Motivational and self-regulated learning components of classroom academic performance. *J Educ Psychol.* 1990;82:33-40.

68. Wigfield A, Eccles JS. The development of competence beliefs, expectancies for success, and achievement values from childhood through adolescence. In: Wigfield A, Eccles JS, eds. *Development of Achievement Motivation.* San Diego, CA: Academic Press; 2002:91-120.

69. Hidi S. Interest, reading, and learning: theoretical and practical considerations. *Educ Psychol Rev.* 2001;13:191-208.

70. Renninger KA. Effort and interest. In: Guthrie JW, ed. *The Encyclopedia of Education.* 2nd ed. New York, NY: Macmillan; 2003:704-709.

71. Renninger KA, Wozniak RH. Effect of interest on attentional shift, recognition, and recall in young children. *Dev Psychol.* 1985;21:624-632.

72. Schiefele U. Interest and learning from text. *Sci Stud Read.* 1999;3(3):257-279.

73. Schiefele U. The role of interest in motivation and learning. In: Collis JM, Messick S, eds. *Intelligence and Personality.* Mahwah, NJ: Lawrence Erlbaum Associates; 2001:163-194.

74. Krapp A, Lewalter D. Development of interests and interest-based motivational orientations: a longitudinal study in school and work settings. In: Volet S, Järvelä S, eds. *Motivation*

in *Learning Contexts: Theoretical Advances and Methodological Implications.* London, UK: Elsevier; 2001:201-232.

75. Renninger KA, Shumar W. Community building with and for teachers: the Math Forum as a resource for teacher professional development. In: Renninger KA, Shumar W, eds. *Building Virtual Communities: Learning and Change in Cyberspace.* New York, NY: Cambridge University Press; 2002:60-95.

76. Snowdon D. *Aging with Grace.* New York, NY: Bantam; 2001.

77. Berninger V, Richards TL. *Brain Literacy for Educators and Psychologists.* New York, NY: Academic Press; 2002.

78. Sansone C, Smith JL. Interest and self-regulation: The relation between having to and wanting to. In: Sansone C, Harackiewicz JM, eds. *Intrinsic and Extrinsic Motivation: The Search for Optimal Motivation and Performance.* San Diego, CA: Academic Press; 2000:341-372.

79. Sansone C, Weir C, Harpster L, Morgan C. Once a boring task always a boring task? Interest as a self-regulatory mechanism. *J Pers Soc Psychol.* 1992;63:379-390.

80. Sansone C, Wiebe DJ, Morgan C. Self-regulating interest: the moderating role of hardiness and conscientiousness. *J Pers.* 1999;67:701-733.

81. Hidi S, Harackiewicz JM. Motivating the academically unmotivated: a critical issue for the 21st century. *Rev Educ Res.* 2000;70(2):151-179.

82. Schraw G, Lehman S. Situational interest: a review of the literature and directions for future research. *Educ Psychol Rev.* 2001;13:23-52.

83. Turner JC, Midgley C, Meyer DK, et al. The classroom environment and students' reports of avoidance strategies in mathematics: a multimethod study. *J Educ Psychol.* 2002; 94:88-106.

84. Meyer DK, Turner JC. Discovering emotion in classroom motivation research. *Educ Psychol.* 2002;37:107-114.

85. Williams GC, Saizow RB, Ryan RM. The importance of self-determination theory for medical education. *Acad Med.* 1999;74(9):992-995.

86. Sobral DT. What kind of motivation drives medical students' learning quests? *Med Educ.* 2004;38:950-957.

87. Kusurkar RA, Ten Cate TJ, van Asperen M, Croiset G. Motivation as an independent and a dependent variable in medical education: a review of the literature. *Med Teach.* 2011;33(5):e242-e262.

88. Kusurkar RA, Croiset G, Ten Cate TJ. Twelve tips to stimulate intrinsic motivation in students through autonomy-supportive classroom teaching derived from self-determination theory. *Med Teach.* 2011;33(12):978-982.

89. Ten Cate TJ, Kusurkar RA, Williams GC. How self-determination theory can assist our understanding of the teaching and learning processes in medical education. AMEE Guide No. 59. *Med Teach.* 2011;33(12):961-973.

90. Schraw G, Bruning R, Svoboda C. Sources of situational interest. *J Read Behav.* 1995;27:1-17.

91. Dweck CS, Chiu C, Hong Y. Implicit theories and their role in judgments and reactions: a world from two perspectives. *Psychol Inq.* 1995;6:267-285.

92. Dweck CS. Motivational processes affecting learning. *Am Psychol.* 1986;41(10):1040-1048.

93. Dweck CS. *Mindset: The New Psychology of Success.* New York, NY: Random House; 2006.

94. Mindset Works. Mindset Assessment; 2017. Available at: http://blog.mindsetworks.com/what-s-my-mindset?view= quiz.

95. Blackwell LS, Trzesniewski KH, Dweck CS. Implicit theories of intelligence predict achievement across an adolescent transition: a longitudinal study and an intervention. *Child Dev.* 2007;78(1):246-263.

96. Yeager DS, Dweck CS. Mindsets that promote resilience: when students believe that personal characteristics can be developed. *Educ Psychol.* 2012;47(4):302-314.

97. Dweck CS. *Self-Theories: Their Role in Motivation, Personality, and Development.* Philadelphia, PA: Psychology Press; 2000.

98. Gross-Loh C. How praise became a consolation prize. *The Atlantic;* December 2016. Available at: https://www .theatlantic.com/education/archive/2016/12/howpraise-became-a-consolation-prize/510845/. Accessed August 15, 2018.

99. Dweck CS. Mindsets and human nature: promoting change in the Middle East, the schoolyard, the racial divide, and willpower. *Am Psychol.* 2012;67(8):614-622.

100. Mueller CM, Dweck CS. Praise for intelligence can undermine children's motivation and performance. *J Pers Soc Psychol.* 1998;75(1):33-52.

101. Romero C, Master A, Paunesku D, Dweck CS, Gross JJ. Academic and emotional functioning in middle school: the role of implicit theories. *Emotion.* 2014;14(2):227-234.

102. Stipek D, Gralinski JH. Children's beliefs about intelligence and school performance. *J Educ Psychol.* 1996;88(3):397-407.

103. Burnette JL, O'Boyle EH, VanEpps EM, Pollack JM, Finkel EJ. Mind-sets matter: a meta-analytic review of implicit theories and self-regulation. *Psychol Bull.* 2013;139:655-701.

104. Dweck CS, Leggett EL. A social-cognitive approach to motivation and personality. *Psychol Rev.* 1988;95:256-273.

105. Stephens NM, Hamedani MG, Destin M. Closing the social-class achievement gap: a difference-education intervention improves first-generation students' academic performance and all students' college transition. *Psychol Sci.* 2014;25:943-953.

106. Walton GM, Logel C, Peach JM, Spencer SJ, Zanna MP. Two brief interventions to mitigate a "chilly climate" transform women's experience, relationships, and achievement in engineering. *J Educ Psychol.* 2015;107:468-485.

107. Walton GM, Cohen GL. A brief social-belonging intervention improves academic and health outcomes of minority students. *Science.* 2011;331:1447-1451.

108. Aronson J, Fried CB, Good C. Reducing the effects of stereotype threat on African American college students by shaping theories of intelligence. *J Exp Soc Psychol.* 2002;38(2):113-125.

109. Steele CM, Aronson J. Stereotype threat and the intellectual test performance of African Americans. *J Pers Soc Psychol.* 1995;69:797-811.

110. Paunesku D, Walton GM, Romero C, Smith EN, Yeager DS, Dweck CS. Mind-set interventions are a scalable treatment for academic underachievement. *Psychol Sci.* 2015;26(6):784-793.
111. Feeley AM, Biggerstaff DL. Exam success at undergraduate and graduate-entry medical schools: is learning style or learning approach more important? A critical review exploring links between academic success, learning styles, and learning approaches among school-leaver entry ("Traditional") and graduate-entry ("Nontraditional") medical students. *Teach Learn Med.* 2015;27(3):237-244.
112. Jegathesan M, Vitberg YM, Pusic MV. A survey of mindset theories of intelligence and medical error self-reporting among pediatric housestaff and faculty. *BMC Med Educ.* 2016;16:58.
113. Scott SD, Hirschinger LE, Cox KR, McCoig M, Brandt J, Hall LW. The natural history of recovery for the healthcare provider "second victim" after adverse patient events. *Qual Saf Health Care.* 2009;18:325-330.
114. Klein J, Delany C, Fischer MD, Smallwood D, Trumble S. A growth mindset approach to preparing trainees for medical error. *BMJ Qual Saf.* 2017;26:771-774.
115. Ng B. The neuroscience of growth mindset and intrinsic motivation. *Brain Sci.* 2018;8:E20.
116. Moser JS, Schroder HS, Heeter C, Moran TP, Lee YH. Mind your errors: evidence for a neural mechanism linking growth mind-set to adaptive posterror adjustments. *Psychol Sci.* 2011;22:1484-1489.
117. Myers CA, Wang C, Black JM, Bugescu N, Hoeft F. The matter of motivation: striatal resting-state connectivity is dissociable between grit and growth mindset. *Soc Cogn Affect Neurosci.* 2016:11:1521-1527.
118. Good C, Aronson J, Inzlicht M. Improving adolescents' standardized test performance: an intervention to reduce the effects of stereotype threat. *Appl Dev Sci.* 2004;24(6):645-662.
119. Response: Applying a Growth Mindset in the Classroom. Education Week Teacher; December 21, 2015. Available at: http://blogs.edweek.org/teachers/classroom_qa_with_larry_ferlazzo/2015/12/response_applying_a_growth_mindset_in_the_classroom.html. Accessed August 18, 2018.
120. Cooley JH, Larson S. Promoting a growth mindset in pharmacy educators and students. *Curr Pharm Teach Learn.* 2018;10:675-679.
121. De Kraker-Pauw E, Van Wesel F, Krabbendam L, Van Atteveldt N. Teacher mindsets concerning the malleability of intelligence and the appraisal of achievement in the context of feedback. *Front Psychol.* 2017;8:1594.
122. Perrella A. Room for improvement: palliating the ego in feedback-resistant medical students. *Med Teach.* 2017;39(5):555-557.
123. Elliott S, Murrell K, Harper P, Stephens T, Pellowe C. A comprehensive systematic review of the use of simulation in the continuing education and training of qualified medical, nursing and midwifery staff. *JBI Libr Syst Rev.* 2011; 9(17):538-587.
124. Cooper JB, Singer SJ, Hayes J, et al. Design and evaluation of simulation scenarios for a program introducing patient safety, teamwork, safety leadership, and simulation to healthcare leaders and managers. *Simul Healthc.* 2011;6(4): 231-238.
125. Fried MP, Satava R, Weghorst S, et al. Identifying and reducing errors with surgical simulation. *Qual Saf Health Care.* 2004;13(suppl 1):i19-i26.
126. Sanderson B, Brewer M. What do we know about student resilience in health professional education? A scoping review of the literature. *Nurse Educ Today.* 2017;58:65-71.
127. Earvolino-Ramirez M. Resilience: a concept analysis. *Nurs Forum.* 2007;42(2):73-82. doi:10.1111/j.1744-6198.2007. 00070.x.
128. Britt TW, Shen W, Sinclair RR, Grossman MR, Klieger DM. How much do we really know about employee resilience? *Ind Organ Psychol.* 2016;9(2):378-404.
129. Kalisch R, Baker DG, Basten U, et al. The resilience framework as a strategy to combat stress-related disorders. *Nat Hum Behav.* 2017;1:784-790.
130. American Psychological Association. *The Road to Resilience.* Washington, DC: APA; 2010. Available at: http://www.apa .org/helpcenter/road-resilience.aspx.
131. Chmitorz A, Kunzler A, Helmreich I, et al. Intervention studies to foster resilience—a systematic review and proposal for a resilience framework in future intervention studies. *Clin Psychol Rev.* 2018;59;78-100.
132. Ungar M, Ghazinour M, Richter J. Annual research review: what is resilience within the social ecology of human development? *J Child Psychol Psychiatry.* 2013;54(4):348-366.
133. Tempski P, Santos IS, Mayer FB, et al. Relationship among medical student resilience, educational environment and quality of life. *PLoS One.* 2015;10(6):e0131535.
134. Wood DF. Mens sana in corpore sano: student well-being and the development of resilience. *Med Educ.* 2016;50(1): 20-23.
135. Lazarus RS, Launier R. Stress-related transactions between person and environment. In: Pervin LA, Lewis M, eds. *Perspectives in Interactional Psychology.* Boston, MA: Springer; 1978:287-327.
136. Leppin AL, Bora PR, Tilburt JC, et al. The efficacy of resiliency training programs: a systematic review and meta-analysis of randomized trials. *PLoS One.* 2014;9(10): e111420.
137. Southwick SM, Charney DS. The science of resilience: implications for the prevention and treatment of depression. *Science.* 2012;338(6103):79-82.
138. Hobfoll SE, Stevens NR, Zalta AK. Expanding the science of resilience: conserving resources in the aid of adaptation. *Psychol Inq.* 2015;26(2):174-180.
139. Fletcher D, Sarkar M. Psychological resilience: a review and critique of definitions, concepts, and theory. *Eur Psychol.* 2013;18:12-23.
140. Maddi SR, Harvey RH, Khoshaba DM, Lu JL, Persico M, Brow M. The personality construct of hardiness, III: relationships with repression, innovativeness, authoritarianism, and performance. *J Pers.* 2006;74:575-598.
141. Steinhardt M, Dolbier C. Evaluation of a resilience intervention to enhance coping strategies and protective factors

and decrease symptomatology. *J Am Coll Health*. 2008;56: 445-453.

142. Windle G, Bennett KM, Noyes J. A methodological review of resilience measurement scales. *Health Qual Life Outcomes*. 2011;9(1):8.

143. Connor KM, Davidson JR. Development of a new resilience scale: the Connor-Davidson Resilience Scale (CD-RISC). *Depress Anxiety*. 2003;18:76-82. doi:10.1002/da.10113.

144. Friborg O, Hjemdal O, Rosenvinge JH, Martinussen M. A new rating scale for adult resilience: what are the central protective resources behind healthy adjustment? *Int J Methods Psychiatr Res*. 2003;12:65-76.

145. Smith BW, Dalen J, Wiggins K, Tooley E, Christopher P, Bernard J. The brief resilience scale: assessing the ability to bounce back. *Int J Behav Med*. 2008;15:194-200.

146. Cassidy S. The Academic Resilience Scale (ARS-30): a new multidimensional construct measure. *Front Psychol*. 2016; 7:1787.

147. Martin AJ. Academic buoyancy and academic resilience: exploring 'everyday' and 'classic' resilience in the face of academic adversity. *Sch Psychol Int*. 2013;34:488-500.

148. Dyrbye LN, Thomas MR, Massie FS, et al. Burnout and suicidal ideation among U.S. medical students. *Ann Intern Med*. 2008;149:334-341.

149. Dyrbye L, Shanafelt T. A narrative review on burnout experienced by medical students and residents. *Med Educ*. 2016;50:132-149.

150. West CP, Shanafelt TD, Kolars JC. Quality of life, burnout, educational debt, and medical knowledge among internal medicine residents. *JAMA*. 2011;306:952-960.

151. Daskivich TJ, Jardine DA, Tseng J, et al. Promotion of wellness and mental health awareness among physicians in training: perspective of a national, multispecialty panel of residents and fellows. *J Grad Med Educ*. 2015;7(1):143-147.

152. Shanafelt TD, Boone S, Tan L, et al. Burnout and satisfaction with work-life balance among US physicians relative to the general US population. *Arch Intern Med*. 2012;172(18): 1377-1385.

153. West CP, Dyrbye LN, Erwin PJ, Shanafelt TD. Interventions to prevent and reduce physician burnout: a systematic review and meta-analysis. *Lancet*. 2016;388:2272-2281.

154. Panagioti M. Controlled interventions to reduce burnout in physicians a systematic review and meta-analysis. *JAMA Intern Med*. 2017;177(2):195-205.

155. Maslach C, Jackson SE, Leiter MP. *Maslach Burnout Inventory Manual*. 3rd ed. Palo Alto, CA: Consulting Psychologists Press; 1996.

156. Shanafelt TD, Hasan O, Dyrbye LN, et al. Changes in burnout and satisfaction with work-life balance in physicians and the general US working population between 2011 and 2014. *Mayo Clin Proc*. 2015;90(12):1600-1613.

157. McAllister M, McKinnon J. The importance of teaching and learning resilience in the health disciplines: a critical review of the literature. *Nurse Educ Today*. 2009;29:371-379.

158. Zwack J, Schweitzer J. If every fifth physician is affected by burnout, what about the other four? Resilience strategies of experienced physicians. *Acad Med*. 2013;88(3):382-389.

159. Dunn LB, Iglewicz A, Moutier C. A conceptual model of medical student well-being: promoting resilience and preventing burnout. *Acad Psychiatry*. 2008;32(1):44-53.

160. Dyrbye LN, Power DV, Massie FS, et al. Factors associated with resilience to and recovery from burnout: a prospective, multi-institutional study of US medical students. *Med Educ*. 2010;44(10):1016-1026.

161. Delany C, Miller KJ, El-Ansary D, Remedios L, Hosseini A, McLeod S. Replacing stressful challenges with positive coping strategies: a resilience program for clinical placement learning. *Adv Health Sci Educ Theory Pract*. 2015;20:1303-1324.

162. Epstein RM, Krasner MS. Physician resilience: what it means, why it matters, and how to promote it. *Acad Med*. 2013;88(3):301-303.

163. Rogers D. Which educational interventions improve healthcare professionals' resilience? *Med Teach*. 2016;38(12):1236-1241.

164. Peng L, Li M, Zuo X, et al. Application of the Pennsylvania resilience training program on medical students. *Pers Individ Dif*. 2014;61:47-51.

165. Fox S, Lydon S, Byrne D, Madden C, Connolly F, O'Connor P. A systematic review of interventions to foster physician resilience. *Postgrad Med J*. 2018;94:162-170.

166. Montgomery A. The inevitability of physician burnout: implications for interventions. *Burn Res*. 2014;1:50-56.

167. Montgomery A, Georganta K, Doulougeri K, et al. Burnout: why interventions fail and what we can do differently. In: Karanika-Murray M, Biron C, eds. *Derailed Organizational Interventions for Stress and Well-Being*. Dordrecht: Springer; 2015:37-43.

168. Dunn PM, Arnetz BB, Christensen JF, Homer L. Meeting the imperative to improve physician well-being: assessment of an innovative program. *J Gen Intern Med*. 2007;22:1544-1552.

169. Stanford Medicine. Chief Wellness Officer Course. Available at: https://wellmd.stanford.edu/center1/cwocourse.html. Accessed December 14, 2018.

170. Deakin Crick R. Learning how to learn: the dynamic assessment of learning power. *Curriculum J*. 2007;18(2):135-153.

171. Davis DA, Mazmanian PE, Fordis M, Van Harrison R, Thorpe KE, Perrier L. Accuracy of physician self-assessment compared with observed measures of competence: a systematic review. *JAMA*. 2006;296:1094-1102.

172. Mylopoulos M, Regehr G. How student models of expertise and innovation impact the development of adaptive expertise in medicine. *Med Educ*. 2009;43:127-132.

Which Cognitive Processes Are Involved in the Master Adaptive Learner Process?

Klara K. Papp, PhD, and Patricia A. Thomas, MD

LEARNING OBJECTIVES

1. Identify the cognitive processes of the master adaptive learner.
2. Describe three broad areas of investigation into the nature of expertise.
3. Enumerate cognitive skills that a master adaptive learner adopts to effectively learn and solve clinical problems.
4. When provided with a description of a learner's behaviors in approaching an unfamiliar problem, identify whether they are aligned with expert-like approaches to learning.

CHAPTER OUTLINE

CHAPTER SUMMARY

When considering the cognitive processes of the master adaptive learner, specific patterns emerge. The master adaptive learner is defined as a person who achieves expertise. The beauty of this definition is that it is simple and logical. The cognitive processes of the master adaptive learner are manifest in the learners' approaches to solving problems or making decisions. Master adaptive learners distinguish themselves by going into a "theory-building mode" to build new schemas when the features of a problem do not fit their knowledge structures. They go through the effort of asking "why" questions and seeking to understand what is not explained by what they know. They go through the mental effort of trying to understand all of the features of unknown problems rather than attempting to fit problems into existing schemas. It is this approach to learning and problem solving that effectively leads to the development of expertise. When it comes to qualifying the nature of expertise, we assert that individuals have areas of expertise that enable them to function, sometimes as adaptive and other times as routine (or automatic) experts.

Through master adaptive learning strategies, individuals develop effective executive cognitive or metacognitive functions to know whether routine or adaptive expertise is called for and which is appropriate to the situation at hand.

The research in this area is challenging. Cultivating master adaptive learning in the classroom, as well as in clinical settings, requires paying attention to and monitoring attitudes, skills, and behaviors of learners. Additionally, role modeling and engaging learners is important. Asking learners to explain their reasoning behind decisions and to "think aloud" in going through their reasoning is a way to open thinking to direct observation. This must be done in a learning climate willing to accept uncertainty and with the intellectual humility to recognize contradictory evidence. There will always be a clear mandate to educate doctors who are able to think critically about patient problems and recognize and avert errors of all kinds. The Master Adaptive Learner model provides an important framework illuminating the ways to achieve these goals.

INTRODUCTION

A new type of learner, the master adaptive learner, is described as an individual who adopts specific and identifiable approaches to learning that effectively lead to the development of expertise. There are some implicit assumptions in this definition—for example, that everyone learns, more or less continuously, throughout life. Yet not everyone learns in ways that lead to the development of expertise. Some learners start medical school and never finish; mastery is not pursued. Other learners take more time than allotted to master the important concepts in the curriculum. They need help from faculty, learning specialists, and tutors to identify better approaches to learning. Not everyone starts medical school with the skills of the master adaptive learner that effectively lead to the development of expertise. Some do; these are the learners who do well on their examinations, effectively mastering the learning objectives identified, and who also have the capacity to participate in extracurricular activities. It is the thought patterns or thinking processes of these medical students—of master adaptive learners—that we wish to describe.

In this chapter, we delineate ways that master adaptive learners think, not just about problems but, more broadly, about learning new skills and adopting them in the clinical setting. It is an ambitious goal given that thinking is a private matter and not open to direct observation. Despite the challenges, in recent decades there have been great advances in cognitive psychology, specifically in the research on how physicians think.

BACKGROUND ON THE RESEARCH ON EXPERTISE

Mastering an enormous body of knowledge is necessary for the master adaptive learner. Research shows that expertise requires a substantial, well-compiled, highly organized knowledge base. The importance of this is not to be underestimated. Information is readily accessible, yet the master adaptive learner must be able to go beyond available knowledge and have the skills to know, interpret, apply, understand, and synthesize the knowledge in order to make correct decisions.

Research on expertise has deep roots in several fields. It first and foremost aims toward an empirical and theoretical understanding of the processes that occur in the mind (i.e., cognition). Special attention is given to expertise and problem solving, including how expertise develops, how it is maintained, and factors that impede its development. Expertise is extraordinarily complex, and the processes involved in high-quality patient care are dependent upon it. A wide variety of cognitive skills are needed for the master adaptive learner in the development of expertise. This includes the thinking that occurs before, throughout, and after situations that enable him to prepare before, to process and appropriately respond during, and to reconstruct the problem space and learn from it following the event.[1] An often overlooked yet important aspect of expertise is habit formation, that is, the development of beneficial habits or ways of being consistent with a professional identity of continual personal and system improvement.

Cognitive psychology distinguishes between routine and adaptive expertise. Routine expertise is at play when the situation is so familiar and frequently encountered that the correct response and course of action are apparent without significant effort or thought. In these situations, problems are successfully resolved through practiced routines. In contrast, when a situation is unfamiliar, it necessitates that the expert slow down to think through the problem because practiced routines do not fit the situation at hand. This is where adaptive expertise comes into play.[2]

We prefer the term *expertise* to describe the skills and abilities of an individual rather than the term *expert*, a noun that describes a person. Each individual who gains expertise in medicine has highly developed expertise that may be considered routine in some cases and adaptive in others. They may not have expertise in areas outside of their discipline or even in some branches within it.

Generic and Context Specific

The concepts and principles that derive from this research are generic. They pertain to all fields and are not specific to one. The studies pertain to how we humans learn, process information, and adapt to our environments to solve problems. Whether the groups studied are emergency medicine physicians seeing a variety of patients in the emergency department or ophthalmologists diagnosing patients in the office setting, the processes and procedures have highly similar features.

These features are embedded in the context in which the individuals have gained expertise. Studying these features, researchers have formed generalizable concepts, despite different contexts, that apply to situations involving expertise. It is important for the reader to remember during review of the subsequent sections of this chapter that the nature of expertise described in the Master Adaptive Learner model, irrespective of the learner's specialty, is dependent on the contexts and problems in which her expertise is situated. This situated cognition has been well described and contends that all thinking and learning must be viewed as situated within the physical and social context of the environment. Durning and colleagues defined context as "the weaving together of participants, within a setting, to create meaning (which evolves)."[3] It may be instructive to educators in all disciplines seeking to understand expertise and the processes engaged in by the master adaptive learner to bear in mind the context and the situation in which the problem occurs.

Interdisciplinary and Multidisciplinary

The research pertaining to cognitive processes is by nature interdisciplinary. Methods and ideas span traditional boundaries. Philosophers, neuroscientists, cognitive psychologists, developmental psychologists, medical educators, primary care physicians, and subspecialists have all added to our rich understanding of this field.

COGNITIVE PROCESSES OF THE MASTER ADAPTIVE LEARNER

There is a clear mandate to educate doctors to be able to think critically about patient problems and recognize and avert errors of all kinds, particularly errors in diagnosis in the clinical setting. Yet uncovering thought processes behind the wide array of decisions in the clinical setting is exceedingly difficult. This is mirrored in the extensive training required to develop and maintain expertise. The Master Adaptive Learner model is an acknowledgment of this complexity and the increasing need for the adaptive facet of medical expertise. In this section, we identify the processes involved in adaptive expertise through the Master Adaptive Learner conceptual framework. There are characteristics of both states and traits that influence adaptive expertise. We will delineate cognitive, attitudinal, and personal processes that contribute to adaptive

expertise and the cognitive processes of the master adaptive learner.

Critical Thinking as Observed in Clinical Decision Making

Critical thinking is defined as "the ability to apply higher-order cognitive skills (conceptualization, analysis, evaluation) and the disposition to be deliberate about thinking (being open-minded or intellectually honest) that lead to action that is logical and appropriate."[4] Knowledge, skills, abilities, and behaviors are foundational to the critical thinking required to assess, diagnose, and care for patients. Critical thinking encompasses the entire range of actions and decisions that are not automatic and innate but rather require thought and mental processing. Critical thinking in medicine is referred to by a variety of names: clinical reasoning, clinical judgment, medical problem solving, diagnostic thinking, medical decision making, situated cognition, diagnostic reasoning, and therapeutic reasoning. The absence of critical thinking can result in delayed or missed diagnoses, cognitive errors, and mismanagement.[5] More specifically, critical thinking includes all conscious thought that goes into establishing a clinical diagnosis and deciding on a plan of action specific to a patient's circumstances and preferences.[6] While the quality and safety movement has focused on eliminating systems errors in the past decade, until recently there has been a surprising lack of attention to critical thinking in this area of medicine.[5] There are numerous reasons for this. For one, it is often difficult to operationalize and measure critical thinking itself. For another, it can be difficult to identify the etiology of errors. There is a surprising lack of feedback on diagnostic performance in many health care settings. The Institute of Medicine has called for renewed attention to and accelerated progress toward effective strategies in health care to improve diagnosis.[5]

Critical thinking informs every phase of the Master Adaptive Learner process from planning the learning through its systematization into clinical practice. There are three divergent lines of research in the critical thinking literature that help illuminate this important domain of physician competence: case studies illustrating diagnostic acumen, representational theories of the mind, and studies of decisions gone awry. By understanding each perspective, master adaptive learners can better reflect on and improve their own expertise, development, and monitoring.

Illustrations of Diagnostic Acumen

One group of studies consists of narratives or reports of interesting or puzzling cases that are solved by the reasoning of an expert clinician. The narratives include both the challenging case and the clinician's account of how it was solved.[7] This line of research is well illustrated by the series of case reports in widely read journals such as the *New England Journal of Medicine, JAMA,* and the *Journal of General Internal Medicine,* among others, as well as stories in the best-selling books *How Doctors Think*[8] and *Every Patient Tells a Story: Medical Mysteries and the Art of Diagnosis.*[9] The emphasis in this line of pursuit is specifically on diagnostic acumen in highly selected challenging cases. A master clinician is given challenging and rather puzzling facts of a patient's case with the goal of demonstrating the skills of the master clinician in asking the right questions, identifying key attributes of the case, thinking it through, and arriving at the correct diagnosis from which all may learn. The master clinician is thorough, efficient, and knowledgeable and uses heuristic thinking and deductive reasoning along with all of his intellectual and intuitive reasoning powers.[10-12] This literature motivates master adaptive learners to aspire to mastery, to struggle with unknown problems, to think deeply and challenge the obvious assumptions one makes, to be humble in knowing that a person cannot know all the answers or even which questions are the right ones to ask, and to activate their resources when reaching an impasse.

Representational Theories of the Mind

Another group of studies within the fields of cognitive psychology and medicine involves analyzing the mental structures that support decision making as well as analyzing patterns of performance of physicians along the continuum of medical education.[13-16] This model of decision

making, dual process theory, has received much attention in social and cognitive psychology since the 1970s.[17] It was popularized in the lay literature by Kahneman in *Thinking, Fast and Slow*[17a] and in the medical literature most prominently by Patrick Croskerry, psychologist and emergency medicine physician at Dalhousie University. Its tenets have gone through many changes over time. At its core, it amounts to a view of two types of concurrent cognitive processes: intuitive (type 1) and analytic (type 2). When faced with a clinical problem, the clinician's pattern processor sorts the problem according to whether it is recognized. If it is, type 1 is the path taken to a solution. Type 1 is intuitive, automatic, fast, nonconscious, effortless, and contextualized. If the problem is not recognized, type 2 is the path chosen to reach a solution. Type 2 is slower, conscious, effortful, reflective, deliberate, cogitative, decontextualized, and conceivably normatively correct[18] (Fig. 5.1).

The Distinction Between Intuitive (Type 1) and Analytic (Type 2) Approaches

This model distinguishes between the inferential mode of discursive or analytic thinking and a nondiscursive or intuitive mode.[14] The various approaches can be located along a continuum with unconscious, intuitive approaches clustering at one end and deliberate, analytic approaches at the other.[13,19-21] There is growing support to conceive of these as a continuum rather than as dichotomous categories.[22] This schema proposes two general classes of cognitive operations to explain human reasoning. One of the

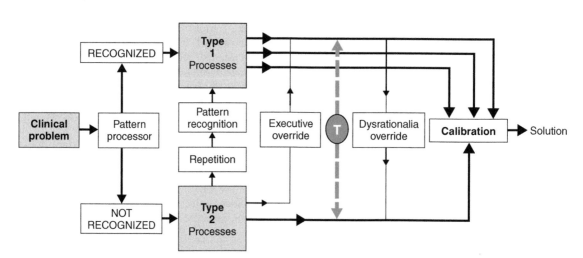

Fig. 5.1 Dual Process Theory Model of Clinical Decision Making. The toggle function (T) enables the decision maker to move back and forth between type 1 and type 2 processes. (From Croskerry P, Singhal G, Mamede S. Cognitive debiasing 1: origins of bias and theory of debiasing. *BMJ Qual Saf.* 2013;22(suppl 2): ii58-ii64. doi:10.1136/bmjqs-2012-001712.)

implicit underlying assumptions of the model is that these two paths represent two possible ways of approaching decisions. Which path is the most effective one is dependent upon many circumstances. In some cases, the intuitive (type 1) is preferred, and in other cases, the analytic (type 2) is more likely to lead to the correct decision or diagnosis. Intuitive (type 1) clinical decision making was portrayed as suspect and more likely to lead to errors. This view has been challenged from two fronts, first by those who maintain that this is not a dichotomy (fast versus slow) but rather a continuum along which a person's problem-solving strategies may lay. Second, some have asserted that clinical reasoning errors are due to a lack of medical knowledge or to cognitive bias rather than to type 1 and type 2 problem-solving approaches.[23-25]

The key point about the relationship between the type 1 and type 2 systems thinking that many have come to recognize is that effective clinical decision making depends upon the ability to toggle between the two, that is,

to have a highly functioning toggle switch, which is depicted in Fig. 5.1 as the "T" shown in blue. This ability to fluidly apportion appropriate cognitive resources of different types is known under the umbrella term *executive functions* in the cognitive psychology literature.[26] According to Croskerry, it is critical that a clinician be able to recognize the need to switch whenever the process she is using to approach the problem appears to not fit the situation. The switch may occur in either direction. A seemingly puzzling problem may crystallize and appear familiar and known. More frequently, a seemingly familiar problem may have features that do not fit the expected pattern and require switching to the analytic mode. It can be said that at times a blend of the two (type 1 and type 2 systems) may be optimal. The notion that the two systems are distinct (Fig. 5.2A) or that one is categorically better than the other has been contentious.[23-25] The prevailing notion is that there may be a continuous line between the two types of thinking (Fig. 5.2B) and that there may, in

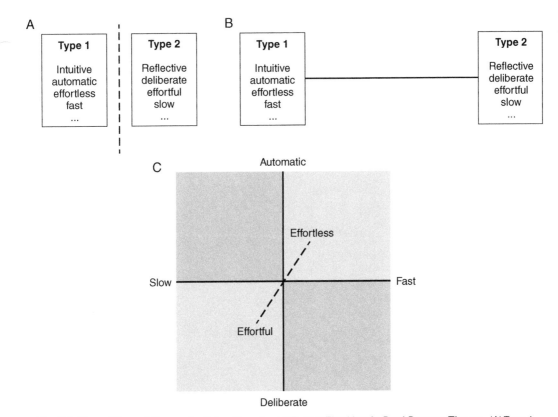

Fig. 5.2 Three Ways of Conceptualizing Type 1 and Type 2 Thinking in Dual Process Theory. (A) Type 1 and type 2 processes—the dichotomy. (B) Type 1 and type 2 processes—the continuum. (C) Tri-dimensional processing. (From Varga AL, Hamburger K. Beyond type 1 vs. type 2 processing: the tri-dimensional way. *Front Psychol.* 2014;5:993. http://doi.org/10.3389/fpsyg.2014.00993.)

fact, be continuous oscillation between the two modes when it comes to approaching even the most familiar problems.[27] Another way of conceptualizing the relationship was suggested by Varga and Hamburger, who graphed it in three dimensions (see Fig. 5.2C).[28]

The Continuum of Intuitive (Type 1) and Analytic (Type 2) Cognitive Processes

The example in Table 5.1 may serve to illustrate the three dimensions involved in problem solving using the dual process theory. The first dimension is the continuum between type 1 and type 2 approaches. One end of the spectrum involves immediate pattern recognition of the symptoms observed (e.g., shingles). The patterns presented are increasingly more ambiguous features that are unrecognizable to the point that, on the other end of the spectrum, the pattern is completely foreign, has not been seen before, and requires systematic review not available in the individual's knowledge base. Thus careful analysis of the pattern and

complete review of the symptoms are required to enable the clinician to solve the problem.

Time is the second dimension, whether the solution is fast or slow. On one end, the clinician may retrieve knowledge from memory or pull a textbook from the shelf knowing exactly on which page to find the correct answer. At the other end of this continuum, the clinician may have to search the literature and review several articles to make correct decisions regarding the patient. The third dimension is the amount of cognitive effort required to retrieve the information needed for the solution. The clinician may retrieve the information from memory effortlessly or exert a great deal of effort, consulting all available resources to arrive at the solution. The examples provided in Table 5.1 display these dimensions. They are highly intercorrelated, but may not necessarily coincide. As one increases, it is not necessarily true of the others. Take, for example, the case in which a clinician chooses to consult a colleague about a problem. The effort on the part of the clinician may be low,

TABLE 5.1   An Example Illustrating the Continuum of Intuitive (Type 1) and Analytic (Type 2) Cognitive Processes.

	Cognitive Process			Clinical Presentation	Instructional Methods
(Type 1) Intuitive	(Fast) Quick	(Effortless) Recalls from rote memory		Make a diagnosis of skin rash [shingles]	• Repetitive practice with cases and non-cases with clear feedback.
Mostly automatic	Quickly finds reference	Knows exactly where to look it up		Compare and contrast two similar skin rashes [shingles and eczema herpeticum]	• Repetitive practice with cases and non-cases with clear feedback. • Focus on exceptions • Learns rules for probabilistic diagnosis of shingles and eczema herpeticum
Blended automatic and analytic	Requires searching; the answers can be found	Takes some time to search and is able to identify		Learn all familiar vesicular rashes	• Recognizing cases that look like known skin rashes but are ambiguous prototypes • Scaffolding
Mainly analytic	Searching takes time and answers are not easily found	Information needs processing; hard to master without help		Review *New England Journal of Medicine* Case Reports to learn new, rarely seen skin rashes	• Coaching • Cognitive debriefing
Purely analytic (Type 2)	Takes deliberate thought and original research (Slow)	Requires careful review and analysis (Effortful)		Study case series; review randomized controlled trials	• Metacognition across cases • Statistical/heuristic approaches

but the time to achieve a response may be either fast or slow (depending upon how soon the colleague responds).

The benefit of identifying these factors as separate dimensions on a continuum as depicted by Varga and Hamberger[28] is that recognition of one's usual level of operation in solving problems may provide opportunities for growth. If the clinician is continually in the intuitive, fast, and effortless mode, the challenges are minimal. All problems are routine, and the expertise called upon in these situations is routine expertise. The problems are not challenging to the clinician, and decisions made under these circumstances may eventually be considered mundane and boring. On the other hand, if the clinician is continuously operating on the opposite end of spectrum (i.e., all problems require analytic, slow, and exerted effort to solve), this may lead to stress and the clinician may be on the trajectory toward burnout and depersonalization. The optimum functioning is in the middle ranges, with challenges occasionally and opportunities for numerous successful encounters with patients. This may be considered the Optimal Adaptability Corridor.[29,30]

Factors That Influence Critical Thinking

The line of research concerned with mental structures that support decision making identifies factors that can directly influence critical thinking. These may be viewed as being both "states and traits," that is, both stable and transitory or situational. The relatively stable ones are intelligence and knowledge,[13,14,16] age,[31-33] and prior experience.[15,34,35] The transitory or situational qualities are emotions, sleep loss, fatigue, and mental well-being,[36-38] as well as the contextual factors or case and context specificity.[39,40]

Six clusters of factors include the cognitive demand of the case: whether the problem presented in the case requires the clinician to recognize features he repeatedly previously encountered, or the case may be considered "high demand" and associated with rigorous processing and analysis to achieve success in approaching a case not seen before or not recognized. These factors are modulated by the context of the situation—for example, the presence of supportive, knowledgeable other people on the team and whether available information technology has a bearing on the case.

Decisions Gone Awry

The third line of research may be found in the patient safety literature analyzing what happens when errors in diagnostic and therapeutic decisions occur and identifying interventions that may decrease the likelihood of their occurrence.[21,41-43] Studies in this category identify the numerous errors involved in decision making and, by articulating and disseminating them, seek to increase consciousness and thereby decrease the likelihood of their occurrence and recurrence.[13,14,19-21,39,41,44-46] Croskerry stressed the importance of ongoing cognitive debiasing, which is arguably the most important feature of the critical thinker and the well-calibrated mind.[46] He has suggested ways to intervene that will mitigate cognitive errors, including educational strategies, workplace strategies, and forcing functions. He stressed the influence of transitory and situational contextual influences on the quality of individual decision making and the importance of identifying and educating clinicians about the factors known to influence, cloud, or impair decision-making judgment.

Whether inspired by examples of master clinicians' skillful diagnostic acumen, thinking about the representational models of the mind, or reflecting on the processes that cause decisions to go awry leading to problems that may have been averted, the master adaptive learner processes these approaches and is humbled by the fact that adaptive expertise is indeed specific to content and context. She considers the vastness of each discipline and the expansiveness of the growth in knowledge. There is always more to learn. There are always ways to improve.

METACOGNITIVE SKILLS OF THE MASTER ADAPTIVE LEARNER

A key quality of master adaptive learners is possession of metacognitive skills, often referred to as the ability to think about one's own thinking. This involves awareness of or vigilance for cues that things could be better and a sense that they can be improved. Learners might think of metacognitive skills as "balcony views" of their own behaviors, attitudes, thoughts, and emotions. Metacognitive processes depend upon a complex interplay of executive functions. Metacognition includes concepts of metacognitive monitoring (processes one engages in when monitoring behaviors, thoughts, emotions, and skills). Metacognitive knowledge is an important subset of metacognitive monitoring or may be thought of as a category in its own right (knowing what one knows and what one does not know).[47,48]

In these metacognitive skills, attention is important. The key skills are attention and reflection in and on action. Identifying and improving metacognitive skills will help learners become well calibrated to achieve continuous self-improvement and identify opportunities for practice-based learning and improvement resulting in higher-quality patient care.

FORMATION OF EFFECTIVE HABITS

A third process important to the master adaptive learner is habit formation. Habits are behaviors that have been practiced to become ingrained, a way of being.[49] Habits are "the choices that all of us deliberately make at some point and stop thinking about but continue doing, often every day."[49] Habits are distinct from the type 1 automatic thinking processes involved with medical decision making as explained earlier. Habits are well-practiced routines that become habituated and involve three elements: an environmental cue, a behavior, and a reward. Habit formation includes repetitive rehearsal of the cognitive process under consistent conditions until it becomes progressively more efficient and, crucially, requires less active planning effort.[50] An effective and well-established habit is invoked not by conscious effort by the individual, but rather in response to a cue in the environment that triggers a set of behaviors. When the cue is present, it is difficult for the master adaptive learner to not carry out the ingrained behavior.

In the Master Adaptive Learner model, there are a number of aspects that would benefit a clinician when ingrained as a habit. Consider, for example, the potential habit of seeking feedback. If the learning clinician is trained to be attentive to cues in the environment ("from each clinic session, choose the patient whose diagnosis caused you the most trouble") and in response to the cue, to invoke a behavior ("call them 1 week later") with the potential reward delineated ("you became a better clinician"), then the friction for invoking this adaptive behavior is decreased with each successive application until it becomes second nature. A well-developed habit is associated with a craving, such that not invoking it results in cognitive dissonance. In short, not knowing how the case turned out puts the clinician into an ego-dystonic state.

Another example of master adaptive learner habits may include literature searches in response to standardized cues ("error reports in clinic") or targeted patient follow-up from specialist colleagues ("every rash sent to dermatology"). Habits can also be incorporated into the clinical microsystem. The important element is their consistency and eventual decreased need for planning.

MASTER ADAPTIVE LEARNERS' APPROACHES TO LEARNING

Our society's well-being depends upon its capacity to innovate and improve. Health professionals must possess not only the knowledge and skills to provide excellent individual patient care by learning the clinical and basic sciences, but also to innovate and recognize opportunities to improve the health care system as well.[51-53] It is critical to educate health professionals to continuously learn so as to improve their level of expertise in their profession and also to have the capacity to make improvements in the

health care systems in which they work, balancing efficiency and innovation.[29] Health professionals face a formidable challenge in mastering up-to-date knowledge in their chosen specialties and being able to participate in innovating—that is, creating new knowledge (individually and also for the profession as well as the health care system in which they function)—as part of their daily professional lives. Drucker stated it well: "Innovation must be part and parcel of the ordinary, the norm, if not routine."[54] This is challenging because the status quo may often be more comfortable than innovation.[55]

The perspectives of the master adaptive learner require careful consideration of the developmental trajectory that learners pass through on their way to developing adaptive expertise. What is the nature of this trajectory, and how do we ensure that our learners are guided to it and move along the stages leading to optimal adaptive expertise?

One often-cited model of the progression through the learning process proposes that there are five (or six) stages of development.[56] This model of expertise suggests that on the way to expertise or mastery, individuals progress through five (or six) levels: novice (advanced beginner), competent, proficient, expert, and master. (The sixth stage, advanced beginner, was added later and was not part of the original model.) In this framework, developmental progression is conceived as a gradual transition from rigid adherence to rules and procedures to a largely intuitive/automatic mode of operation that relies on deep, implicit knowledge.[56] The model has its critics, those who believe that this fits only a restricted range of expertise and is not applicable to clinical skills acquired for the practice of medicine:

> Although the Dreyfus model may partially explain the acquisition of some skills, it is debatable if it can explain the acquisition of clinical skills. The complex nature of clinical problem-solving skills and the rich interplay between the implicit and explicit forms of knowledge must be taken into consideration when we want to explain acquisition of clinical skills. The idea that experts work from intuition, not from reason, should be evaluated carefully.[57]

Though there is no empirical evidence for these stages, the labels are effective and are widely used in describing the developmental progression and when speaking about the nature of expertise. The Accreditation Council for Graduate Medical Education (ACGME) used this framework in identifying the ACGME competencies, which have become the cornerstone of the competency-based movement in medicine in the United States.[58] Many have built upon this framework, describing milestones for assessing achievement of competencies at the resident physician level using the Dreyfus labels.[58-60]

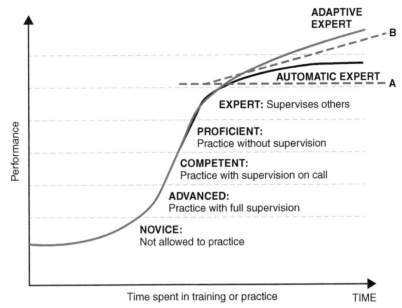

Fig. 5.3 Building upon Dreyfus and Dreyfus stages from novice to expert, showing differentiation in expertise and among experts (automatic and adaptive). (From Pusic MV, Santen SA, Dekhtyar M, et al. Learning to balance efficiency and innovation for optimal adaptive expertise. *Med Teach.* 2018;40:820-827. doi:10.1080/0142 159x.2018.1485887.)

This perspective on acquiring master adaptive expertise is the framework that has been extended by Kalet and Pusic.[60a] Fig. 5.3 depicts the developmental progression of adaptive expertise along the dimension of time and shows the differentiation of expertise, identifying adaptive expertise as the highest attained. A learner may not experience the stage of automatic expert at all, because differentiation of adaptive and automatic expertise occurs earlier (at the intersection of lines A and B in Fig. 5.3). We have asserted throughout this chapter that these classifications are useful if we accept that individuals have areas of expertise enabling them to function, sometimes as adaptive and other times as routine or automatic experts. Few, if any, function exclusively at the routine or automatic level unless they have chosen not to adopt lifelong learning in their practice.

When conceptualizing the needs of the master adaptive learner, Croskerry adapted the Dreyfus' framework to the dual process theory model of clinical decision making (Fig. 5.4). In this schema, when the clinical problem features are recognized, the type 1 (intuitive) mode of decision making comes into play. If the problem is not recognized, the clinician's thinking might take three possible routes. First, the clinician might approach this as an experienced nonexpert by following routines (left column in Fig. 5.4); if clinicians "have unquestioning, passive attitude, using rote learning with minimal insight, they will accumulate

experience but may not acquire expertise, i.e., they become experienced non-experts."[61] If the clinician is active and engaged, expending effort to build a knowledge structure to comprehend the reasons for decisions, the clinician is well on her way to gaining competence and proficiency and demonstrating the abilities of the routine expert (middle column in Fig. 5.4). This is likely to occur during the final stages of residency or early years of independent practice.[61]

Finally, if the clinician continues to pursue deeper understanding and expertise, he may demonstrate adaptive expertise, which occurs with deep understanding of routine expertise together with the ability to innovate and recognize atypical cases and respond with appropriate action (right column in Fig. 5.4). This expertise is contextualized, as noted earlier, and the person may still be a novice or competent in other clinical problems. We should guard against drifting into overattributing expertise to an individual in all domains rather than restricting it to the content- and context-specific domains the evidence supports. Croskerry suggested that this may be time dependent, that is, adaptive expertise may occur and develop following "five to ten years of deliberate practice."[61] The question this raises is whether the adaptive expertise (executive functioning) emerges after sufficient steeping in cases or whether it can be taught. We all have a prefrontal cortex, so we do have executive functioning. The model in

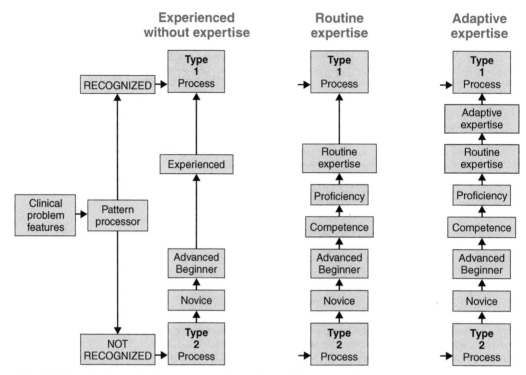

Fig. 5.4 General schema for development of experience without expertise, routine (classic) expertise, and adaptive expertise in clinical decision making (based on the Dreyfus model[56]). (Adapted from Croskerry P. Adaptive expertise in medical decision making. *Med Teach.* 2018;40:803-808.)

Fig. 5.4 suggests that when the problem is easily recognized, there is no difference between the levels of experts—between experienced nonexperts, routine experts, and adaptive experts. It is when the clinical problem features are not recognized that an individual approaches the problem with experienced nonexpertise, routine expertise, or adaptive expertise (see Fig. 5.4). In this schema, it is possible to trigger adaptive expertise when the problem is not recognized by conscious deliberate knowledge of adaptive expertise, which in one view can be induced, practice, nurtured, celebrated, and modeled. In short, the question is whether the clinician will develop the disciplined habits of mind necessary to develop the skills of adaptive expertise.

There may be evidence of expert and nonexpert approaches to learning.[62] Tal, as part of her doctoral dissertation, followed four medical students through their clinical training for an entire year. Two of these medical students were identified by the faculty as functioning in ways that resembled experts in the field. Another set of two was identified by the faculty as functioning as typical medical students.[63] Using a "think aloud" protocol, these medical students were recorded while trying to solve difficult diagnostic problems. Tal recorded them both before and after training in the discipline and found that, though they all performed better after training, the two expert-like medical students performed closer to experts even *before* training than did the two nonexpert-like medical students *after* their training. Differences existed in how the two groups of medical students approached a challenging problem. The nonexpert-like medical students treated the challenging problem as if it were an easy one that could be solved by matching the symptoms with existing known patterns. Even though these medical students had relatively undifferentiated knowledge structures when it came to the problems, they worked to fit the symptoms with what they knew and used their best-fit strategy. In contrast, the expert-like medical students, as do the experts, went into a kind of *theory-building mode*. They tried to construct an explanation that accounted for all the symptoms.[62] It is plausible that adaptive expertise is gained through this kind of progressive problem-solving approach to build a new schema rather than attempting to fit the problem to existing schemas. These contrasting adaptation styles were first proposed by Piaget in describing assimilation (fitting new experience into existing schemas) versus accommodation (creating new schemas to fit new experiences).[64] It is possible that these habits of mind may exist in the earliest learners and demonstrate the path toward better understanding the master adaptive learner.

Bereiter and Scardamalia caution us not to overinterpret expertise in learning, exaggerate its scope, or take too narrow a view of it.[62] In some real way, comparing and contrasting expert-like and nonexpert-like learning behaviors implies a type of approach to learning, that is, a learning style. One is tempted to generalize this style across problems. The research on learning styles has not gained much traction because it suffers from a lack of empirical evidence.[65,66] The benefit of recognizing individual differences between expert-like and nonexpert-like learners is to reflect on one's approach to problems in given situations and identify which attitudes and behaviors dominate in the contrasting styles illustrated in Table 5.2. In fact, the real contrasts between the expert-like learner and the nonexpert-like learner may be ascribed to underlying attitudes or habitual ways of approaching problems that could be addressed, challenged, and eventually changed. All learners, even learners using maladaptive strategies, could cultivate the attitudes and develop the skills of the master adaptive learner.

Vignette 1

A 61-year-old patient with a history of uncontrolled hypertension and chronic schizophrenia presents to the clinic with a complaint of high blood pressure readings at home. She was hospitalized 2 months ago for "urgent hypertension" and discharged on a complex regimen, including five classes of antihypertensive medications, two of which are taken twice a day. She checks her blood pressure readings at home and has systolic BP readings at 160 to 170 mm Hg. Today her blood pressure is 200/95 mm Hg. The resident presents the case to the attending with the assessment that the reason for uncontrolled blood pressure is most likely nonadherence to the regimen. Her plan is to address nonadherence to the care plan with specific counseling, written instructions, and use of a pill pack from the pharmacy.

1. Using the dual process theory of clinical decision making, in which system may the resident be processing (type 1 or type 2) in her approach to the clinical problem?
2. Is the information in the patient's presentation consistent with nonadherence? Is there any contradictory evidence? (intellectual humility)
3. What other explanations could there be for uncontrolled hypertension? (open-mindedness, curiosity)

TABLE 5.2 Contrasts Between Expert-Like and Nonexpert-Like Learners.		
Expert-Like Learners	**Nonexpert-Like Learners**	**Significance**
There is probably more to be learned than I might imagine at the outset.	I give no thought to how much more there is to learn and jump to conclusions on the basis of what I already know.	Magnitude/Openness
I may be unable to distinguish what is important from what is not, and so I will err on the side of assuming everything is important.	I make subjective judgments of what is important, ignoring events or statements that do not stand out as important in their own right.	Priorities
Words that I think I already know may turn out to have different meanings in the new discipline.	I assume that words mean what I am used to having them mean.	Semantics
My initial understanding may be simplistic, and so I had better be on the watch for complicating factors.	I quickly construct simplistic interpretations, which are retained in the face of contradicting evidence.	Humility
No matter how unappealing the discipline might seem, there are intelligent people who find it fascinating and so I should watch for what it is that arouses the intellectual passions of people in this discipline.	I dismiss the whole topic as boring, without attempting to discover what might be interesting about it, while allowing myself to be captivated by items of tangential interest.	Social awareness

Adapted from Bereiter C, Scardamalia M. *Surpassing Ourselves: An Inquiry into the Nature and Implications of Expertise*. Chicago, IL: Open Court Publishing; 1993.

The attending notes the unusual nature of a nonadherent patient presenting with concern for uncontrolled hypertension and prompts the resident to consider alternative explanations for uncontrolled hypertension. In the discussion, the resident is able to name alternative explanations: secondary causes of hypertension, inappropriate medications for this patient (low renin on ACE inhibitors), fluid retention in the face of volume-active medications, over-the-counter medications with drug interactions.

4. What cognitive process is the resident demonstrating in this discussion with the attending?

Vignette 2

A 45-year-old patient presents for her third visit for hypertension management. Six months ago, the patient presented for a routine physical and was found to have a BP of 160/95 mm Hg. She has a family history of hypertension. After initial laboratory evaluation and counseling for lifestyle management, the decision was made to start medication. She was seen in follow-up after the start of medication with BP 121/72 mm Hg. Results were shared with the patient, and she was counseled to continue lifestyle changes and medication and return in 6 months. At today's 6-month visit, BP is 172/95 mm Hg. When questioned, the patient reports that she was very stressed when she first presented but is feeling much less "tense" and assumed she no longer needed the "antihypertensive" medication.

1. What error did the clinicians make in the management of this patient?
2. How would the dual process model of thinking clarify the patient's perspective on her diagnosis and possibly have avoided this outcome?

Vignette 3

An intern is called in the middle of the night to evaluate a patient for chest pain and shortness of breath. The patient is a 39-year-old woman admitted with acute DVT and on a heparin drip. She appears acutely ill and uncomfortable with a low blood pressure, rapid heart rate, tachypnea, and diaphoresis. The intern is concerned that this represents an acute pulmonary embolus. A protocol is initiated with an ECG, arterial blood gases, complete blood count, coagulation test, and metabolic panel. The patient is treated with fluids, oxygen, and eventually pressors to maintain blood pressure. While initial diagnostics are collected, the blood pressure continues to fall and the patient experiences a cardiac arrest. The blood count is returned showing a decline in the hematocrit from admission. The intern needs to consider alternative explanations for low hematocrit in this situation but is also actively engaged in resuscitation. A senior resident arrives and assesses the situation as a potential intraabdominal bleed; the anticoagulant is stopped and the patient is resuscitated with additional blood products.

1. Using Croskerry's clusters involved in clinical decision making (Fig. 5.5), what clusters affected the intern's decision making in this situation? Which of these factors are transitory and which are stable?
2. What factors affected the resident's decision making in this situation?
3. How does the structure of the team support critical thinking in acute situations?

Vignette 4

A 35-year-old woman is seen by her primary care physician for evaluation of chronic abdominal pain. Her initial evaluation, including laboratory and imaging, has not revealed a diagnosis. A referral to gastroenterology resulted in endoscopy and colonoscopy studies with no diagnosis. The physician has prescribed antispasmodics and elimination diets with little improvement in symptoms. The patient frequently calls the practice asking for urgent visits and becomes well known to the staff. The clinic visits are uncomfortable for the physician, with a sense that the patient is feeling angry about the failure to diagnose, and the physician feels frustrated with no other therapeutic options. She recognizes that she is using avoidance behaviors at times with this patient and is concerned about her own professionalism.

1. How does the use of metacognition assist the physician in managing this problem?

The physician discusses her emotions in working with this patient with a colleague who recalls a similar situation in which a patient had a history of abuse and recent psychosocial issues that presented as physical pain. At a follow-up visit with the patient, the primary care physician reviews the evaluation to date and suggests that both the patient and the physician broaden their understanding of the symptoms and the impact on the patient's life by bringing in additional expertise of behavioral health and social work. The physician urges the patient to include family members in visits and plans for care. The social worker uncovers financial stressors that have led to marital discord and begins to work with the patient and her spouse in marital counseling. Behavioral

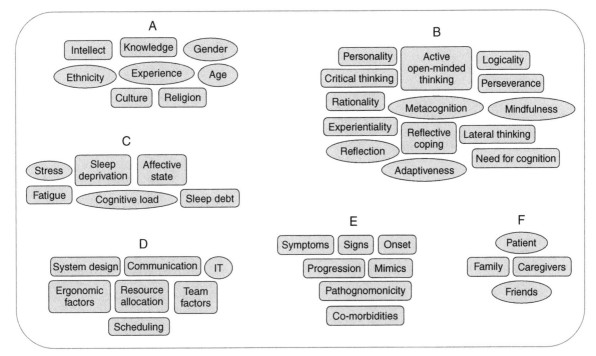

Fig. 5.5 Six Clusters Involved in Clinical Decision Making. The six clusters in clinical decision making are clinician factors (A), metacognition (B), emotional factors (C), systems factors (D), illness factors (E), and patient factors (F). (From Croskerry P. Adaptive expertise in medical decision making. *Med Teach.* 2018;40:803-808. doi:10.1080/0142159x.2018.1484898.)

health instructs the patient in relaxation and mindfulness exercises.

2. What habit of mind did the physician use to find an alternative approach to this problem?

3. What metacognitive factors were demonstrated in this physician's approach to the problem?
4. What system factors did the physician engage in approaching this problem?

TAKE-HOME POINTS

1. Master adaptive expertise involves many cognitive processes, including critical thinking, metacognitive skills, self-monitoring, self-reflection, and habits.
2. Adaptive expertise manifests on occasions when challenging situations call it forth. It is arguable whether all clinicians attain adaptive expertise and sustain it throughout the life of their medical practice.
3. Though adaptive expertise manifests on occasions of challenging situations, it is limited by contextual factors, knowledge, and patient factors.
4. Early in a physician's education, in some cases perhaps even prior to medical education, individuals develop master adaptive learning habits that endure through residency and solidify the skills of developing master adaptive expertise.

QUESTIONS FOR FURTHER THOUGHT

1. How might adaptive expertise be modeled for learners?
2. Is the occurrence of master adaptive expertise in medicine frequent enough that it can be identified and role-modeled in educational settings for learners of all levels?
3. How might qualities of master adaptive learning be better identified and reinforced to ensure that a culture of master adaptive expertise becomes a cultural norm?

ANNOTATED BIBLIOGRAPHY

1. Croskerry P. A universal model of diagnostic reasoning. *Acad Med.* 2009;84(8):1022-1028.
   In this article, the dual process theory of clinical decision making is described.
2. Croskerry P. Adaptive expertise in medical decision making. *Med Teach.* 2018;40:803-808.
   In this paper, the author explains the concepts of adaptive expertise using the Dreyfus model and dual process theory.
3. Daniel M, Rencic J, Durning SJ, et al. Clinical reasoning assessment methods: a scoping review and practical guidance. *Acad Med.* 2019;94(6):902-912. doi:10.1097/ACM.0000000000002618.
   The authors performed a scoping review to identify existing measures available to assess different components of clinical reasoning. Valid measures of clinical reasoning are clinically and educationally important.
4. Pusic MV, Santen SA, Dekhtyar M, et al. Learning to balance efficiency and innovation for optimal adaptive expertise. *Med Teach.* 2018;40:820-827.
   This article describes the necessity of learning to balance routine and adaptive expertise for successful and effective functioning and provides examples at the individual as well as the organizational level.

REFERENCES

1. Cutrer WB, Miller B, Pusic MV, et al. Fostering the development of Master Adaptive Learners: a conceptual model to guide skill acquisition in medical education. *Acad Med.* 2017;92:70-75.
2. Moulton CA, Regehr G, Mylopoulos M, MacRae HM. Slowing down when you should: a new model of expert judgment. *Acad Med.* 2007;82:S109-S116.
3. Durning SJ, Artino Jr AR, Pangaro LN, van der Vleuten C, Schuwirth L. Perspective: redefining context in the clinical encounter: implications for research and training in medical education. *Acad Med.* 2010;85:894-901.
4. Scriven M, Paul R. Critical thinking as defined by the National Council for Excellence in Critical Thinking. 8th Annual International Conference on Critical Thinking and Education Reform. Sonoma State University in Rohnert Park, California; 1987. https://www.criticalthinking.org/.
5. Ball JR, Balogh EP, Miller BT. *Improving Diagnosis in Health Care.* Washington, DC: National Academies Press; 2015.
6. Cook DA, Sherbino J, Durning SJ. Management reasoning: beyond the diagnosis. *JAMA.* 2018;319:2267-2268.
7. Ericsson KA, Simon HA. How to study thinking in everyday life: contrasting think-aloud protocols with descriptions and explanations of thinking. *Mind Cult Act.* 1998;5:178-186.
8. Groopman J. *How Doctors Think.* Boston: Houghton Mifflin Company; 2007.
9. Sanders L. *Every Patient Tells a Story: Medical Mysteries and the Art of Diagnosis.* New York: Broadway Books; 2009.
10. Lurie JD, Sox HC. Principles of medical decision making. *Spine (Phila Pa 1976).* 1999;24:493-498.
11. Owens DK, Sox HC. Medical decision-making: probabilistic medical reasoning. In: Shortliffe EH, Perreault LE, eds. *Medical Informatics.* New York, NY: Springer; 2001:76-131.
12. Sox HC, Blatt MA, Higgins MC, Marton KI. *Medical Decision Making.* Philadelphia: American College of Physicians Press; 2007.
13. Croskerry P. The cognitive imperative: thinking about how we think. *Acad Emerg Med.* 2000;7:1223-1231.
14. Croskerry P. Clinical cognition and diagnostic error: applications of a dual process model of reasoning. *Adv Health Sci Educ Theory Pract.* 2009;14(suppl 1):27-35.
15. Brush Jr JE, Sherbino J, Norman GR. How expert clinicians intuitively recognize a medical diagnosis. *Am J Med.* 2017;130:629-634.
16. Coderre S, Mandin H, Harasym PH, Fick GH. Diagnostic reasoning strategies and diagnostic success. *Med Educ.* 2003;37:695-703.
17. Evans JSB, Wason P. Rationalisation in a reasoning task. *Br J Psychol.* 1976;67:479-486.
17a. Kahneman D. *Thinking, Fast and Slow.* New York, NY: Farrar, Straus and Giroux; 2011.
18. Croskerry P. A universal model of diagnostic reasoning. *Acad Med.* 2009;84:1022-1028.
19. Croskerry P. Achieving quality in clinical decision making: cognitive strategies and detection of bias. *Acad Emerg Med.* 2002;9:1184-1204.
20. Croskerry P. Cognitive forcing strategies in clinical decision-making. *Ann Emerg Med.* 2003;41:110-120.
21. Croskerry P. Advances in patient safety diagnostic failure: a cognitive and affective approach. In: Henriksen K, Battles JB, Marks ES, Lewin DI, eds. *Advances in Patient Safety: from Research to Implementation (Volume 2: Concepts and Methodology).* Rockville, MD: Agency for Healthcare Research and Quality; 2005.
22. Custers EJ. Medical education and cognitive continuum theory: an alternative perspective on medical problem solving and clinical reasoning. *Acad Med.* 2013;88:1074-1080.
23. McLaughlin K, Eva KW, Norman GR. Reexamining our bias against heuristics. *Adv Health Sci Educ Theory Pract.* 2014;19:457-464.
24. Norman GR, Monteiro SD, Sherbino J, Ilgen JS, Schmidt HG, Mamede S. The causes of errors in clinical reasoning: cognitive biases, knowledge deficits, and dual process thinking. *Acad Med.* 2017;92:23-30.
25. Sherbino J, Norman GR. Reframing diagnostic error: maybe it's content, and not process, that leads to error. *Acad Emerg Med.* 2014;21:931-933.
26. Diamond A. Executive functions. *Annu Rev Psychol.* 2013;64:135-168.
27. Hammond KR. *Human Judgment and Social Policy: Irreducible Uncertainty, Inevitable Error, Unavoidable Injustice.* New York: Oxford University Press; 1996.
28. Varga AL, Hamburger K. Beyond type 1 vs. type 2 processing: the tri-dimensional way. *Front Psychol.* 2014;5:993.
29. Pusic MV, Santen SA, Dekhtyar M, et al. Learning to balance efficiency and innovation for optimal adaptive expertise. *Med Teach.* 2018;40:820-827.

30. Cutrer WB, Atkinson HG, Friedman E, et al. Exploring the characteristics and context that allow Master Adaptive Learners to thrive. *Med Teach.* 2018;40:791-769.

31. Durning SJ, Artino AR, Holmboe E, Beckman TJ, van der Vleuten C, Schuwirth L. Aging and cognitive performance: challenges and implications for physicians practicing in the 21st century. *J Contin Educ Health Prof.* 2010;30:153-160.

32. Singer T, Verhaeghen P, Ghisletta P, Lindenberger U, Baltes PB. The fate of cognition in very old age: six-year longitudinal findings in the Berlin Aging Study (BASE). *Psychol Aging.* 2003;18:318-331.

33. Small SA. Age-related memory decline: current concepts and future directions. *Arch Neurol.* 2001;58:360-364.

34. Eva KW, Link CL, Lutfey KE, McKinlay JB. Swapping horses midstream: factors related to physicians' changing their minds about a diagnosis. *Acad Med.* 2010;85:1112-1117.

35. Ilgen JS, Humbert AJ, Kuhn G, et al. Assessing diagnostic reasoning: a consensus statement summarizing theory, practice, and future needs. *Acad Emerg Med.* 2012;19:1454-1461.

36. Croskerry P, Abbass A, Wu AW. Emotional influences in patient safety. *J Patient Saf.* 2010;6:199-205.

37. Lajoie SP, Zheng J, Li S. Examining the role of self-regulation and emotion in clinical reasoning: Implications for developing expertise. *Med Teach.* 2018;40:842-844.

38. McConnell MM, Monteiro S, Pottruff MM, et al. The impact of emotion on learners' application of basic science principles to novel problems. *Acad Med.* 2016;91:S58-S63.

39. Croskerry P. Context is everything or how could I have been that stupid? *Healthc Q.* 2009;12 Spec No Patient:e171-e176.

40. McBee E, Ratcliffe T, Schuwirth L, et al. Context and clinical reasoning : understanding the medical student perspective. *Perspect Med Educ.* 2018;7:256-263.

41. Croskerry P. More on the causes of errors in clinical reasoning. *Acad Med.* 2017;92:1064.

42. Croskerry P, Abbass AA, Wu AW. How doctors feel: affective issues in patients' safety. *Lancet.* 2008;372:1205-1206.

43. Croskerry P, Shapiro M, Campbell S, et al. Profiles in patient safety: medication errors in the emergency department. *Acad Emerg Med.* 2004;11:289-299.

44. Croskerry P. Perspectives on diagnostic failure and patient safety. *Healthc Q.* 2012;15:50-56.

45. Croskerry P. Bias: a normal operating characteristic of the diagnosing brain. *Diagnosis (Berl).* 2014;1:23-27.

46. Croskerry P. When I say... cognitive debiasing. *Med Educ.* 2015;49:656-657.

47. Colbert CY, Graham L, West C, et al. Teaching metacognitive skills: helping your physician trainees in the quest to 'know what they don't know'. *Am J Med.* 2015;128:318-324.

48. Wokke ME, Cleeremans A, Ridderinkhof KR. Sure I'm sure: prefrontal oscillations support metacognitive monitoring of decision making. *J Neurosci.* 2017;37:781-789.

49. Duhigg C. *The Power of Habit: Why We Do What We Do in Life and Business.* New York: Random House; 2012.

50. Lally P, Van Jaarsveld CH, Potts HW, Wardle J. How are habits formed: modelling habit formation in the real world. *Eur J Soc Psychol.* 2010;40:998-1009.

51. Gonzalo JD, Graaf D, Johannes B, Blatt B, Wolpaw DR. Adding value to the health care system: identifying value-added systems roles for medical students. *Am J Med Qual.* 2017; 32:261-270.

52. Gonzalo JD, Haidet P, Papp KK, et al. Educating for the 21st-century health care system: an interdependent framework of basic, clinical, and systems sciences. *Acad Med.* 2017;92:35-39.

53. Gonzalo JD, Wolpaw T, Wolpaw D. Curricular transformation in health systems science: the need for global change. *Acad Med.* 2018;93:1431-1433.

54. Drucker PF. The discipline of innovation. *Harv Bus Rev.* 1998; 76:149-157.

55. Samuelson W, Zeckhauser R. Status quo bias in decision making. *J Risk Uncertain.* 1988;1:7-59.

56. Dreyfus SE, Dreyfus HL. *A Five-Stage Model of the Mental Activities Involved in Directed Skill Acquisition.* Berkeley, CA: University of California Berkeley Operations Research Center; 1980.

57. Peña A. The Dreyfus model of clinical problem-solving skills acquisition: a critical perspective. *Med Educ Online.* 2010; 15:4846. doi:10.3402/meo.v15i0.4846.

58. Batalden P, Leach D, Swing S, Dreyfus H, Dreyfus S. General competencies and accreditation in graduate medical education. *Health Aff (Millwood).* 2002;21:103-111.

59. Green ML, Aagaard EM, Caverzagie KJ, et al. Charting the road to competence: developmental milestones for internal medicine residency training. *J Grad Med Educ.* 2009;1:5-20.

60. Friedman KA, Balwan S, Cacace F, Katona K, Sunday S, Chaudhry S. Impact on house staff evaluation scores when changing from a Dreyfus- to a Milestone-based evaluation model: one internal medicine residency program's findings. *Med Educ Online.* 2014;19:25185.

60a Kalet A, Pusic M. Defining and assessing competence. In: Kalet A, Chou CL, eds. *Remediation in Medical Education: A Mid-Course Correction.* New York, NY: Springer; 2014:3-15.

61. Croskerry P. Adaptive expertise in medical decision making. *Med Teach.* 2018;40:803-808. doi:10.1080/0142159x.2018.1484898.

62. Bereiter C, Scardamalia M. *Surpassing Ourselves: An Inquiry into the Nature and Implications of Expertise.* Chicago, IL: Open Court Publishing; 1993.

63. Frankel Tal N. *Diagnostic reasoning of difficult internal medicine cases: expert, proto-expert, and non-expert approaches.* Unpublished doctoral dissertation, University of Toronto, Toronto, Ontario. 1992.

64. Flavell JH. Piaget's Legacy. *Psychol Sci.* 1996;7:200-203.

65. Cook DA. Learning and cognitive styles in web-based learning: theory, evidence, and application. *Acad Med.* 2005;80: 266-278.

66. Cook DA. Revisiting cognitive and learning styles in computer-assisted instruction: not so useful after all. *Acad Med.* 2012; 87:778-784.

6

What Is the Role of Self-Assessment in the Master Adaptive Learner Model?

Margaret Wolff, MD, MHPE, and Sally A. Santen, MD, PhD

LEARNING OBJECTIVES

1. Explore the role that a learner's self-assessment has on identifying and prioritizing gaps in knowledge, skills, and attitudes.
2. Guide learners through the process of informed self-assessment.

3. Identify learners exhibiting master adaptive learner behaviors.

CHAPTER OUTLINE

CHAPTER SUMMARY

Self-assessment is a critical part of being a master adaptive learner. In order to embark on learning using the Master Adaptive Learner (MAL) process, trainees must identify their gaps in performance. Unfortunately, self-assessment is difficult to do accurately and may lead to misjudgments in abilities; poor prioritization of gaps in knowledge, skills, and attitudes; and ineffective implementation of learning goals. In this chapter, we describe the role self-assessment plays in the MAL process and explore the challenges of self-assessment. Then we focus on the model of *informed* self-assessment where trainees seek complementary external information to provide a more accurate concept of their own knowledge, skills, and attitudes, and we describe strategies to promote informed self-assessment.

Vignette

Sue is the attending physician on an inpatient internal medicine rotation with a fourth-year medical student, Miriam. This is Miriam's second subinternship. Sue notes that although Miriam connects with patients and demonstrates good communication skills, her medical knowledge is only average. On rounds Miriam's differentials are off base and incomplete, and she is not able to interpret results to align with her differential. After gentle correction on rounds, Sue is disappointed that the following day, Miriam again asserts the same wrong information and has not studied to fill in the gaps in her medical knowledge on her patients. Sue pulls Miriam aside after rounds to talk about the rotation. When asked how the rotation is going, Miriam says "This is a great subinternship. I am so glad that I decided to be an internist because it matches my strengths of clinical reasoning. I love the field! I feel like I am a natural internist. The patients are complicated, but I understand the patient presentations, and I am able to use the information to make the right diagnosis and plan."

Miriam is clearly confident in her medical knowledge, patient presentations, and data interpretations. She does not remember that on rounds the team corrected these aspects of assessment and management of her patients. She has not been reading about her patients because she does not recognize that there are gaps in her knowledge and practice. Sue realizes that Miriam represents a senior trainee experiencing a self-assessment disconnect resulting in failure to recognize knowledge gaps. This inaccurate self-assessment leading to her faulty overconfidence in her abilities has resulted in her not launching into the MAL process.

1. How can the faculty member help this trainee improve the accuracy of her self-assessment so that she might see her deficits?
2. What methods of feedback assist all trainees to move in the direction of informed self-assessment?

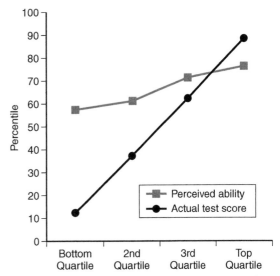

Fig. 6.1 In this figure, participants were ranked according to their test scores (*black line* and quartiles). They were also asked what they *perceived* their test scores to be (*blue line*). More novice (less competent) participants perceived themselves to be less competent than those ahead of them *but* not by as much as was actually the case. The gap was worse the more novice they were, with the thought being that novices do not yet have the ability to diagnose themselves accurately. Notice the interesting phenomenon at the top end of the ability scale where those who could have the most accurate self-perception actually carry an *adaptive* underestimation of their abilities, with the thought being that this allows them to be sensitive to signals for improvement. (From Kruger J, Dunning D. Unskilled and unaware of it: how difficulties in recognizing one's own incompetence lead to inflated self-assessments. *J Pers Soc Psychol.* 1999;77[6]:1121-1134. doi:10.1037/0022-3514.77.6.1121.)

THE ROLE OF SELF-ASSESSMENT IN THE MASTER ADAPTIVE LEARNER PROCESS

Self-assessment—the evaluation of one's own knowledge, skills, and attitudes in order to identify gaps in performance—is a crucial determinant in the acquisition of new skills as well as the maintenance and improvement of performance for a physician. The capacity to seek performance-related information, recognize performance gaps, and address deficits is the basis of the MAL process. Unfortunately, research demonstrates that people, including physicians and trainees, are often unable to independently and accurately assess their performance and identify areas of weakness in order to focus further development efforts[1-7] (Fig. 6.1). This can result in physicians being unaware of existing gaps, thereby rendering them unable to fill those gaps.

Unfortunately, the maladaptive bias in unguided self-assessment also works to undermine the gaps that providers

do identify. Physicians often incorrectly identify areas of relative strength as areas of weakness and subsequently focus learning opportunities on these areas of relative strength.[2] This process is further complicated by the finding that physicians who are the least skilled have the largest gap with their (relatively inflated) self-perceptions.[1,3] Together, this results in individuals spending the limited time they have on areas where they need the least development. However, despite these limitations, self-assessment is necessary for the initiation and monitoring of the learning process.[4,8] An individual's self-assessment determines learning gaps and drives any personal development plan.[9-11]

In consideration of this, we propose that an essential component of becoming a master adaptive learner is to augment *unguided* self-assessment with *informed* self-assessment. Informed self-assessment, proposed by Sargeant and colleagues,[4] is a process of seeking and integrating external

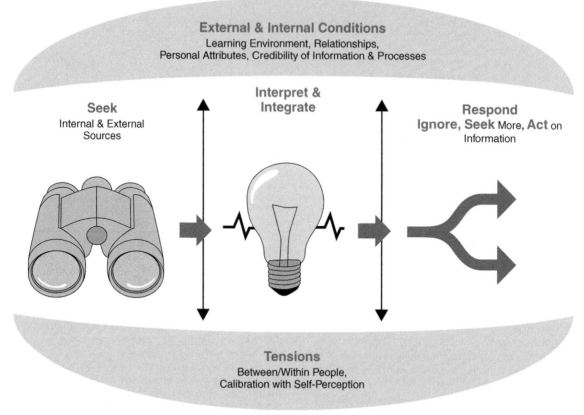

External & Internal Conditions
Learning Environment, Relationships,
Personal Attributes, Credibility of Information & Processes

Seek
Internal & External
Sources

**Interpret &
Integrate**

Respond
Ignore, Seek More, **Act** on
Information

Tensions
Between/Within People,
Calibration with Self-Perception

Fig. 6.2 The Process of Informed Self-Assessment. (Modified by Kenneth Warren Foster, EdD, from Sargeant J, Armson H, Chesluk B, et al. The processes and dimensions of informed self-assessment: a conceptual model. *Acad Med.* 2010;85[7]:1212-1220. doi:10.1097/ACM.0b013e3181d85a4e.)

feedback and performance information into a more complete self-assessment (Fig. 6.2). What follows is a description of the three steps in informed self-assessment as well as how it can be integrated into the MAL process.

THREE STEPS IN THE PROCESS OF GUIDED, INFORMED SELF-ASSESSMENT

Step 1: Commit to Guided, Informed Self-Assessment

Unguided self-assessment is the process whereby a trainee makes a judgment on her performance without examining external information about that performance. The unguided self-assessment is formed by one's self-concept or internal mirror, which may tend to focus on the positive aspects instead of acknowledging negative performance. The self-assessment process can threaten one's self-perception in an ego-dystonic fashion so that, for example,

negative performance might be dismissed as outside of the individual's control. This bias, to the positive, leads most people to think they are above average, while in reality they may not be.[6,7] The opposite bias, of minimizing one's performance, is also possible with some trainees experiencing more of an imposter syndrome, but it is less common.[12]

Informed self-assessment moves beyond the weaknesses of traditional self-assessment in isolation and describes a multidimensional approach that can serve as the basis for the MAL process. Informed self-assessment involves collecting information concerning one's performance from both internal and external sources (Table 6.1). Internal sources are the individual's self-assessment of his skill or performance, which includes both cognitive and emotional inputs related to doing the task, recognizing that he may be prone to a positive bias. External sources include information gathered from both formal and informal sources, such as patient feedback, patient outcome data, summative assessments, and informal discussions or

TABLE 6.1 Sources of Information for Informed Self-Assessment.

Internal Sources	External Sources
Emotional inputs	Objective performance data
Cognitive inputs	Workplace clinical assessments
	Formative feedback from peers, interprofessional team members, and supervisors
	Patient feedback

interactions with peers, supervisors, or other members of the care team.

From an individual trainee's perspective, seeking external data to inform a more realistic self-assessment is a crucial part of this process. The source of the external data will vary depending on the practice setting. It can be provided verbally, through nonverbal communication, or written. It can also be performance feedback in the form of a score on an examination, workplace-based assessment, or data from a self-assessment module. Furthermore, it can be from the learner following up on a patient at some later time and discovering that the patient had a different diagnosis than had been considered, a different management plan, or other patient outcome, including quality and safety reporting data. Although all of these sources of external information will play a role, critical to this process is clear, timely, and specific feedback from trusted and credible sources in a safe environment.[4,13,14] Perhaps most importantly for the master adaptive learner is the ability to actively seek feedback on gaps based on interactions with the environment (see Chapter 11). A master adaptive learner is an avid feedback seeker who, perhaps counterintuitively, prizes *negative* or surprise feedback above all else. It is the feedback received from this gap-seeking process, wherein the learner recognizes what she knows or does not

know, that informs her self-assessment. Learners may consider developing a habit to collect regular input by following up on at least one patient every shift, seeking feedback once weekly on the same day from supervisors or peers, or following up on specific types of patients.[15]

Step 2: Interpret and Integrate Information

As information is collected, the learner will systematically interpret the information (i.e., all of the sources of feedback listed previously) and relate it to her perception of herself (Table 6.2). During this process, the learner reflects on the information, calibrates it with other information and her self-concept, and then responds to the information (step 3). The interpretation includes calibrating, considering, and then synthesizing information to integrate with one's self-concept.[4] The interpretation and integration are affected by several influences. The first is the perceived quality of the information, which is related to the source as well as the content.[4,16] If the source is trusted, then feedback may be more likely to be integrated into performance changes. If the source is not trusted or there are questions as to the quality of the information, it may be perceived as less "informing" information for the trainee, no matter the actual quality. Aspects that contribute to a source being trusted include treating the individual with respect and approaching feedback in a nonjudgmental manner. Ideally, this process is regular and systematized. The other strong influences are internal, such as emotions, prior experiences, and self-confidence. At times, self-concept makes it difficult to accept, integrate, and act on the external feedback. Learners require opportunities to practice, reflect, and adjust so that interpretation and integration develop over time. Coaching and seeking feedback from trusted sources can facilitate the process. In addition, structured learning activities such as reflective activities, mid-rotation feedback, and supervisors providing performance feedback can promote this step and encourage the trainee to take the opportunity to access and interpret the feedback.

TABLE 6.2 Integrating Feedback With Internal Assessment.

		EXTERNAL ASSESSMENT	
		Positive	**Negative**
INTERNAL ASSESSMENT	**Positive**	Aligned Reinforcing Keep calm and carry on	Most valuable Most threatening Benefits from coaching support
	Negative	Important to calibrate Adaptive bias Feral vigilance for improvement	Aligned Requires action Can be self-initiated

Step 3: Respond to the Integrated Information

Based on the learner's interpretation and willingness to integrate the feedback, the potential responses to this information include ignoring and rejecting the data, seeking more information, or accepting and acting on the information.[4] Older frameworks for feedback information/delivery have used the concept of positive or negative feedback. Current frameworks consider the feedback in terms of whether it is concordant or discordant with the trainee's self-concept.[4,13] Feedback information that is "negative" (critical of performance) but aligns with the trainee's own perception of performance is likely to be interpreted as correct and therefore acted upon. Thus critical but concordant feedback reinforces the need to act. In the same vein, feedback confirming one's perceptions of a positive performance is generally valued and reinforces one's self-image. In contrast, information that is discordant with personal beliefs is, unfortunately, likely to be discounted despite the fact that this situation has the most potential for significant change. For example, even when an individual receives feedback on poor performance, it is natural to discount the negative performance by attributing it to external circumstances beyond his control (e.g., the case was complex) rather than accepting negative performance data and learning from it.[7] An aspiration of the MAL framework is to provide a calibrated, grounded, metacognitive perspective on learning, one that recognizes that discordant feedback is difficult, but potentially the most valuable of all. One factor that likely influences this process is the learner's perspective on learning. Individuals with a growth mindset believe that their abilities and academic potential can be improved with effort rather than remaining fixed and inflexible (see Chapter 4).[17] Therefore individuals with a growth mindset, one of the batteries in the MAL framework (see Fig. 1.1), may be more open to critically assessing their performance in light of negative feedback and thinking about how they can learn from the feedback.

Having established that it is possible to train and improve self-assessment accuracy, we now describe the direct role of informed self-assessment in the MAL process.[18] Self-assessment occurs in each of the four phases of the model and especially in the planning and assessing phases, which depend on external information.

INFORMED SELF-ASSESSMENT IN THE MASTER ADAPTIVE LEARNER PROCESS

Informed Self-Assessment in the Planning Phase

In the development of a master adaptive learner, a critical first capacity is the accurate recognition of the knowledge or performance gap that would launch the learner into the MAL cycle. The planning phase of the MAL process starts with identification of gaps in knowledge, skills, and attitudes followed by prioritization of the gaps, creation of learning goals, and selection of learning resources and opportunities. The steps in the process of informed self-assessment discussed earlier describe how a learner may launch into this phase.

After a learning gap is identified, an individual must prioritize this gap and decide if he will spend the time and cognitive energy necessary to engage in learning to fill this gap. Many factors contribute to this decision, including competing demands, external pressures, perceived amount of effort required to complete the task, self-efficacy to complete the task, and degree of cognitive dissonance experienced regarding the learning gap.[19-21] As Fox and colleagues described, goals requiring a large effort are less likely to be completed.[19] This phenomenon was recently observed in learners participating in a clinical skills examination.[10] The learners with the lowest global perception of their performance were the least likely to follow through on their learning goals. Conversely, students with higher general/global perception of their performance perceived a larger cognitive dissonance and were motivated by it. They put more energy into grappling with feedback and into subsequently incorporating feedback into their learning goals, and they were more likely to have taken action on their learning goals.[9,10] This suggests that the more deeply an individual feels cognitive dissonance, the more motivated she is to take action, thereby prioritizing filling that learning gap.[22] This is to say that learners have certain dispositions, such as not automatically attempting to achieve effortful goals; therefore becoming a master adaptive learner requires recognizing these leanings and facing them. It is not easy.

Informed Self-Assessment in the Learning Phase

The learning phase consists of the implementation and follow-through for achieving learning goals. Even during the learning phase, informed self-assessment continues to play a role, dynamically monitoring the effectiveness of the learning and its sufficiency and, indeed, continuously refining the prioritization of the learning goal. Despite the next phase being termed "assessing," there is a considerable amount of necessary assessment *within* the learning phase. The importance of external sources of assessment applies even during the learning phase, wherein frequent check-ins with a coach can ensure that the learner remains on track.

Informed Self-Assessment in the Assessing Phase

In this phase, learners try out their newly developed knowledge, skills, and attitudes to address the initial problem and decide to accept or reject new ideas. This process will be influenced by self-assessment that is informed by both internal and external sources of feedback. Given that self-assessment is a natural and automatic process that is at times subconscious, learners must maintain "an almost feral vigilance to detect personal biases,"[23] including the subconscious bias toward overestimating one's abilities.[6] As described earlier, a learner's confidence and self-efficacy will affect the willingness to address considerations of effort, implementation, and disconfirming feedback. We are asking a great deal of the developing clinician—sufficient confidence to seek out potentially difficult feedback, self-efficacy to engage with that feedback, and finally resilience to be able to countenance the occasions when the entire effort does not work out as anticipated.

Informed Self-Assessment in the Adjusting Phase

In this phase, learners incorporate positively assessed learning into practice. They use their newly gained knowledge and skills to better address routine or novel problems at an individual or system level. For individual-level changes, the change in practice results in either routines that are more efficient and effective or a better capacity to innovate in response to unique or complex clinical problems. Furthermore, informed self-assessment can be a system-level attribute. As an example, consider the emergency physician who must decide whether to perform a potentially difficult procedure himself or to activate a resource-intensive escalation of care: "Am I the right person in the hospital to be doing this procedure?" For these decisions, there is always a gray zone requiring self-assessment. The calibration of that system of care invokes many of the themes we have enumerated in advocating for external information to inform individual-level self-assessment so that it is available when necessary. Just as the level of cognitive dissonance, relative importance, and perceived effort required influence the likelihood that an individual would engage with a learning gap, these influences will determine the implementation and maintenance of these changes in practice.

STRATEGIES TO PROMOTE INFORMED SELF-ASSESSMENT IN TRAINEES

Ultimately, the goal is to develop learners into master adaptive learners who incorporate informed self-assessment into their routine practice to address both routine and novel problems. Returning to the vignette, initially mentors or coaches such as Sue can walk learners such as Miriam through the MAL process by helping them seek out feedback, filter and weigh it, prioritize gaps, and develop learning goals, and by modeling appropriate growth-oriented behavior. Specifically for Miriam, working to gain her trust and helping her accept and integrate the disconfirming

feedback is critical (see Chapter 13). Learners may need encouragement to seek out feedback to overcome the tension between the desire to improve and the desire to seem knowledgeable and competent, particularly in settings where they are being assessed.[24] Faculty can support this process by providing specific, timely, direct, and respectful feedback based on valid sources of evidence, including direct observation of performance. Verbal or narrative rather than quantitative feedback is generally preferred.[25-27] Just as faculty modeling professionalism, clinical skills, and systems-based practice can teach learners ideal behaviors through the cognitive apprenticeship model, faculty can help teach this process by modeling the desired MAL behaviors and are more likely to be viewed as credible if they walk the walk.[28,29] Beneficial curricular approaches that support this process include supplying clear performance standards with explicitly and clearly stated competencies to provide explicit benchmarks for learners to measure themselves against. In addition, faculty need development in providing feedback and forming individualized learning plans. However, there will be situations in which explicit benchmarks are not possible. Here, one can argue that informed self-assessment is even *more* important. Whereas in the absence of external benchmarks one might otherwise hide behind the uncertainty, the informed self-assessment process underlying master adaptive learning would encourage the clinician to in fact work even harder to collect and interpret signals that we are doing all that we can for our patients. Although self-assessment is difficult, inculcating and modeling the intrinsic motivation to improve requires the difficult work of rationalizing what can be opposing forces.

INFORMED SELF-ASSESSMENT IN ADAPTIVE EXPERTISE

The MAL model provides an advance organizer for trainees to use as a metacognitive schema and as a faculty guide for reinforcing the same schema (see Chapter 2). This advance organizer helps learners engage in the process of developing adaptive expertise, whereby the expert clinician is able to adapt optimally to the clinical situation. When problems are routine, the learner reaches for the usual approaches. However, when problems are not routine, he reaches for innovative approaches in the moment. It is the informed self-assessment and self-monitoring that helps him determine which approach is appropriate. Moreover, the adaptive master adaptive learner also recognizes that at times she will be overconfident in her ability and at other times will underestimate it, and therefore she must be especially/continually vigilant. Thus the MAL learning process can be applied (transferred) in future, novel situations.

Developing a deep understanding (mastery) of learning, with attention to informed self-assessment, will enable the clinician to better resolve problems deep into the future. She knows that the highest level of clinical expertise includes adaptability and an appropriate level of vigilance for situations in which her expertise is, in fact, inadequate to the situation. And once identified, the adaptive expert would know to mistrust her early developing competence, especially as viewed through self-assessment. The result would be a clinician who recognizes a gap earlier, appropriately prioritizes learning resources (including the necessary time), effectively monitors the implementation of the newly required competence, and, finally, maintains an ongoing vigilance for its appropriate use and adaptation to the system. Our hope is that this discussion of informed self-assessment is in the spirit of the MAL philosophy, wherein we promote a deep mechanistic understanding of *learning* so as to advantage learning transfer both in the moment and in the future.

In summary, informed self-assessment is the basis for the MAL process. This should be intentionally taught and modeled, and feedback-seeking behaviors should be developed in trainees.

TAKE-HOME POINTS

1. Despite how difficult it can be, self-assessment plays an essential role in the planning and assessing phases of the MAL framework.
2. Unguided self-assessment is flawed and should be discouraged.
3. The informed self-assessment framework can be used to foster master adaptive learning.

QUESTIONS FOR FURTHER THOUGHT

1. How will you change how you deliver feedback to increase the likelihood that a learner will act on your feedback?
2. How will you incorporate informed self-assessment into your own practice and pursuit of becoming a master adaptive learner?

ANNOTATED BIBLIOGRAPHY

1. Bounds R, Bush C, Aghera A, Rodriguez N, Stansfield RB, Santen SA. Emergency medicine residents' self-assessments play a critical role when receiving feedback. *Acad Emerg Med.* 2013;20(10):1055-1061. doi:10.1111/acem.12231.
   This paper demonstrates that, following feedback on an oral examination, trainees generated the majority of their learning goals from their own self-assessments.
2. Wolff M, Stojan J, Cranford J, et al. The impact of informed self-assessment on the development of medical students' learning goals. *Med Teach.* 2018;40(3):296-301. doi:10.1080/0142159X.2017.1406661.
   This paper demonstrates that learners who created learning goals based on feedback were more likely to implement learning goals than those goals based on self-assessment.
3. Sargeant J, Armson H, Chesluk B, et al. The processes and dimensions of informed self-assessment: a conceptual model. *Acad Med.* 2010;85(7):1212-1220. doi:10.1097/ACM.0b013e3181d85a4e.
   This paper describes the model of informed self-assessment and explores the influencing factors.
4. Guardiola A, Barratt MS, Omoruyi EA. Impact of individualized learning plans on United States senior medical students advanced clinical rotations. *J Educ Eval Health Prof.* 2016; 13:39. doi:10.3352/jeehp.2016.13.39.
   This study demonstrates that the majority of medical students perceive the individualized learning plan to be helpful and highlights the need for trained faculty to support these efforts.

REFERENCES

1. Davis DA, Mazmanian PE, Fordis M, Van Harrison R, Thorpe KE, Perrier L. Accuracy of physician self-assessment compared with observed measures of competence: a systematic review. *JAMA.* 2006;296(9):1094-1102. doi:10.1001/jama.296.9.1094.
2. Peterson LE, Blackburn B, Bazemore A, O'Neill T, Phillips RL. Do family physicians choose self-assessment activities based on what they know or don't know? *J Contin Educ Health Prof.* 2014;34(3):164-170. doi:10.1002/chp.21247.
3. Sadosty AT, Bellolio MF, Laack TA, Luke A, Weaver A, Goyal DG. Simulation-based emergency medicine resident self-assessment. *J Emerg Med.* 2011;41(6):679-685. doi:10.1016/j.jemermed.2011.05.041.
4. Sargeant J, Armson H, Chesluk B, et al. The processes and dimensions of informed self-assessment: a conceptual model. *Acad Med.* 2010;85(7):1212-1220. doi:10.1097/ACM.0b013e3181d85a4e.
5. Schneider JR, Verta MJ, Ryan ER, Corcoran JF, DaRosa DA. Patient assessment and management examination: lack of correlation between faculty assessment and resident

self-assessment. *Am J Surg.* 2008;195(1):16-19. doi:10.1016/j.amjsurg.2007.08.050.

6. Kruger J, Dunning D. Unskilled and unaware of it: how difficulties in recognizing one's own incompetence lead to inflated self-assessments. *J Pers Soc Psychol.* 1999;77(6):1121-1134. doi:10.1037/0022-3514.77.6.1121.

7. Eva KW, Regehr G. "I'll never play professional football" and other fallacies of self-assessment. *J Contin Educ Health Prof.* 2008;28(1):14-19. doi:10.1002/chp.150.

8. Cutrer WB, Miller B, Pusic MV, et al. Fostering the development of master adaptive learners. *Acad Med.* 2017;92(1):70-75. doi:10.1097/ACM.0000000000001323.

9. Bounds R, Bush C, Aghera A, Rodriguez N, Stansfield RB, Santen SA. Emergency medicine residents' self-assessments play a critical role when receiving feedback. *Acad Emerg Med.* 2013;20(10):1055-1061. doi:10.1111/acem.12231.

10. Wolff M, Stojan J, Cranford J, et al. The impact of informed self-assessment on the development of medical students' learning goals. *Med Teach.* 2018;40(3):296-301. doi:10.1080/0142159X.2017.1406661.

11. Chang A, Chou CL, Teherani A, Hauer KE. Clinical skills-related learning goals of senior medical students after performance feedback. *Med Educ.* 2011;45(9):878-885. doi:10.1111/j.1365-2923.2011.04015.x.

12. LaDonna KA, Ginsburg S, Watling C. "Rising to the level of your incompetence." *Acad Med.* 2018;93(5):763-768. doi:10.1097/ACM.0000000000002046.

13. Sargeant J, Eva KW, Armson H, et al. Features of assessment learners use to make informed self-assessments of clinical performance. *Med Educ.* 2011;45(6):636-647. doi:10.1111/j.1365-2923.2010.03888.x.

14. Lockyer J, Armson H, Chesluk B, et al. Feedback data sources that inform physician self-assessment. *Med Teach.* 2011;33(2):e113-e120. doi:10.3109/0142159X.2011.542519.

15. Crommelinck M, Anseel F. Understanding and encouraging feedback-seeking behaviour: a literature review. *Med Educ.* 2013;47(3):232-241. doi:10.1111/medu.12075.

16. Mann K, van der Vleuten C, Eva K, et al. Tensions in informed self-assessment: how the desire for feedback and reticence to collect and use it can conflict. *Acad Med.* 2011;86(9):1120-1127. doi:10.1097/ACM.0b013e318226abdd.

17. Dweck CS, Leggett EL. A social-cognitive approach to motivation and personality. *Psychol Rev.* 1988;95(2):256-273. doi:10.1037/0033-295X.95.2.256.

18. Keister DM, Hansen SE, Dostal J. Teaching resident self-assessment through triangulation of faculty and patient feedback. *Teach Learn Med.* 2017;29(1):25-30. doi:10.1080/10401334.2016.1246249.

19. Fox R, Mazmanian PE, Putnam R. *Changing and Learning in the Lives of Physicians.* New York, NY: Prager; 1989.

20. Bandura A. Perceived self-efficacy in cognitive development and functioning. *Educ Psychol.* 1993;28(2):117-148. Available at: https://www.uky.edu/~eushe2/Bandura/Bandura1993EP.pdf. Accessed August 15, 2018.

21. Wolff M, Stojan J, Buckler S, et al. Improving implementation of learning goals with coaching. 2018.

22. Cordes D. Relationship of motivation to learning. In: Green JS, ed. *Continuing Education for the Health Professions.* San Francisco, CA: Jossey-Bass; 1984:52-71. Available at: https://eric-ed-gov.proxy.lib.umich.edu/?id=ED247785. Accessed March 17, 2017.

23. Croskerry P. ED cognition: any decision by anyone at any time. *Can J Emerg Med.* 2014;16(1):13-19. doi:10.2310/8000.2013.131053.

24. Balmer DF, Tenney-Soeiro R, Mejia E, Rezet B. Positive change in feedback perceptions and behavior: a 10-year follow-up study. *Pediatrics.* 2018;141(1):e20172950. doi:10.1542/peds.2017-2950.

25. Sargeant J, Lockyer JM, Mann K, et al. The R2C2 model in residency education: How does it foster coaching and promote feedback use? *Acad Med.* 2018;93(7):1055-1063. doi:10.1097/ACM.0000000000002131.

26. Ericsson KA. Deliberate practice and acquisition of expert performance: a general overview. *Acad Emerg Med.* 2008;15(11):988-994. doi:10.1111/j.1553-2712.2008.00227.x.

27. Telio S, Ajjawi R, Regehr G. The "Educational Alliance" as a framework for reconceptualizing feedback in medical education. *Acad Med.* 2015;90(5):609-614. doi:10.1097/ACM.0000000000000560.

28. Lyons K, McLaughlin JE, Khanova J, Roth MT. Cognitive apprenticeship in health sciences education: a qualitative review. *Adv Heal Sci Educ.* 2017;22(3):723-739. doi:10.1007/s10459-016-9707-4.

29. Merritt C, Daniel M, Munzer B, Nocera M, Ross J, Santen S. A cognitive apprenticeship-based faculty development intervention for emergency medicine educators. *West J Emerg Med.* 2018;19(1):198-204. doi:10.5811/westjem.2017.11.36429.

7

How Do You Measure the Master Adaptive Learner?

JK Stringer, PhD; Margaret Wolff, MD, MHPE; and Sally A. Santen, MD, PhD

LEARNING OBJECTIVES

1. Apply Miller's framework for assessment of a master adaptive learner.
2. Select appropriate instruments and methods to measure potential underlying constructs of master adaptive learning.
3. Design programmatic assessment using multiple sources and types of assessments at multiple times to measure various aspects of master adaptive learning.

CHAPTER OUTLINE

CHAPTER SUMMARY

In order to cultivate traits associated with the Master Adaptive Learner (MAL) model, educators need to measure the characteristics of the learner, the processes and observable behaviors in which a master adaptive learner engages, and the outcomes of MAL performance. There are multiple methods of assessment that measure what trainees know, show, and do. Different methods have different strengths depending on the desired outcome, so these should be aggregated to create a clear picture of the skills, performance, and outcomes of the master adaptive learner.

INTRODUCTION

Our ability to understand the MAL process is directly related to how we are assessing our learners.[1] Assessment of MAL processes and outcomes has three main goals: (1) to provide formative feedback to the trainee for optimizing her capabilities by promoting motivation and direction for future learning, (2) to make summative judgments about performance, and (3) to evaluate the educational program using an aggregate of assessments as evidence of achieving objectives.[2,3] Ultimately, master adaptive learning is a multidimensional continuum and, by developing assessment, we can help move our learners along it.

We see MAL measurement occurring in three domains: (1) characteristics of the individual, (2) observable behaviors, and (3) outcomes (Fig. 7.1). Trainees have characteristics or disposition toward engaging in MAL processes that lead to observable behaviors such as goal setting, learning, and readjusting. This engagement with master adaptive learning leads to learning or skill outcomes that are measurable as well. Ultimately, our goal in training and supporting the development of master adaptive learners is improved patient care, and recognizing and assessing the master adaptive learner in the three domains will be an important step. By detailing assessments that provide opportunities for observations of MAL behaviors and cognitions and also describing instruments for measuring these MAL outcomes, this chapter outlines some of what a master adaptive learner is and how we can measure it.

We propose assessments that take different forms for each of these three domains (characteristics, observable behaviors, and outcomes). Individual characteristics might be captured through self-reported survey instruments and would be used to provide descriptive information about learners.[4] Observable behaviors could be assessed through a range of methods designed to capture different levels of performance.[5] The assessments might serve formative roles by providing feedback to learners about the observed behaviors. An aggregate of behavioral assessments might inform a summative decision. Finally, assessing learning outcomes serves a summative role and can be used to understand the overall quality of the skills and practices of the assessed learners.[6] There is overlap between the three domains, indicating that they influence each other. For example, if a learner has the individual characteristic of curiosity, this will likely also influence her observable behaviors, and she will achieve her learning outcome with more expertise. Each of these three categories is discussed further in the sections that follow.

If we wish to answer the question of "How do you measure the master adaptive learner/learning?", we need to provide our interpretations of the MAL framework in concrete ways. Master adaptive learning is a process through which a learner engages in self-reflection and self-regulation to improve his practice and, in this context, patient outcomes. This process, however, is complex and difficult (if not impossible) to measure as a whole. Our work as educators is to identify tangible parts of this whole that we can use to observe individual learners' master adaptive learning processes.

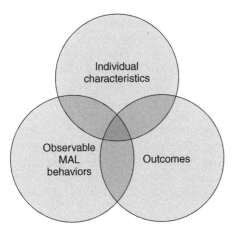

Fig. 7.1 MAL Measurement Model. It is possible to measure each of these domains. The assessment instruments differ accordingly.

Vignette

As a coach working with trainees, your role is to both review the assessments of these trainees and assess their ability to be master adaptive learners. You understand that MAL skills will manifest in many different ways, and you seek evidence of these skills. Because we see master adaptive learning as a process, differentiating between MAL domains for the trainees you work with is an important step. You are currently working with three trainees: Sarah and Jason, first-year medical students (M1s); and Maggie, a third-year medical student (M3).

1. How will you determine if the trainee is approaching learning with a MAL approach?
2. On what domains of the master adaptive learner do you want to focus?
3. What assessment will provide evidence that the trainee is successfully implementing master adaptive learning and becoming a master adaptive learner?

Your school administers surveys across medical students' undergraduate medical education to better understand the relationship between medical students' performance and their individual differences. You aim to capture information about the individual characteristics of MAL domains on the annual survey. One instrument that is collected each year captures information about goal orientation: a medical student's orientation toward achievement situations. Sarah and Jason both completed this instrument during matriculation, while Maggie's most recent completion occurred prior to the beginning of her clinical rotations. Sarah's responses suggest a learning orientation, in which she is driven to develop her own competencies, whereas Jason's suggest an avoidance orientation. His orientation tends toward avoiding, displaying a lack of competence rather than developing one. Maggie's pre-clerkship responses indicate a change. She, like Sarah, began the program with a learning orientation but has since moved to a different performance orientation. Her interests are in demonstrating her competence to others rather than developing competence for herself.

INDIVIDUAL MASTER ADAPTIVE LEARNER CHARACTERISTICS

We believe that MAL assessment begins with an adequate understanding of our learners and how they are approaching their learning experiences. Collecting data (most frequently self-reported) about beliefs, motivation, and personality helps us frame learners' experiences. Self-assessments (see Chapter 6) and attitudinal scales may provide this framework on which we can build behavioral and outcome assessment.

The survey responses such as those described in the vignette allow us to see how medical students are approaching their learning experiences. By themselves, these data do not indicate whether a medical student is demonstrating master adaptive learning, but, given the motivational components of the framework, we can see that Sarah and Maggie are exhibiting attitudes that are closer to a MAL approach than Jason is.

There are numerous attitudinal scales that may demonstrate a learner's attitudes or inclinations toward the MAL model domains (Table 7.1). Each of these domains is a broad area, so scales in this table represent only a sampling of potential instruments that could be used to capture trainee

TABLE 7.1	Self-Report or Attitudinal Instruments of Master Adaptive Learning (MAL).		
MAL Phase	**Outcome**	**Instrument**	**Description**
Planning	Motivation	Motivated Strategies for Learning Questionnaire[13]	An instrument developed to capture academic motivation, including elements of learner affect, value, and efficacy.
Planning	Lifelong learning	Jefferson Scale of Physician Lifelong Learning—Medical Students[14]	Scale designed to measure medical students' orientations toward continuous knowledge development.
Learning	Critical thinking	Critical Thinking Disposition Scale[15]	Scale indicates individuals' disposition toward critical thinking, defined as critical openness and reflective skepticism.
Learning	Strategy use	Motivated Strategies for Learning Questionnaire[13]	An instrument developed to capture specific learning strategy use by learners relating to resource management as well as cognitive and metacognitive strategies.
Assessing	Self-assessment	Emotion Regulation Questionnaire[16]	Highlights individual differences in managing emotional stress, based on one's evaluation of a situation and a response to that situation.
Assessing	External feedback	Feedback Environment Scale[17]	Instrument made up of seven subscales (including source credibility, feedback quality, and feedback delivery) that provides information on feedback and context.
Adjusting	Self-reflection	Self-Reflection and Insight Scale[18]	Focuses on the frequency with which individuals engage in self-reflection, their level of insight and introspection, and their valuing of self-reflective thought.
Adjusting	Attribution	Revised Causal Dimension Scale[19]	Scale for use in defining an individual's attributions for success or failure (internal vs. external, stable vs. unstable, controllable vs. uncontrollable).

attitudes and cognitions to inform our understanding of these trainees as master adaptive learners. It is important for educators to note that, given the early nature of our conceptual understanding of master adaptive learning, the instruments described in this table were not developed with the specific measurement of master adaptive learning in mind. They have varying validity evidence. Therefore if choosing to employ one of the scales found in Table 7.1, we should refer to the literature for updated information about their use, recent validity evidence for the specific construct we want to measure, and the population it has been used for.

The scales provide a basis to understand and compare learners' attitudes. They can be used in several ways. First, as we create curricula to support trainee MAL development, determining if trainees have characteristics related to master adaptive learning can be useful for program evaluation. For example, if a school institutes team-based learning modules to promote master adaptive learning, administering a self-regulated learning scale before and after the curriculum intervention might help to evaluate whether it was effective. Second, an attitudinal survey at application might guide the selection of trainees who are predisposed to be master adaptive learners. This is entirely theoretical because the evidence for MAL scales is not robust. Third, in the nascent field of master adaptive learning, examining cohorts of trainees' attitudes toward master adaptive learning and academic outcomes may be useful to better understand MAL development. Finally, educators may find it helpful to provide trainees with reports of their own MAL-related attitudinal scales. If self-report or self-assessment is a foundation for learner feedback, the master adaptive learner will find it helpful to incorporate external data and feedback to provide an informed self-assessment (see Chapter 6). It might be helpful to provide learners and their coaches with the results of their attitudinal scales so they might reflect on their approach to learning. By combining this self-assessment information, intentional assessment data, and individual difference information, we stand to better understand our trainees.

Significant research work is needed in these areas before scales to measure MAL attitudes can be recommended. The American Psychological Association and the American Educational Research Association have published standards that identify five sources of validity evidence[7]:

1. Content—ensuring that content matches the purpose of the test
2. Response process—ensuring that learners, raters, or both are responding in the desired manner
3. Internal structure—degree to which individual items within the instrument fit the underlying constructs
4. Relation to other variables—relationship between scores and other variables relevant to the construct being measured
5. Consequences—impact of using the assessment method.

These sources of validity evidence should be considered when choosing or designing an assessment and making appropriate inferences and judgments about learners.

Given that assessments capturing individual differences will all be self-reported, the measurement of individual MAL domains will not differ methodologically, but educators need to select appropriate instruments for the desired domain. Also significant is that constructs of interest may vary by the educational level of the learner being assessed. For example, expectations and attitudes toward learning may differ between M1s and M3s. To use the example of goal orientation, an M1 might be more learning oriented by nature of the preclinical environment, while an M3 might be more performance oriented because of the social nature of the clinical space. Potential scales presented in Table 7.1 represent a broad selection of MAL-related constructs, but they may not answer questions as well for learners at different levels.

Vignette Continued

Your observation of these trainees' place on the MAL continuum began with understanding their individual characteristics, but can be supported by examining what behaviors they exhibit in their learning environments. Sarah and Jason have both recently completed a pre-clinical-phase exam and neither performed to the level he or she wanted. Their exam scores illustrate a lack of knowledge, but in your coaching sessions Sarah clearly indicates she has identified a key area where she needs to put more attention, and asks for your help in seeking out resources to support her learning in this area. Jason attributes his struggles to the overall difficulty of the exam and does not recognize that his lack of understanding some core concepts is the foundation for his missed items. You provide support to both trainees to help their learning, but where Jason wants to "do better," Sarah clearly articulates where she plans to focus her energy and her desired outcomes.

At the same time, Maggie is completing a third-year clerkship and is interested in developing her skills as much as possible during the experience. On her previous rotation, an attending had suggested that she work on improving her history-taking skills. Using a real-time feedback delivery tool, Maggie requests that residents and attendings observe her history and physical examinations and provide assessment and feedback, which she uses to make changes to her practice.

OBSERVABLE MASTER ADAPTIVE LEARNER BEHAVIORS

Although self-reported survey instruments can give us some information about our learners, they do not provide much concrete information about what our learners do. To capture this kind of information about our learners and their learning, it is necessary to use a greater range of assessments. In the preclinical and clinical settings, faculty can observe MAL behaviors in learners' approaches to learning. Do they identify their gaps in knowledge, set goals for learning, and the like? To measure observable behaviors, Miller's framework describes a series of levels moving from factual knowledge to using that knowledge in practice.[8] Just as the MAL framework moves through the stages of planning, learning, assessing, and adjusting, understanding types of assessments using Miller's framework (Fig. 7.2) allows us to look at increasingly complex and rich demonstrations of MAL behaviors. Returning to the vignette, we can observe and assess Maggie's MAL behaviors as she reviews with you her action plan for developing her communication skills for the next week. She has achieved the "knows" and "knows how" stages and through her action plan she "shows how" to engage in the MAL process to improve. With the next session, you might be able to assess if she "does" successfully engage in the MAL process through discussion of how her action plan was implemented. As we explore the different stages of the MAL framework, we describe observations and outcomes of various levels that may help educators make decisions about their learners.

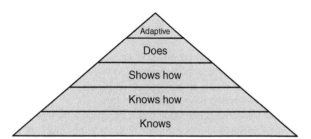

Fig. 7.2 Miller's Framework Expanded to Include Adaptability. Miller's framework is a model for assessing clinical competence. At the lowest level, learners know and then know how to do activities. At the higher levels, learners are able to show how to do things and then do the activities. Finally, as we consider master adaptive learning, we believe there is yet a higher level—the ability to adapt knowing, showing, and doing to the context.

OUTCOMES AND PROCESSES OF MASTER ADAPTIVE LEARNING

The third component of the MAL assessment model we propose relates to learner outcomes. As learners engage in theory-based processes of master adaptive learning, the outcomes of their endeavors will improve. For example, a medical student who recognizes her gaps in knowledge in a course will use her MAL skills to fill that gap. As a result, assessments of that content knowledge will be improved. Similarly, a resident in the emergency department will recognize that he has a skill deficit in suturing a wound or resuscitation of a neonate and seek to fill that gap. The outcomes of these MAL processes can be measured by assessment of patient care. The outcomes can range from examination scores in medical school to potential patient outcomes as our learners engage with the community in practice.

Therefore, when we examine observable behaviors we are assessing both the process of master adaptive learning and the outcomes of master adaptive learning. This is the overlap of observable behaviors and outcomes that we see on the Venn diagram for the process of master adaptive learning (see Fig. 7.1). Do we see evidence that the learner is engaging in master adaptive learning behavior? For the outcomes of master adaptive learning, do we see evidence that the learning outcomes are improving as a result of the learner's MAL process? We can use Miller's assessment framework to measure both the process of master adaptive learning and the outcomes of master adaptive learning as described next.

BRINGING IT BACK TOGETHER: MASTER ADAPTIVE LEARNING AND MILLER'S PYRAMID

Knows/Knows How

Through questions and essays, assessment can make visible learners' knowledge and learners' application of that knowledge. These levels of the framework mainly capture learners' cognitions and their ability to gather, interpret, and apply information. Examples of assessment methods might be oral examinations, short- and long-answer questions, multiple-choice questions, extended matching items, or a key features test. Assessing Sarah's and Jason's course-specific learning with multiple-choice tests or capturing Maggie's experiences in the clerkships with essays would be one way to observe master adaptive learning–related information at the "knows/knows how" level. For the most part assessment at this level is measuring the outcomes of master adaptive learning. However, there are "knows/knows how"–level assessments that demonstrate the process. For example, does a trainee know which resources to use to fill a knowledge gap? Does a trainee know that self-quizzing is an effective way to learn through the testing effect?

Shows How

Trainees may have a range of knowledge that could apply to a given situation, but their own critical appraisal of skills and context is what will guide them to a successful or unsuccessful outcome. The "shows how" level allows trainees to demonstrate their learning and to prove base levels of competence prior to engaging with clinical behaviors. Assessments at this level include short and long cases, objective structured clinical examinations (OSCEs), and other simulated patient encounters. Sarah and Jason may engage with simulated patients in their preclinical coursework, while Maggie might complete an OSCE as an element of her overall clerkship performance. In these examples, the medical students are demonstrating the outcomes of master adaptive learning through improvement in performance. In addition, a faculty member or coach working with a trainee may also be able to assess how that trainee "shows how" to set learning goals or other processes of master adaptive learning.

Does

Assessment here is where a learner can see and demonstrate the development of her skills and reflect on events as they happen. Learners at this stage also incorporate feedback from a wider variety of sources that can often be of greater depth. These assessments allow us to see the integration of medical students' learning into their practice and will represent their day-to-day practice. Examples of such tools include direct observation, workplace-based assessment, and portfolios of learning and performance. Although much of this is clinically bound and would be less relevant to medical students in preclinical phases of the curriculum, we can still observe the integration of learning in earlier medical students such as Jason and Sarah, whereas for medical students such as Maggie, we can observe at the "does" level during acting internships or other advanced fourth-year electives.

Adaptive: Does According to Contexts—A Distinctly Master Adaptive Learner Assessment

Up until now we have described a portfolio of conventional measures and how they can be used to develop insight as to the degree to which a learner has successfully incorporated the lessons of the MAL conceptualization. However, there are newer less conventional measures that in many respects are even more aligned with the MAL message. For these assessments, the context matters—the learner is required to adapt in order to perform well. In this section we discuss "adaptive" in various contexts, balancing innovation and efficiency, and preparation for future learning.

We believe the assessment of the master adaptive learner should not end with learners' completion of tasks in familiar environments but should address some level of adaptability—in other words, how learners perform in varied clinical contexts. By observing behaviors using methods similar to those described earlier, it will be important for us to understand how students perform in contexts that are different from those in which they trained in order to assess adaptive learning. For example, we might assess a new intern's ability to adjust patient care plans as he adapts to novel environments and situations with each new rotation.

While "adaptive" is not in the original Miller framework, we propose that beyond "does," there is adaptability. It is defined as the ability of the learner to innovate appropriately to the novelty of the context. Adaptive learners have the ability to innovate through learning and changing their process, which takes significant energy and resources. The master adaptive learner has both the ability to innovate and the ability to recognize when efficiency and getting work done become the priority. In many ways adaptability is the process of a fully functioning master adaptive learner who learns; plans; assesses; adjusts in series and in parallel as well as at the appropriate times, contexts, or subjects; and chooses to be efficient and minimize the effort associated with the MAL model in those dimensions. This process focus lends itself to consideration of what might be an expanded version of Miller's "does," where learners are not only to complete a task in the real world, but to complete a task in a context that varies greatly from the one in which they were trained.

Preparation for future learning is a foundational principle for the MAL framework. A master adaptive learner learns in a fashion that may be less efficient in the moment but that is paid back with differentially better learning in the future (see Chapter 2). For example, practicing informed self-assessment–seeking behavior will take more time in clerkship but will result in a resident who is more assiduous from day 1 of residency. It is difficult to assess preparation for future learning because it requires temporally distant measures of differential learning. As more and more process and outcome data are digitized and available for learning analytic analysis, the capacity to link today's educational data with future performance in this way is not far off in the future.[9-11] Assessments of the "adaptive" level might include repeated assessments in different contexts to demonstrate transfer and adaptive learning. In addition, they might assess whether new learning is more efficient and less effortful based on intentional MAL learning.

BRINGING IT ALL TOGETHER

The value of Miller's framework is to provide opportunities for educators to identify different examples of content knowledge and skill development in the MAL model. Table 7.2 includes a range of assessment examples from all of Miller's levels that we have associated with distinct domains of the MAL framework. The range of methods

for assessing medical students in the preclinical and clinical learning environments is wide, but when master adaptive learning specifically is considered, it becomes that much more important to pick an instrument that allows a medical student to demonstrate the desired MAL phase directly. As operationalized now, master adaptive learning consists of four phases: planning, learning, assessing, and adjusting. Many of the methods described in

TABLE 7.2   Assessment Methods for Different Phases of Master Adaptive Learning (MAL).

Assessment Methods	Planning	Learning	Assessing	Adjusting
Multiple-choice questions, extended matching, short-answer questions—tend to measure "knows" and "knows how." They can be used to assess the master adaptive learner's knowledge and application in various domains. If the question is open book, it also allows the opportunity to assess the master adaptive learner's ability to search.	×	×		
Long and short essay questions—tend to measure "knows," "knows how," and "shows." They can allow the assessment of the learner on multiple levels. An essay can demonstrate knowledge, application of knowledge, and "shows how." These questions might ask the learner how to approach a problem and, thus, demonstrate the learner's ability to question, prioritize, and search as well as goal set. Similarly, an essay question that documents learning in practice can demonstrate "does."	×	×	×	×
Oral examination—similarly assesses all of the dimensions of the planning stage at "knows," "knows how," or "shows how" levels. Furthermore, an oral examination, when performed in the clinical setting, can assess how the learner "does" and apply the planning stage of master adaptive learning.	×	×	×	×
Objective Structured Clinical Examination (OSCE)—tends to measure "shows how," but also demonstrates "knows" and "knows how." OSCEs are usually used for clinical skills of history and physical examination, but can be applied to clinical reasoning and the ability to conduct a problem-focused history and physical examination. An OSCE can include time for the learner to engage in MAL planning as well as learning. The OSCE demonstrates "knows," "knows how," and "shows how."	×	×		
Evidence-based medicine cases—such as the Fresno-based cases, questions, and scoring rubric. These tend to measure "shows how" as well as "knows" and "knows how."	×	×		
Paper or video vignette cases—tend to be "shows how." These can be models of cases that allow the learner to show the phases of master adaptive learning.	×	×		
Patient-based long and short cases—tend to measure "shows how" and "does." These are the direct observation of a trainee during an entire case or a portion of a case (such as the mini–Clinical Evaluation Exercise [mini-CEX]). During this process, the observer can assess the searching for information through the history and physical, the prioritization of history questions, and physical examination.	×	×		
Reflection (essay)—tends to measure "does." These can measure multiple MAL levels depending on the prompt. One might ask the learner about responses to feedback as well as the actions and goal setting that occur as a response, which demonstrate this phase of master adaptive learning.	×	×	×	×

TABLE 7.2 Assessment Methods for Different Phases of Master Adaptive Learning (MAL).—cont'd

Assessment Methods	Planning	Learning	Assessing	Adjusting
Reflection via a talk (aloud or chart-stimulated recall)—tend to be "does" level. In these methods, one asks the learner to reason through or talk aloud her thought process to make visible the MAL assessing.	×	×	×	×
Direct observation—through watching a learner in workplace-based assessments, the faculty can see that learner adjusting her practice based on the patient, information, and feedback. Direct observation can take a number of forms, including mini-CEX, a checklist observation form, and direct observation of an entrustable professional activity or another competency.	×	×	×	×
Oral case presentations—tend to demonstrate "does" as well as "knows" and "knows how." Through presenting patients in rounds, the master adaptive learner's approach to learning may be seen as along with other phases of master adaptive learning.	×	×	×	×
Global assessment forms—tend to measure "does." These are another form of direct observation, but they are based on multiple encounters and require the assessor to aggregate those observations into a single assessment form.	×	×	×	×
360-degree or multisource feedback—tends to demonstrate "does." This method provides input from multiple sources that might include the patient, interprofessional colleagues, and peers. These can be used to assess all phases of master adaptive learning.	×	×	×	×
Log book—tends to demonstrate "does." This method, with appropriate prompts, can demonstrate all phases of master adaptive learning.	×	×	×	×
Portfolio—tends to demonstrate "does." This method, with appropriate prompts, can demonstrate all phases of master adaptive learning.	×	×	×	×
Self-assessment—tends to demonstrate "does." This method is aimed at the assessing phase and can demonstrate whether the self-assessment is informed by external data. It can take the form of a scale assessment or a narrative refection of the learner's own behavior. Self-assessment may be limited in accuracy (see Chapter 6).			×	
Attitudes—tend to demonstrate "does." There are a variety of scales that measure self-reported responses to aspects of the MAL model (see Table 7.1). They have limitations similar to self-assessment because the learner may not have a clear view of herself.	×		×	×
Review of individualized learning plans (ILPs) or case log or portfolio—tends to demonstrate "does." The review specifically of ILPs will provide the opportunity to see the assessing and adjusting phases, especially if this review is cyclic.	×	×	×	×

Table 7.2 can be used to assess any of these four phases, but that is not to say they are a whole measure of master adaptive learning. These phases represent a learner's progress through the learning process, wherein an information need is identified, addressed, and applied. As a process, learners will exhibit some traits associated with master adaptive learning at different points, so the best way to capture the range of evidence to suggest that they are acting in ways consistent with master adaptive learning is to use multiple instruments and to bring together multiple data sources.

It is critical that the assessments occur over time because the key construct of the master adaptive learner is adaptive learning, which means assimilating and improving over time. The complexity of the MAL model requires a diversity of assessment techniques, so that one can measure the process of the learner working through the MAL model, such as: can she identify her gaps in knowledge, frame the right question, and seek appropriate sources to fill the knowledge gap? These might be measured by increased learning, fewer knowledge gaps, or adaptive expertise in clinical care. For example, one might use a series of multiple-choice questions to gauge the demonstration of knowledge about a core science course, while an OSCE could be used as a way for a medical student to show his learning. As our medical students become more capable, matching assessment types that allow them to demonstrate skills and practice will be an important way to promote masterful learning.

Vignette Continued

Several weeks have passed, and Sarah and Jason have both recently completed the next course in their series of basic science courses and received their grades on their most recent exam. Sarah's performance has improved significantly. This grade outcome illustrates the trajectory of Sarah's learning. She recognized a gap in her learning, used resources to fill that gap, tested learning, and finally incorporated it into her base of knowledge. Based on the collected evidence across the three domains of MAL data described, we can say that Sarah exhibits outcomes and behaviors associated with being a master adaptive learner.

Jason's performance on this latest exam has declined from the previous one. He failed to recognize and change the mistakes in his understanding, which only compounded the difficulties in his test-taking for the next exam. Because of this, he was unable to adequately test or incorporate new knowledge into his learning, and his performance declined as a result. Based on the evidence collected about him, we can say that Jason does not exhibit outcomes and behaviors associated with master adaptive learning.

Maggie's request for specific feedback on her history-taking led to additional specific feedback on this skill. Although her orientation toward these encounters was about demonstrating her competence more so than developing it, she was still able to make an improvement to her skills because she tested her skills, applied knowledge, and incorporated this new learning into her practice. Based on this collection of evidence, we can suggest that Maggie exhibits outcomes and behaviors related to master adaptive learning.

These cases begin to illustrate some of the importance of choosing outcomes and assessments carefully when it comes to trying to capture master adaptive learning. For example, asking Maggie to describe the steps required in a history-taking might elicit competence at the "knows" or "knows how" level, but at her level of training we are more interested in her ability to accurately perform such skills. Similarly, trying to have Sarah and Jason demonstrate the basic science knowledge they are learning may not provide information about their learning that is as useful as whether they know certain core concepts.

LONGITUDINAL ASSESSMENT

One of the advantages and opportunities we see in this MAL assessment framework is that there is the opportunity for longitudinal data collection. The core of master adaptive learning is that it is adaptive. Therefore we are looking for evidence of a pattern of MAL cycles with each cycle incorporating learning, self-reflection, and adaptation, not only by the nature of the three domains of outcomes but also, as mentioned in the vignette, the need for developmentally appropriate assessments to capture information about our learners as they grow. Portfolio learning, for example, represents a meaningful opportunity here for such assessment. We would argue that master adaptive learning in learners is not static, but instead is a tendency toward adaptability and the integration of knowledge to practice. These kinds of applications are not measurable in a moment-to-moment way and would need a range of evidence over a range of times and contexts for us to be able to say that a particular student demonstrates more master adaptive learning than another. By actively engaging learners and their instructors in the use of a portfolio, we can build this body of evidence. This is salient to the core of master adaptive learning as a framework about growth. Students who exhibit fewer master adaptive learning–related characteristics or behaviors are not non–master adaptive learners; they simply need more support to develop the skills we suggest are related to better performance.

PROGRAMMATIC ASSESSMENT

When used to observe master adaptive learning, two main purposes of assessment must be kept in mind: the first is to give formative feedback to the trainee to optimize his learning by providing motivation and direction for future learning (assessment for learning), and the second is to use assessments to make a summative judgment about performance (assessment of learning). These two purposes of assessment can be viewed on a continuum as frequently formative assessments are brought together to make a summative judgment. This process of intentional mapping and aggregation of assessment data is programmatic assessment. Finally, the aggregation of assessments provides an evaluation of the educational program to determine if the objectives were achieved.[12]

Programmatic assessment is the intentional collection of key data points from multiple sources for both assessment of learning and assessment for learning. Because each assessment views a portion of the MAL process, aggregating assessment data across methods will provide a clearer picture of the master adaptive learner and her performance. Therefore it is important to use multiple methods, performing various tasks from multiple sources at multiple time points, in order to provide a clearer picture of the learner. Because the goal is lifelong habits of practice, this assessment process must be repeated over time to provide informed feedback and to monitor growth in becoming a master adaptive learner.

CONCLUSIONS

It is important that MAL assessments be chosen thoughtfully to best be connected to medical students' learning, outcomes, and the MAL process. If one thing is taken away from this chapter, it is that the measurement and assessment of a master adaptive learner is complicated. Rather than being a reason to halt our efforts, however, we see this as evidence that we are engaging with this work properly. The assessment of something as complicated as learning and the development of mastery should be complicated. The use of multiple methods allows our understanding to grow with our learners. This chapter represents an early attempt to measure some of the MAL process; future work will be needed to develop instrumentation that is tailored to the medical education context and to build validity evidence for our populations of learners.

TAKE-HOME POINTS

1. Assessment drives learning; so, learners will pay attention to what you are assessing.
2. Assessment of a master adaptive learner includes multiple types and sources of assessment data.
3. Examining the multiple sources of evidence of master adaptive learning, including programmatic assessment, will best demonstrate the learner's skill in master adaptive learning.
4. Longitudinal assessments that include a component of self-monitoring are construct-aligned with the adaptive expertise model.

QUESTIONS FOR FURTHER THOUGHT

1. Given all the different forms of assessment for master adaptive learning, which ones help achieve your goals of formative or summative assessment for your learners?
2. When choosing a method of assessment, what are you trying to measure? Is the purpose of the assessment aligned with what the instrument is measuring? What is the validity evidence of the instrument?
3. What dimensions and what sources of assessment are your learner assessment systems using? Should you add assessments of master adaptive learning in dimensions that are not already measured to add to your learner's programmatic assessment?

ANNOTATED BIBLIOGRAPHY

1. Epstein RM. Assessment in medical education. *N Engl J Med.* 2007;356(4):387-396.
   This article highlights the goals of assessment in medical education along with examples that encourage careful thought about how and why we assess our learners.
2. Miller GE. The assessment of clinical skills/competence/performance. *Acad Med.* 1990;65(9 suppl):S63-S67.
   Miller's framework provides a developmental frame for learner performance that aligns closely to the cyclical nature of the MAL process.
3. White CB, Gruppen LD, Fantone JC. Self-regulated learning in medical education. In: Swanwick T, ed. *Understanding Medical Education: Evidence, Theory, and Practice.* 2nd ed. Chichester, West Sussex, UK: John Wiley & Sons; 2013: 201-211.
   This chapter frames self-regulated learning in four phases that would eventually be adopted into the MAL process and suggests examples of individual characteristics to be measured.

REFERENCES

1. Epstein RM. Assessment in medical education. *New Engl J Med.* 2007;356(4):387-396.
2. Newstead S. The purposes of assessment. *Psychology Learning & Teaching.* 2004;3(2):97-101.
3. Schalock R. *Outcome-Based Evaluation.* 2nd ed. New York, NY: Kluwer Academic/Plenum; 2001.
4. White CB, Gruppen LD, Fantone JC. Self-regulated learning in medical education. In: Swanwick T, ed. *Understanding Medical Education: Evidence, Theory, and Practice.* 2nd ed. Chichester, West Sussex, UK: John Wiley & Sons; 2013:201-211.
5. Amin Z, Chong YS, Khoo HE. *Practical Guide to Medical Student Assessment.* Hackensack, NJ: World Scientific; 2006.
6. Frank JR, Snell LS, Cate OT, et al. Competency-based medical education: theory to practice. *Med Teach.* 2010;32(8):638-645.
7. American Educational Research Association, American Psychological Association, National Council on Measurement in Education. *Standards for Educational and Psychological Testing.* Washington, DC: American Educational Research Association; 2014.
8. Miller GE. The assessment of clinical skills/competence/performance. *Acad Med.* 1990;65(suppl 9):S63-S67.
9. Asch DA, Nicholson S, Srinivas SK, Herrin J, Epstein AJ. How do you deliver a good obstetrician? Outcome-based evaluation of medical education. *Acad Med.* 2014;89(1):24-26.
10. Chan T, Sebok-Syer S, Thoma B, Wise A, Sherbino J, Pusic M. Learning analytics in medical education assessment: the past, the present, and the future. *AEM Educ Train.* 2018;2(2): 178-187.
11. Mylopoulos M, Brydges R, Woods NN, Manzone J, Schwartz DL. Preparation for future learning: a missing competency in health professions education? *Med Educ.* 2016;50(1):115-123.
12. Praslova L. Adaptation of Kirkpatrick's four level model of training criteria to assessment of learning outcomes and program evaluation in higher education. *Educ Assess, Eval Account.* 2010;22(3):215-225.
13. Pintrich PR, Smith DAF, Garcia T, McKeachie WJ. *A Manual for the Use of the Motivated Strategies for Learning Questionnaire (MSLQ).* Washington, DC: Education Resources Information Center; 1991. Available at: https://eric.ed.gov/?id=ED338122.
14. Wetzel AP, Mazmanian PE, Hojat M, et al. Measuring medical students' orientation toward lifelong learning: a psychometric evaluation. *Acad Med.* 2010;85(10):S41-S44.
15. Sosu EM. The development and psychometric validation of a Critical Thinking Disposition Scale. *Think Skills Creat.* 2013;9:107-119.
16. Gross JJ, John OP. Individual differences in two emotion regulation processes: implications for affect, relationships, and well-being. *J Pers Soc Psychol.* 2003;85(2):348-362.
17. Steelman LA, Levy PE, Snell AF. The Feedback Environment Scale: construct definition, measurement, and validation. *Educ Psychol Meas.* 2004;64(1):165-184.
18. Grant AM, Franklin J, Langford P. The Self-Reflection and Insight Scale: a new measure of private self-consciousness. *Soc Behav Pers: An Int J.* 2002;30(8):821-835.
19. McAuley E, Duncan TE, Russell DW. Measuring causal attributions: the revised Causal Dimension Scale (CDSII). *Pers Soc Psychol Bull.* 1992;18(5):566-573.

How and Where Do I Teach My Learners About the Master Adaptive Learner Model?

Nicole K. Roberts, PhD; Richard N. Van Eck, PhD; and Rosa Lee, MD

LEARNING OBJECTIVES

1. Support your learner's development as a master adaptive learner.
2. Create opportunities for low-stakes failures among your learners' experiences.
3. Identify and create opportunities to observe master adaptive learning behaviors in your learners.
4. Model master adaptive learner behaviors yourself.

CHAPTER OUTLINE

CHAPTER SUMMARY

Children become adaptive experts through curiosity, interaction with the world, and a desire for both understanding and results. As educators, it is our responsibility to tap into and encourage these capacities in our learners, to shape their curiosity and desire for results to particular ends. In medical education, that same type of shaping is toward educating physicians who maintain their curiosity and desire for results such that the care of their patients is optimized, and one can hope that the health care system is reformed and optimized as a result. The need for physicians to finish training with the habits of the Master Adaptive Learner (MAL) model well inculcated is hard to debate. It is more difficult to envision how educators in

medical schools can configure teaching and learning activities to ensure learners develop and maintain these habits. Other chapters detail how to adapt MAL strategies to different learning modalities, including lecture classrooms, team-based learning classrooms, and problem-based learning classrooms. In this chapter, we focus on foundational strategies to help promote the MAL mindset, with a focus on how to adapt these strategies for beginning medical students.

Vignette

Taylor is a first-year medical student who has been struggling with the active learning components of her courses. Her teachers/instructors say she seems reluctant to speak out and is content to let the others in the group lead the discussion. She just got her end-of-block test scores back, and they are not as high as she expected based on her prior academic success. She feels that this teaching strategy is putting her at a disadvantage: "I've always done very well in school and I just work better when you lecture on what is most important, point me toward the readings I need, and let me work on my own."

1. What would you say to Taylor?
2. How might you have her use the Master Adaptive Learner (MAL) model to guide her future learning?

WHERE AND HOW TO PROMOTE THE MASTER ADAPTIVE LEARNER MODEL

Part of teaching the MAL model is to make it part of the culture of the school. If all members of the school community are versed in the MAL model, fluent in its language, and visible practitioners, it will be seen as a normal part of teaching and learning. In this chapter, we share some strategies and practices educators may use in any learning setting to foster medical students learning the MAL model and to incorporate it as a part of school culture.

EXPOSURE: DEVELOPING A SHARED LANGUAGE TO PROMOTE METACOGNITION

Metacognition, or thinking about and monitoring one's own thinking and learning, is an essential part of the medical school curriculum and a core tenet of the MAL model. This requires raising the process of metacognition to the same conscious level that is typically devoted to course content. Most learners need help developing metacognition as a habit of mind so that they can use it to assess their strengths and weaknesses.

There are numerous methods educators can use to help learners develop metacognitive approaches. For instance, by providing opportunities to reflect on their learning, as classes or small group sessions occur, an educator sends the clear message that the point of the class is not only to develop knowledge of content but also to pay attention to how it is best learned. Asking learners to specify how they intend to study a particular concept and providing feedback on the plan sends the same message: How you study is important.

Reflecting on the vignette, an educator might encourage Taylor to practice metacognition by asking her, "What is the difference between learning in a lecture and learning in a small group? What skills do you have to develop in the small group that you can't develop in lecture?" A master adaptive learner with more developed metacognitive skills would focus on the fact that she is not successful in participating in the teaching activities, that her level of discomfort is holding her back from learning a new set of skills, and that she could formulate a plan for becoming more successful in this form of learning. Developing this skill early in her medical school career will make it more likely that Taylor will leave school with the ability to reflect on her medical practice.

We propose that teaching the MAL process allows educators and learners to use a shared language about learning. Doing so allows for efficient and effective conversations among learners and between teachers and learners. Furthermore, having this language allows both teachers and learners to engage in diagnostic reasoning about learning when learners are having "other than desirable" difficulties (see Chapter 13).

A school could begin the process of developing a shared language by simply advertising on its website that one of the outcomes expected of its graduates is that they become master adaptive learners, with a brief explanation of the model and its connection to lifelong learning and patient outcomes. Learners interviewed for entry into the program could be given an opportunity to demonstrate some elements of the MAL model. For instance, within a Multiple Mini Interview[1] context, one of the stations could be a complicated puzzle with no easy solution. Does the applicant respond with a growth mindset, pursuing or inventing a solution? Does the applicant give up? This is not intended to mean that the applicant who gives up should not be admitted, of course; a growth mindset can be taught.[2] It is simply a way to understand the learner's current state and to inform the advising and mentoring that the learner may need to be successful moving forward.

Once a student has been admitted, the faculty of the school should continue this process of intentionally articulating and developing the language and understanding of the MAL model. For instance, the MAL model could be both described (e.g., direct lecture) and demonstrated (e.g., active learning) during an orientation week. Educators can stress that learning is a practice, just as sports or theater or chess are practices, and the intent of teaching the MAL process is to make visible the habits of learning the school has adopted as additional learning outcomes.

In the beginning of the curriculum, it will be helpful for faculty to continue to make the MAL model explicit and to provide opportunities for demonstrating the mindset. Echoing what learners have learned from the website, the admissions process and the orientation will begin to establish a goal state for the learner. Educators should also provide frequent and timely support and formative feedback in the beginning (e.g., prior to the first significant assessment), and early intervention is critical. Those who do not do as well on early tests as expected, such as Taylor, need one-to-one support so they can develop a plan for being more successful in cultivating the MAL mindset moving forward.

As the year progresses, educators should repeatedly refer to elements of the MAL model in a way that isolates individual components and concepts across the first year of the curriculum. The focus should be to teach about the components, to stimulate recall of prior knowledge and activate appropriate knowledge schemas. There should also be practice opportunities with feedback in demonstrating the component by, for instance, placing learners in experiences designed to elicit MAL behaviors. Educators should be sure to provide frequent and explicit feedback to assist learners in identifying where they are mastering the concepts and where they require work.

"DO AS I SAY *AND* AS I DO."

Educators can deliberately model their use of the MAL process for their own learning and require the same of learners at increasingly higher levels. For instance, a surgeon might explicitly state, "I have reduced hundreds of inguinal hernias, but I'm still trying to lessen my time to close in my laparoscopic repair for the sake of the comfort and safety of the patient. I'm going to ask Dr. Francis to watch me next time to see if she has any suggestions. Now that I've identified my learning gap and decided what resource to use to address it, I'll be interested to see how much I can improve." Here the surgeon has not only engaged in portions of the MAL model, but she has also identified them by step in the process, and demonstrated a growth mindset by asking how much she could improve. Sharing such examples can be invaluable when counseling medical students such as Taylor about the MAL model. Failing to do so is equivalent to saying "do as I say, not as I do," and turns the MAL model into just another hoop a medical student has to jump through to become a physician, enacting a hidden curriculum that can lead to learner cynicism.

When educators are willing to take a risk, as the surgeon mentioned previously did by publicly revealing a goal for improvement, they can help encourage their learners to do the same. Educators can assess their success at teaching the MAL model in part by recognizing and rewarding when learners take appropriate risks in their learning. As learners develop the tools to address errors and failure, they should become more willing to step outside their comfort zones. This might take the form of speaking up in class more frequently, offering answers, asking questions, or developing learning activities that expose a lack of knowledge. Making note of these behaviors as they begin to emerge is extremely helpful for promoting the MAL mindset. Early attempts may produce what seem like negative results to medical students such as Taylor. It is critical that facilitators

are able to help learners deconstruct those experiences and reclassify them as learning experiences that are necessary for true growth. In addition to simply being unwilling to risk looking like they do not know something, medical students such as Taylor may have made initial attempts at risk taking that were not recognized by their teachers and that they have now classified as mistakes. Taylor's coach could discuss with her how, with a growth mindset, failures are opportunities for further exploration. Furthermore, learning should be hard or she is not learning.

As learners proceed through the curriculum, educators should continue to create opportunities for risk that are commensurate with the growing MAL mindset of learners. For example, simulated ethical dilemmas for which there are no known right answers, played out over a number of sessions, can give learners an opportunity to take risks, innovate, fail, and learn from experience. Learners could also be encouraged to use the MAL model as an analytic tool to assess where in the process the failure originated. For instance, learners could start by asking whether or not they demonstrate curiosity, motivation, a growth mindset, and resilience. They could specifically ask if their coach has noticed their strengths and deficits, and whether the coach feels the learners have been sufficiently receptive to the coaching. They could interrogate their engagement in each phase of the MAL learner cycle (see Chapter 1):

1. Did I identify the gap correctly?
2. Did I select proper opportunities and resources for learning?
3. Did I actively engage my learning process?
4. Did I give my new learning a proper trial, or is it possible that what I see as a failure is in fact simply a need to adjust what was learned to more effectively incorporate it into practice?

Taylor's coach could begin a conversation with her by asking the question about whether or not she allowed herself to reflect on the small group learning process and how she might adjust to make it an effective one for her. All of these questions could be made explicit by defining the associated strategies and providing handouts to which learners can refer as they continue to move through the curriculum—or, in fact, encouraging the learners to determine how they might best remember the strategies and questions.

FOUNDATIONS OF MASTER ADAPTIVE LEARNING

In addition to the previous suggestions for promoting the MAL mindset, there are several other educational concepts and principles that should be brought to bear across the curriculum. Each can be considered a foundational building block of master adaptive learning. As you read about them, consider which of these you think might be most relevant in explaining Taylor's current predicament, in guiding your discussion with her, or in both. Many of the foundational educational theories are listed in Chapter 16.

Priming and Supporting Learners for Master Adaptive Learning

Regardless of learning environment or outcomes, learners should always be encouraged to assess their prior knowledge, identify gaps in their knowledge, develop goals for how they will use learning events to address these gaps, and consider how they can extend their learning beyond the event.[3] This has implications for educators, both in how they *prepare* (prime) learners for success before a learning event and in how they support and encourage MAL behaviors *during* those events. Taylor seems to be demonstrating a need for more or better priming for her classes this session.

Schemas and Mental Models

Schemas, sometimes also called mental models, are cognitive structures that we build over time to represent what we know about something.[4-6] Novices have sparse, ill-structured schemas; expert schemas are well developed and dense.[7] For instance, on the first day of clinic, a learner may be able to report that the patient's heart rate and rhythm are regular, but because he has not developed a robust schema of heart sounds, he may miss the subtle murmur of a stenotic mitral valve. The attending, a cardiologist with decades of experience, has heard this sound many times and can point out the opening snap and diastolic murmur.

If the attending had known of the murmur before sending the learner into the room, she might have primed him to listen for it. The MAL process focuses on building schemas, which in turn requires that we activate them ahead of time.[5] "What do I know?" and "What do I need to know?" are questions designed to activate prior knowledge, find gaps in our schemas, and develop plans to intentionally use that information to manage our own learning (see Chapter 9).

Optimizing Challenge

It is important to create opportunities for students to experience challenge and even failure. This means making the learning hard enough to be worth doing, but not so hard that success is impossible, though success may follow a failure or two. This is what Vygotsky[7] called keeping students in "the zone of proximal development"[8] (ZPD; Fig. 8.1), which has been shown to be the optimal level of challenge for learning, an approach made concrete in enacting the challenge point framework.[9] Thus educators communicate to students that they should expect to fail, and design activities with enough challenge to ensure it. At present, Taylor does not see the active learning as a positive opportunity to challenge herself.

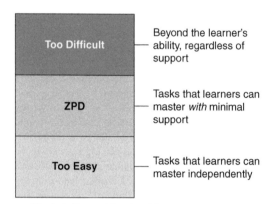

Fig. 8.1 Zone of Proximal Development (ZPD)

Scaffolding

This concept is related to the ZPD. If students are in the ZPD, they will be unsuccessful unless they receive "just enough, just-in-time, and just-for-me" support from their group, instructors, and self-selected resources. A helpful mechanism is to suggest that feedback, whether it comes from peers, instructors, or others in the environment, be aimed at answering the question: "What is the one thing this person could do that would most improve his performance?" This can be asked in most environments and about most activities. For example, peers might suggest to a learner in the problem-based learning environment that the one best thing he could do to improve performance is to consult primary literature and texts as he addresses his learning issues, rather than using a review book. As learners become more cognizant of their learning, they might be explicitly scaffolded on using the MAL process. Rather than pointing to an explicit action for improvement, they might be asked where they are in the learning cycle and what they need to do next. Some structured approaches to teaching have built mechanisms for scaffolding right into the process. For instance, in team-based learning, the Group Readiness Assurance Test used to begin the learning session is designed to provide scaffolding in the form of group support.[10] If Taylor is afraid to challenge herself by participating fully in active learning sessions or if she has made attempts that she feels were unsuccessful, scaffolding her experiences could be a key way to help her take small risks and gradually increase them over time as she matures as a master adaptive learner.

Self-Efficacy

Self-efficacy refers to the beliefs one holds about how successful one can be under adverse circumstances.[11] If self-efficacy is too low, learners believe that no amount of work will allow them to be successful, which leads to learned helplessness. When self-efficacy is too high, it can lead to "superhero syndrome," wherein learners try to go it alone and never reach out for additional resources, help, or coaching. Keeping learning in the ZPD ensures an appropriate amount of failure and supported success, which leads to a healthy self-efficacy. Self-efficacy could easily be what is driving Taylor's desire to study in the way in which she has always been successful before.

Goal Orientation

This refers to the kind of goals that a learner will set for herself, and can be categorized roughly as "performance" and "mastery" orientation.[2] Performance orientation emphasizes success in terms of markers of success outside the individual (grades, promotion, etc.), whereas mastery orientation defines success in terms of how well the knowledge, skills, and abilities have been demonstrated. The MAL process encourages learners to adopt a mastery orientation so that they are always learning, always in the ZPD, and therefore better prepared for the challenges of an unknown future. Educators can enhance the likelihood that learners will adopt a mastery orientation by muting the external markers of success or making them at least as available for those who take risks and fail as they are to students who succeed at low-risk endeavors. Ensuring that the learning environment supports application of learning to new problems and supports adjustment without adverse consequences will further support the appropriate goal orientation. Taylor is clearly not setting a mastery orientation in her goal setting. She is more concerned about not failing than about challenging herself to be the best.

Intrinsic/Extrinsic Motivation

Intrinsic motivators are internal beliefs and dispositions (e.g., satisfaction in a job well done; mastery orientation) that drive performance toward a goal.[12] Extrinsic motivators are those that are external to the individual (e.g., grades, pay, promotion). The MAL process promotes mastery orientation, which relies on intrinsic motivators (one of the four batteries within the model; see Fig. 1.1). Because it is Taylor's performance on the test that has brought her to her coach, we might surmise that she is extrinsically motivated by the test rather than motivated by an intrinsic desire to be the best she can be.

CONCLUSION

We propose that teaching the MAL model should be done explicitly, using a variety of educational approaches. By developing a shared language with students, educators create opportunities for conversations directed at learning how to learn. Keeping educational activities within the zone of proximal development ensures that students have sufficient opportunities to try, fail, and become resilient so as to try again. Educators can be explicit in their use of the MAL model, noting what steps in the process they are using when they do so. Creating a culture where everyone is not only learning, but also talking about learning, helps to create the desired outcome of graduating students who are Master Adaptive Learners.

TAKE-HOME POINTS

1. Opportunities to teach the master adaptive learner exist throughout the medical school learning environment, even beginning with the admissions process.
2. Educators who are deliberate in their own use of the MAL model allow students to see its use and impact and also to see that it is a skill practiced for life.
3. Using the language of learning assists students in practicing metacognition.
4. Students can use the MAL model as a diagnostic tool when encountering difficulties.

QUESTIONS FOR FURTHER THOUGHT

Consider how you would apply these principles to the design of a curriculum over 4 years:

1. At what points in a year would you increase challenge? How about over the full schedule of medical school?
2. How will you know when students are ready for more challenge?
3. How might you integrate overt and covert MAL teaching opportunities into different instructional modalities (lectures, cases, patient encounters, simulations)?
4. What kind of individualized plan would you create for Taylor moving forward over the next instructional block?
5. How might you make use of more advanced students (years 3 and 4) in modeling and supporting the MAL mindset for newer students?
6. How do you get your volunteer/clinical faculty to be comfortable with modeling the MAL approach in their practices?
7. What does the MAL mindset look like during clerkships?

ANNOTATED BIBLIOGRAPHY

1. Hatano G, Inagaki K. Two courses of expertise. In: Stevenson HW, Azuma H, Hakuta K. *A Series of Books in Psychology. Child Development and Education in Japan.* New York, NY: W H Freeman/Times Books/Henry Holt & Co.; 1986:262-272.
   Focused on children, this chapter is the first work to describe the entity of adaptive expertise, how it is developed, and how to foster its development.
2. Carbonell KB, Stalmeijer RE, Könings KD, Segers MR, Van Merrienboer JJG. How experts deal with novel situations: a review of adaptive expertise. *Educ Res Rev.* 2014;12:14-29.
   This paper provides an excellent review of the literature on adaptive expertise, including information about learner, personality, task, training, and learning climate characteristics that influence the development of adaptive expertise.
3. Ericsson KA, Krampe RT, Tesch-Romer C. Deliberate practice and the acquisition and maintenance of expert performance. *Psychol Rev.* 1993;100(3):363-406.
   In this paper the relationships among mindsets, deliberate practice, and the development of expertise become very clear.
4. Dweck C. *Mindset: The New Psychology of Success.* New York, NY: Ballantine Books; 2006.
   This book shows that it is very helpful to have a good understanding of the role of mindsets in learning and also to know that a growth mindset can be taught.

REFERENCES

1. Eva KW, Rosenfeld J, Reiter HI, Norman GR. An admissions OSCE: the multiple mini-interview. *Med Educ.* 2004:38:314-326.
2. Dweck C. *Mindset: The New Psychology of Success.* New York, NY: Ballantine Books; 2006.
3. Bruner JS. *The Process of Education.* Cambridge: Harvard University Press; 1977.
4. Piaget J. *The Psychology of Intelligence.* San Diego, CA: Harcourt Brace; 1950.
5. Piaget J. *The Origins of Intelligence in Children.* New York, NY: International University Press; 1952.
6. Driscoll MP. *Psychology of Learning for Instruction.* 3rd ed. Needham Heights, MA: Allyn & Bacon; 2004.
7. Vygotsky LS. *Mind in Society: The Development of Higher Psychological Processes* (Cole M, John-Steiner V, Scribner S, Souberman E, eds.). Cambridge, MA: Harvard University Press; 1978.
8. Elstein AS. What goes around comes around: return of the hypothetico-deductive strategy. *Teach Learn Med.* 1994;6(2):121-123. doi:10.1080/10401339409539658.
9. Guadagnoli M, Morin, MP, Dubrowski A. The application of the challenge point framework in medical education. *Med Educ.* 2012:46(5):447-453
10. Michaelsen LR, Sweet M. The essential elements of team-based learning. In: Michaelsen LK, Sweet M, Parmelee DX. *Team-Based Learning: Small Group Learning's Next Big Step. New Directions in Teaching and Learning.* Hoboken, NJ: Jossey-Bass; 2009:7-28.
11. Bandura A. Self-efficacy. In: Ramachaudran VS, ed. *Encyclopedia of Human Behavior.* Vol 4. New York, NY: Academic Press; 1994:71-81. (Reprinted in H. Friedman [Ed.], *Encyclopedia of Mental Health.* San Diego, CA: Academic Press, 1998.)
12. Ryan RM, Deci EL. Intrinsic and extrinsic motivations: classic definitions and new directions. *Contemp Educ Psychol.* 2000;25:54-67.

9

How Will the Master Adaptive Learner Process Work in the Classroom?

Amy L. Wilson-Delfosse, PhD, and Leslie H. Fall, MD

LEARNING OBJECTIVES

1. Redesign a traditional content-based curriculum to one that describes and promotes adaptive clinical expertise within a given domain.
2. Use the Master Adaptive Learner Scorecard to evaluate and select the most appropriate classroom pedagogical approach for promoting adaptive expertise in the given domain.
3. Apply the Master Adaptive Learner Classroom Checklist to plan and assess the effective implementation of the selected approach.
4. Design and assess the adaptive expertise of classroom learning teams.
5. Consider the use of virtual patients or other technology-enhanced learning tools to promote coaching for adaptive expertise.

CHAPTER OUTLINE

CHAPTER SUMMARY

The medical education classroom provides an important environment in which learners build mastery of content, concepts, and clinical practice skills that are relevant in their development of clinical mastery and progression toward adaptive expertise. In this chapter, we begin with an overview of how three types of knowledge critical for adaptive expertise are learned, organized, integrated, and continuously honed over time in the mind of a clinical expert. We then evaluate three classroom models (lecture, team-based learning, and problem-based learning) commonly used to establish this clinical knowledge base and propose easily implemented modifications that promote skill development beneficial to the master adaptive learner. We offer tools to assist the teacher in the development of these improved classroom settings. The chapter concludes with a consideration of methods to blend technology-based learning into the classroom to further promote the knowledge and skills of an adaptive expert.

KNOWLEDGE DEVELOPMENT FOR CLINICAL MASTERY

Knowledge Organization and Application in Adaptive Expertise

In addition to having the qualities of compassion, empathy, and technical abilities, a clinician must be smart and wise in order to be effective. Cognitive science research and experience clearly demonstrate that expertise requires deep domain knowledge gained and refined over time through experience and continued learning. Beyond a vast knowledge base of information, research demonstrates that the defining traits of a true expert mind are the deliberate construction of large, highly developed, extremely rich, and intricate mental models (or "schemas") within the domain of expertise and a deep understanding of meaning and how the domain functions as an integrated system.[1,2] For adaptive experts, information that consistently proves to be true, and the routine steps needed to mentally combine and use that information, is effortlessly chunked and encapsulated into tacit understanding in order to free up working memory for more creative endeavors.[3] New learning is thereby efficient and seeks to build out and further enrich known schemas and connections and to continuously enlarge the comprehensive picture of the domain. Ongoing experience teaches the adaptive expert when and how to act on this understanding—the essence of wisdom.

This robust mental framework and ongoing practice allow prior knowledge to be effectively and efficiently transferred and applied to new and progressively more complex situations—and creates a virtuous cycle of new learning that furthers adaptive expertise.[2,4] Expert understanding goes beyond obvious surface features of a problem and sees deeper characteristics and meaningful patterns. This understanding enables expert perception to be particularly keen and purposeful. Patterns are accurately perceived as specific problems to be solved. Experts quickly extract relevant from irrelevant details, freeing up mental resources to creatively attack the problem at hand. Information retrieval is fluent and strategic, and proposed solutions are flexible and adapted to the unique circumstance.[1] Most

importantly, experts are able to leverage their knowledge to see how recent events will create impending events and, thus, more accurately project and predict future events and outcomes. This ability to run multiple mental experiments prior to acting enables adaptive experts to take the calculated risks necessary to creatively solve complex and ambiguous problems even when the stakes are high. This grand knowledge organization—and the ability to flexibly leverage it as needed—is what gives adaptive expertise so much power.

Three Types of Knowledge

Knowledge is generally considered by cognitive psychologists to be organized into three categories: content knowledge (facts and information stored in memory), conceptual knowledge (deeper understanding using schemas and mental models), and procedural knowledge (knowledge applied to a given problem or task so as to effect a desired outcome) (Fig. 9.1). Effective procedural knowledge—knowing how to solve commonly encountered problems through appropriately balanced application of content and conceptual knowledge—is the desired end point for routine expertise.

Content knowledge, also known as declarative knowledge, refers to the vast amount of information that must be learned and effectively organized so that it may be gathered quickly into working memory and applied through procedural knowledge as clinical skills to solve routine problems. For experts, a vast content knowledge base serves both as the grounding scaffold upon which the mental models required for conceptual knowledge are constructed and a resource to be interrogated as needed when solving more complex problems. Novices, on the other hand, must rely on content knowledge and working memory to solve even simple problems, and therefore cognitive load is initially quite high and can be mentally exhausting. With enough practice with routine problems, relevant content knowledge is encapsulated (or "chunked") in memory, becoming interwoven with relevant procedural knowledge, and can be pulled (rather than constructed each time) with virtually no cognitive cost. This is how experts know routinely what to do.[1]

Conceptual knowledge enables content knowledge to be understood in the context of a variety of known problems within the practice domain, providing direction regarding appropriate application, as well as supporting creative thought required for newly encountered problems. Concepts (e.g., regulation of glucose homeostasis) move learners to consider content knowledge (e.g., cellular mechanisms for ATP generation) at a deeper level, thereby bringing context (e.g., starvation, pregnancy), meaning (e.g., disease vs. growth state), and purpose (e.g., need to

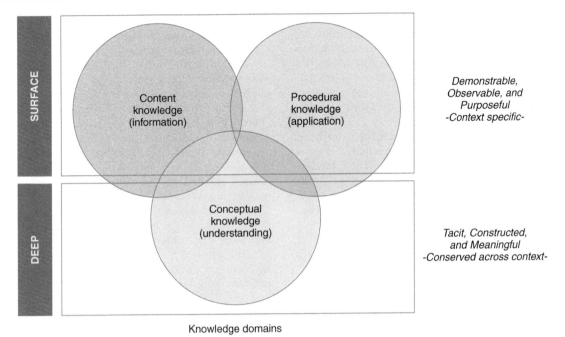

Fig. 9.1 **Knowledge Domains.** (Used with permission of Leslie Fall, MD. Copyright Aquifer.)

provide diagnosis, treatment, or prevention strategies) to bear on the problem.[5,6] Concepts lead to enduring understanding by drawing meaningful connections between seemingly disparate content knowledge (e.g., mechanisms of glycolysis and of fatty acid metabolism), thereby deepening and enriching understanding. In this manner, conceptual knowledge binds content and procedural knowledge together as a requisite for the eventual development of adaptive expertise. A clinician with deep conceptual understanding unsupported by robust mastery of relevant content knowledge or sufficiently tested procedural knowledge remains a promising novice. A clinician with sufficient content or procedural knowledge, or both, without the relevant deeper conceptual understanding is a practitioner who risks making poor decisions in complex new problems or contexts, such as the glycemic management of a pregnant woman with a toxic liver injury.

Procedural knowledge is the type of knowledge exercised in the performance of a clinical skill or task. Classic examples include knowing how to take a history of present illness, knowing how to palpate the fundus of a pregnant uterus, and knowing how to start an intravenous (IV) line. Often this type of knowledge may be taught in very disparate places throughout the medical school curriculum. In the case of a pregnant, diabetic woman presenting to a primary care office feeling unwell, the procedural knowledge related to IV insertion will be less impactful without

the deep conceptual understanding of glucose homeostasis, honed over time and experience, combined with the content knowledge needed to take the appropriate medication, dietary, and gynecologic history and to interpret a fingerstick glucose level, which will allow an expert clinician to understand the urgency of inserting an IV line to address the unforeseen clinical problem at hand. This is the essence of the clinical wisdom that training for master adaptive learners is designed to achieve.

Concept-Based Medical Education

In medicine, development of a scientific content knowledge base traditionally occurs in the classroom and begins long before medical school. Therefore classroom educators must begin instruction with a clear understanding of how content knowledge is stored and retrieved in the mind of an expert clinician, and then ensure that medical students' foundational knowledge base and conceptual scaffold is robust and well organized to allow for the inevitable encapsulation and continuous growth required for adaptive clinical expertise. Unfortunately, although medical students have been selected to become physicians largely through demonstrating their grasp of scientific information, this same process often promotes a poorly (and often haphazardly) constructed knowledge base, provides limited deep conceptual understanding, ingrains many ineffective study habits, and rewards knowledge application to the constrained problems presented on many entrance examinations. In order to develop the effective tripartite deep domain knowledge described earlier, classroom educators must push and reward learners for unpacking and reorganizing their knowledge (often unlearning and re-learning foundational information and schemas) and for taking calculated mental risks, in order to prepare for effective adaptive expertise in clinical practice.

Conceptual knowledge is the most difficult to teach and acquire, because understanding is never acquired de novo. A teacher cannot pour concepts directly into a learner's head, nor can concepts be memorized the way declarative content knowledge can be. Teaching and learning driven by overarching concepts necessitates that learners transfer their content knowledge to new and more complex problems and mandates critical thinking and problem solving at increasingly higher orders of complexity and application (i.e., levels of the Bloom taxonomy). Learning new concepts (e.g., glucose homeostasis) will increasingly depend on prior conceptual understanding (e.g., cellular metabolism) and must build upon something medical students already know (i.e., structure and function of carbohydrates, amino acids, and proteins). If a medical student fails to gain conceptual understanding at the right time in the curriculum—or fails to effectively encapsulate prior content knowledge—the student will be progressively more challenged to catch up as the new conceptual knowledge builds on prior understanding. Such medical students will become more and more likely to simply memorize content knowledge (e.g., Krebs cycle and gluconeogenesis) and procedural knowledge (e.g., algorithms for management of diabetic ketoacidosis) and apply them with limited understanding.

Because true conceptual knowledge is difficult to learn, it requires the in-depth study of just a few core concepts at a time. Faculty should be sure to sequence content knowledge development such that the distance between core concepts is initially small and, when learning new concepts, that the application and utility of previously learned concepts is clear and obvious (e.g., cellular and whole-body glucose homeostasis). As conceptual knowledge grows, the distance between related concepts (e.g., glucose homeostasis and nitrogen balance) can expand.[7]

As learned concepts become more complex, explicit examples become harder to generate and the use of a common analogy in the medical student's life (e.g., the concept of work-life balance as an analogy for whole-body glucose homeostasis), as a compare-and-contrast activity between the concept and the analogue, becomes helpful.[8-10] Evidence shows that several principles make analogies especially effective: familiarity, vividness, making the alignment

plain, and ease of continuing to reinforce the concept. It is also useful for a medical student to learn a single analogy to which she returns again and again.

Concepts, by their nature, bring purpose and meaning by connecting content to the bigger picture. Concepts are not intended to replace content or procedural knowledge, and all three should be taught simultaneously to promote effective knowledge organization and transfer. For example, a course in biochemistry should be structured such that learners are continuously returning to the concept of glucose homeostasis as an underlying mental model for both learning glycolysis and fatty acid metabolic pathways and for applying this knowledge to the lifetime management of a patient with diabetes.[6] Concept-based instruction therefore must necessarily begin with a base level of content knowledge and contextual understanding. Consequently, relatively equal emphasis should be placed on both content and concepts throughout the process. As learners incrementally gain knowledge (content) and understanding (concepts), the knowledge supports the understanding and vice versa. Content knowledge is no guarantee of conceptual understanding, and conceptual understanding alone may lead to an invention of the facts to support it. Learners must understand that real fluency with procedural and factual retrieval and recall is important. It frees their minds to be curious, to think about more complex problems, to create new solutions, and to further deepen their conceptual understanding. This requires rigor in appropriate memorization and ample and effective retrieval practice.[11] It also requires a high degree of restraint in the educator to first laser focus the curricular objectives on the most important core concepts required for adaptive clinical expertise and only then to build out the supporting content needed to be taught and assessed. This illustrates the preparation for future learning concept explored in Chapter 2.

Cognitive practice through application entails a critically important virtuous cycle in the development of content expertise: (1) an ever-expanding and more nuanced foundational content knowledge base and (2) construction of progressively higher order and deeper conceptual understanding. The human brain is an eager and natural problem solver and so, done well, conceptual knowledge development can become relatively easy and enjoyable for the emerging adaptive expert once the relative pains of novicehood are breached.

Thus core concepts should be introduced early and readdressed throughout the curriculum. For example, the core concepts of laminar and turbulent flow could be introduced in an early course on the cardiovascular system and revisited throughout the year in later courses on the gastrointestinal and urinary systems. This spiraling process of recurring concepts allows medical students to elaborate and enrich their understanding, making it "sticky" for new content. Deliberate practice activities should be designed that integrate the concept(s) into medical student learning as new content is added and implement problem-solving and applications sessions that force the application and transfer of the concept to new problems.[6,12] This is why multiple examples that require comparing and contrasting commonalities are so useful when introducing a new concept and provide practice for similar cognitive activities critical to clinical reasoning.[13] These activities further hone conceptual understanding by encouraging learners to determine which properties of the problem are essential to the solution and which properties are incidental. Additionally, regular attention to examining and exploring single concepts in multiple ways or introducing problems that force medical students to integrate multiple concepts to solve new problems are also effective. Yes, these strategies take more effort, but they lead to master adaptive learning that is deeper and more durable and to the broad and flexible knowledge base required for adaptive clinical expertise (see Figs. 2.3 and 9.1).

EVALUATING THE CLASSROOM

As educators of future physicians, we have a responsibility to ensure that our medical students acquire the foundational sciences knowledge base needed for competent clinical practice. A variety of pedagogical approaches can be used toward this end, including the traditional and still common large group lecture. If we pause to consider, however, the more inclusive learning opportunities that may exist within our classroom settings, we can foster not only the acquisition of medical knowledge but also development in a number of other important competencies. It does not require much pedagogical imagination to add exercises in reflective practice to almost any curricular activity, nor is it hard to see how teamwork and professionalism are already part of so many of the commonly practiced small group pedagogical approaches. Our learning opportunities in the basic science classroom span beyond the development of competencies of clinical practice and include development of expertise.[14,15] Although routine expertise is an important aspect of any health professions practice, fostering the development of adaptive expertise in future physicians is critical. The following sections describe an approach to critique current and future learning approaches using a Master Adaptive Learner (MAL) Classroom Checklist (Fig. 9.2) and the potential for these pedagogical approaches to more effectively foster the development of the master adaptive learner.[16]

Lecture Classroom

Although current trends in medical education would seem to disfavor the traditional grand rounds–style lecture, it remains an efficient approach that many use in an attempt to teach large numbers of medical students with limited faculty. As summarized in the MAL Classroom Scorecard (Table 9.1), the traditional lecture does not fare well when evaluated for alignment with the MAL model. Specifically, not all lectures are created equal. The typical, passive lecture does not directly encourage the learner to identify gaps that exist in its content, conceptual, and/or procedural knowledge types, nor does it prioritize the learner filling those gaps with self-identified resources (planning phase). The passive consumption of a traditional lecture does not provide obvious opportunities for critical appraisal of prior content knowledge or conceptual frameworks and fails to employ effective learning strategies (e.g., knowledge retrieval practice, spaced repetition, calibration, elaboration, or concept interleaving) that are an essential part of the learning phase in the MAL model. The often large learner audiences and lack of interaction between the learner and lecturer preclude the delivery of meaningful external feedback, thereby diminishing the learner's ability to self-assess (assessing phase). Although the lecturer may attempt to lay the foundation of conceptual understanding or to demonstrate the transfer of information presented to a new situation, or both, these important cognitive developments are not necessarily happening in the mind of the learner (adjusting phase).

The traditional lecture does not score well with regard to the four phases of the MAL model and also has the potential to drain the learner's "batteries" by too often failing to foster curiosity, development of growth mindset, motivation, and resilience. Although the teacher efficiency of the lecture is a significant reason for its continued practice, the poor learner-teacher ratio precludes individual coaching. It is interesting to consider, though, that the lecture format and lack of individual feedback may actually promote self-coaching by necessity. The role that the lecturer may play in coaching the large team should not be discounted.

Team-Based Learning Classroom

Team-based learning (TBL) as created and described by Michaelsen is an increasingly popular teaching method as evidenced by the increasing number of studies that have demonstrated its effectiveness.[17,18] On our MAL Classroom Scorecard (see Table 9.1), TBL rates quite well, particularly in the learning and assessing phases. The major deficits of this method, as it relates to fostering the development of the master adaptive learner, lie within the planning phase.

Does this classroom setting provide opportunities for:

- **Planning**
  - Identify gaps
  - Select opportunities for learning
  - Search for learning resources

- **Learning**
  - Critically appraise
  - Practice effective learning strategies (e.g., knowledge retrieval practice, spaced repetition, calibration, elaboration, concept interleaving)

- **Assessing**
  - Self-assess
  - Receive feedback

- **Adjusting**
  - Transfer learning to a routine and/or novel application involving individuals or system

Coaching Rheostat
  - Recharge, or at least minimize the drain on, the batteries of the learners

  Battery

  - *Curiosity*
    - Construct important questions
    - Encourage use of nontechnical expertise

  - *Mindset*
    - Develop a growth mindset

  - *Motivation*
    - Focus the learners on their own continual growth (and not judge by comparison to others)

  - *Resilience*
    - Manage uncertainty

Fig. 9.2 MAL Classroom Checklist

TBL does not specifically encourage learners to identify gaps in content, concept, or procedural knowledge or select opportunities for learning. In fact, one of the hallmarks of TBL is that learners work on the same problem, thereby precluding individualized learning plans but maximizing opportunities for diverse group learning. Specific preparation is dictated by the faculty so learners have little choice in selecting learning resources.

TBL is itself an effective learning strategy that requires learners to demonstrate their preparatory learning (individual readiness) and provides robust opportunities for self-assessment through the Individual Readiness Assurance Test, the Group Readiness Assurance Test, interteam debates, and peer feedback (learning and assessing phases).[18] Application exercises that build upon each other and require the learner to transfer what was learned in the

TABLE 9.1 MAL Classroom Scorecard			
	SETTING		
	Lecture	TBL	PBL
Planning	Low	Low	High
Learning	Low	High	Medium
Assessing	Low	High	High
Adjusting	Low	Medium	Medium
Status of batteries	Draining	Neutral	Charging
Knowledge development	Content > Concept > Procedural	Concept > Content > Procedural	Procedural > Content > Concept
Coaching rheostat	Coaching team; promotes self-coaching	Coaches pathway through uncertainty	Coaches team and individual; gets out of way of curiosity; effective feedback

MAL, Master Adaptive Learner; *PBL*, problem-based learning; *TBL*, team-based learning.

preparatory work to new situations have the potential to support the adjusting phase. The focus on new unsolved problems and managing uncertainty and ambiguity within application exercises also establishes TBL as a strong method for further developing conceptual understanding and practicing transfer.

Multiple MAL-friendly aspects of TBL should keep the learner's batteries charged or at least prevent them from overdraining. Curiosity may be promoted by the very nature of an effective application exercise that forces learners to consider many possible solutions to a problem. A growth mindset may be fostered by embracing robust feedback provided by peers. Resilience is robustly encouraged in TBL as learners are forced to encounter uncertainty in what are the most effective application exercises. Faculty provide critical coaching to walk learners through the process of managing uncertainty. Finally, motivation may be the weakest charge provided to the learners' batteries if assessment focuses more on competition than learning.

Although some educators have chosen to truncate the original method, each of the phases of TBL (Individual Readiness Assurance Test, Group Readiness Assurance Test, with use of immediate feedback, assessment technique scratch-off forms, application exercises, and peer feedback) fulfills important elements of the MAL model and is therefore predicted to be beneficial in the development of cognitive competence and expertise.

Problem-Based Learning Classroom

Problem-based learning (PBL) has been adopted and adapted by schools around the world and is perhaps the classroom method that most closely aligns with the priorities of the MAL model.[19,20] In the PBL model, small

teams of learners identify learning objectives that will help them understand a clinical case. Following self-study, teams reassemble and discuss their learning. Planning, learning, assessing, and adjusting are all promoted in PBL. The expectation of this method is that learners will select opportunities for learning and identify appropriate resources to fill knowledge gaps (planning phase). Critical appraisal of selected resources may take place organically as team members discuss their learning, but may also be glossed over if not made a specific expectation. For example, elaboration of concepts is diminished if learning objectives generated by team members are answered within a group using a divide and conquer approach and subsequently presented back to the team in a passive manner. This would short-circuit individual participation in the entire problem and impoverish the interchanges between learners, across the material. The PBL method permits robust opportunities to interleave concepts if the method is consistently practiced in a longitudinal fashion and case authors pay attention to intentionally spiraling important content.

Informed self-assessment is a bedrock component of the MAL process (see Chapter 6). Given the advantageous faculty-learner ratio commonly used in the PBL small group approach, opportunities abound for learners to receive the external feedback required to optimally self-assess. Particular attention therefore should be paid to develop the skills of faculty in providing effective feedback. Because PBL is a self-directed approach to learning and the facilitator generally is not well positioned to accurately judge medical knowledge (the content), the primary role of the teacher may be to coach the learners' development through regular feedback about competencies such as their metacognitive approach (indeed, the features of the MAL model) as well as professionalism, collaboration, and leadership. As was the case with TBL, PBL cases hold potential for promoting learning transfer if attention is paid to providing cases that support the need to consider concepts in multiple contexts (adjusting phase).[8,9]

The curiosity and growth mindset batteries are charged during a well-functioning PBL session. All kinds of questions are expressed by learners as they encounter a clinical case. Some of these questions are detail oriented and technical, whereas others demonstrate a learner's emerging ability to ask deep, concept-based questions. PBL demands that learners take control of their own learning and work to fill their individual gaps and, ultimately, the gaps of the team. Given the diversity of competency areas that can be addressed in PBL, it is tempting to speculate that the method may encourage a growth mindset that benefits not only knowledge and skill acquisition but also professional identity formation.[21]

The motivation battery may be charged during PBL, but this is more likely to occur when the learner is in a criterion-referenced, competency-based assessment system. Ideally, the learner will focus on his own continual growth and not judge his progress by comparison to others. Finally, resilience may be fostered as learners take more control of their learning and faculty get out of the way of learner curiosity.

OPTIMIZING THE MASTER ADAPTIVE LEARNING CLASSROOM

The methods considered here vary with regard to how well they align with the phases of the MAL model and how they charge or drain the learner's battery. Relatively simple changes or additions to these pedagogies can improve alignment with the core MAL principles, as evidenced by the MAL Classroom Scorecard (see Table 9.1), and improve the likelihood that an environment will foster the development of master adaptive learners.

Lecture Opportunities for Master Adaptive Learning

A relatively straightforward way to encourage learners to identify gaps prior to coming to lecture is to include self-assessment questions with other assigned preparatory work. Well-written learning objectives that are specific, measurable, and phrased like short answer or essay questions, and that balance and integrate relevant content and conceptual understanding with a clear focus on how this knowledge is clinically applied, may serve this function if they are well-aligned to the pre-lecture assignments. Often our session learning objectives reflect what we are going to talk about in the lecture and may not drill down into the

foundational work that medical students need to do to prepare themselves to enter the lecture classroom. More likely, lectures rehash what medical students have already read at our insistence, resulting in the time spent in lecture being unintentionally redundant with any prework they may have accomplished. The result is that learners make a choice between reading or attending a lecture because there does not seem to be any added value to doing both.[22] However, if time in seat with learners focuses on setting them up with a conceptual framework for further learning or helps them to clarify gaps in content knowledge identified before entering the classroom, the large group lecture can make at least some inroads in coaching learners into the planning phase of the MAL model.

Large-scale studies of undergraduate learning, recent scoping reviews, and meta-analyses support the value of the active learning approach to lectures.[23-29] A number of effective active learning strategies exist to make time during the lecture more interesting for medical students and assist them in learning and self-assessing.[30,31] The use of audience response systems (low or high tech) has been widely adopted and is a low-effort approach for teachers to increase engagement/active participation of learners during lectures.[32] Committing to answering self-assessment questions can identify for the teacher content or conceptual knowledge areas, or both, where learners need the most help and, perhaps more importantly, identify for the learner where her individual gaps lie. Think-pair-share and mini-brainstorming sessions during which learners segment off into pairs or small clusters within their seats in the lecture hall and address a particular topic or problem are approaches that facilitate knowledge retrieval, advance group conceptual understanding, or repair prior misunderstandings.[30,32] Such practices may also permit learners to self-assess as they discuss concepts with peers. The inclusion of case scenarios that challenge medical students to apply prior learning and transfer that learning to a new situation or to the development and critique of a common analogy that facilitates solving a new problem (or explaining a clinically relevant concept to a patient) also enhances medical student interest and engagement and begins to build skills within the adjusting phase of the MAL model.

Regardless of the specific approach offered for large group classroom sessions led by content experts, teachers can help prime their learners through course description and communication so that learners can make the best determination about attendance and the best plan for addressing their own learning needs. MAL components can be explicitly labeled in learning objectives and preparatory materials, and during in-class activities and instructor coaching. Class activities and timing should allow for metacognition, and the instructor can model and make these opportunities explicit verbally, through activity handouts and assessments, or both. Debriefing at the end of such activities will also help learners determine how to make the best use of what has been learned and enhance retention and transfer of learning in the future. Reflection, in particular, is an underutilized technique for promoting metacognition.

Learners can optimize their experience in the large group classroom and prepare for the development of MAL skills by intentionally preparing themselves for engagement in educational experiences. Prior to coming to the classroom, medical students should learn to think deliberately about what they intend to achieve there:

1. What do I know about this topic? What do I need to know? Could I accurately explain what I know to a patient if needed?
2. How will this expert help me fill a gap in my knowledge?
3. Goal setting and preparation to interact with the content expert: What do I want to know or be able to do at the end of this session? What are my expectations and needs?
4. Thinking critically: How can I make the most robust use of the fact that there is a content expert in front of the room? What learning gaps can this person uniquely help me address?

Although the traditional lecture may never inspire curiosity, mindset, motivation, and resilience as effectively as other classroom teaching approaches, there are excellent efficiency reasons for why schools continue to offer this pedagogical approach. To think that this historic approach to education will become extinct in the near future is probably unrealistic. The easy modifications described earlier can convert the typical lecture from an approach that drains learners' MAL batteries to experiences where learners can begin to practice many of the skills needed of a mature master adaptive learner.[30-32] Such lecture adaptations do not have to take a lot of time or teacher effort and may, in fact, help to recharge the teachers' batteries.

Team-Based Learning Opportunities for Master Adaptive Learning

TBL is an approach that aligns well on our MAL Classroom Scorecard (see Table 9.1) but, as was the case with lecture, TBL can also be enhanced to more effectively foster the development of MAL skills. As with lectures, TBL as a method suffers from a weak planning phase because all decisions are made for the learning. Once again, self-assessment questions can be provided for TBL learners as they are working to ready themselves for the TBL session. This should help learners identify learning gaps in all three types of knowledge. If they do not fill these gaps prior to

coming to the session, they may have the opportunity to fill them with assistance from their peers during the Group Readiness Assurance Test or during discussion of an application exercise. If during the session, learners are provided with some opportunity to look up information, this also may promote skills of selecting quality resources. Perhaps the greatest limitation to fostering the planning phase and inquiry during TBL may be the time limitations of the actual session. It is therefore important that learning continues beyond the in-seat session.

Because TBL provides many opportunities to self-assess in a way that is informed by external feedback, medical students should have a good sense of their own individual needs for further growth in knowledge, teamwork, professionalism, and the like. Perhaps incorporating an opportunity for a "minute paper" (intensive reflective writing for 1 minute) at the end of TBL with prompts such as "Describe one concept that you feel comfortable with, following participation in today's TBL" followed by "What questions, curiosities or confusion remain for you?" followed by "What resources will you use to address your questions, curiosities or confusion?" or "Can you develop a common analogy to explain this concept to a patient?" would enhance opportunities for both self-assessment and planning (identification of gaps, selection of learning opportunities, and resources for learning).[31] To close the loop on learning and minimize the requirement for in-class time, the learners could be encouraged or required to share their minute papers and the results of their further learning with their TBL team members through use of an online discussion board where learners could elaborate on concepts that had previously been confusing. Finally, the inclusion of application exercises that highlight the conceptual underpinning of the problem and utilize the "gallery walk" approach wherein learners review and vote on the best constructed responses to application exercise challenges holds the potential to promote creativity and application of concepts to new settings, thereby encouraging the MAL adjusting phase.

As is the case with other classroom settings, learners can contribute to their success in development of MAL skills by preparing themselves metacognitively to engage in learning within the TBL classroom. Teachers can coach learners in this priming process by taking the following steps:

1. Prime learners (or encourage them to prime themselves) to consider what the purpose of the task is.
2. Ask learners to document what they know, what they do not know, what they need to get out of the task (goals), and how they plan to do so.
3. Set the stage for learners taking on metacognitive tasks. Prime them to ask, "Why are we doing this, what are we thinking, what resources do we have, and what do we

need?" These questions can take the form of pre-course communication, assigned pre-course worksheets, or in-class handouts/activity records.

4. Optimize challenge to the TBL teams by designing tasks that are beyond the ability of any single learner to achieve and that require strong conceptual foundations in order to solve. Give tasks that have nebulous boundaries and have no obviously right answers to encourage risk taking. Ensure that the grading does not punish failure due to legitimate risk taking.

TBL as a method is generally a positive force when it comes to maintaining or charging learners' batteries. Care should be taken to avoid negative impacts on mindset and motivation that can result from a perception of competing with others for the best grade. Where possible, a pass-fail approach to assessment is preferred so that competition is reduced while collegiality is advantaged.

Problem-Based Learning Opportunities for Master Adaptive Learning

In its most traditional form, PBL was a method that encouraged learner curiosity and identification and filling of knowledge gaps.[19] Learners in PBL encounter problems just as professionals would, using real-world problems to focus inquiry. In medicine, PBL is built around patient cases in which clinical reasoning is learned and practiced. Medical students must use prior content and conceptual knowledge and build upon them to solve previously unseen problems by applying procedural knowledge, identifying learning gaps, and finding approaches to addressing these problems. They then reinforce the learning of their peers through shared learning activities in the group setting. The development of the master adaptive learner can be even further promoted in this method by paying close attention to the following:

1. As with small group discussion, learners should prime themselves (or be primed) to consider what they know, what they do not know, and how to make the best use of the upcoming experience. A focus on current conceptual understanding is particularly effective at this stage.

2. Because the nature of the interaction is problem based, learners must also consider what the *group* knows and does not know and how the *group* plans to address those gaps and make the most out of the experience. Advancing the *group's* understanding of core concepts promotes further refinement, elaboration, and retention at this stage.

3. PBL is also generally among the most difficult educational experiences, so failure will be more frequent than success. Learners should expect this, and teachers should remind them of this along the way. Reframing

or reconstructing faulty conceptual understanding at this stage may help medical students understand that this approach sets them up for future clinical success.

4. Metacognition is perhaps the most important skill set for successful PBL. Unfortunately, learning groups are prone to "group think," making it difficult to recognize individual or collective gaps in reasoning through the case. Particular to master adaptive learning is learning how to learn. Learners and facilitators should emphasize this regularly, modeling and demonstrating the use of probing and open-ended questions such as "Are we sure we understand this? How do we know? Can we really explain the underlying core concepts or mechanism of action?"

5. Determining how to make the most of the experience for retention and transfer of content and conceptual knowledge is also a challenge in PBL because of the number of people involved and the tremendous variety of patient case analogs for any given case. Medical students should ask (or be reminded to ask) "How would we have approached the case differently, knowing what we know now? How typical is this case? What are the key variations that could have led us to a very different conclusion? Why didn't we understand/consider (some aspect of the case)? How could we prevent that in the future? What pearls do you want to take away from this case?"

6. As learners acquire familiarity with the PBL process, facilitators can prepare to "fade," offering fewer interventions that direct the discussion and occasional interventions that offer reflections on the process. Learners will take on the role of asking, "Why are we thinking this and not that?" The facilitator can assist in reflecting on the process: "I noticed you were very concerned about organizing the learning objectives for study. What accounts for that concern? What do you accomplish by organizing the learning objectives appropriately?"

A number of iterations of the PBL method have been implemented since its first introduction. In fact, when discussing PBL, one typically needs to inquire for a full description of the method to understand exactly how it is practiced at any given school. Although even its earliest forms were user friendly to the emerging master adaptive learner, some 21st-century improvements are worth discussing because they have the potential to more effectively foster the development of the adaptive expert. In 2005, a revised approach to PBL was introduced at McMaster University School of Medicine.[20] The new method moves away from the presentation of one long, unfolding case to consideration of multiple shorter cases that exist in single parts and do not unfold over the course of the week. The opportunity for learners to juxtapose multiple examples of related content areas holds the potential to promote transfer and the adjusting phase of the MAL model.[8,9]

Unlike many approaches to PBL wherein learners divide and conquer team-identified learning areas and return to make formal or semiformal presentations to their peers on the subject areas, the newest McMaster model insists on all learners studying all identified learning points. The result is that collaborative discussion can take place about all learning areas with an opportunity for all learners to retrieve their own knowledge during discussion, self-calibrate based on input from multiple teammates, and work collaboratively to elaborate knowledge. In the absence of all learners being prepared to discuss all learning areas, such results seem less likely.

The newest McMaster approach to PBL was adapted by Case Western Reserve University School of Medicine with the launch of the Western Reserve2 Curriculum in 2006. Enhancements that further enrich the PBL environment for the growth of master adaptive learners have been introduced.

In an effort to specifically promote critical appraisal, medical students dedicate approximately 10 minutes during one of their three weekly PBL sessions to critically appraising a study from the primary literature that relates to their learning for the cases of the week.[33] In the early months of the first year, medical students are presented with critical appraisal templates, and papers are assigned. All learners in each team complete the requested information in the template and discuss the content in-person as a team. After approximately 4 months of learning how to critically appraise the literature, medical students then move on to incorporating their skills of critical appraisal into a brief (5-minute) presentation based on the "ask," "acquire," "appraise," and "apply" steps of the evidence-based practice cycle.[34] This exercise supports medical students in their development within the planning, learning, and adjusting phases of the MAL model.

Promotion of self-assessment and mindset are other areas of PBL that can be enhanced. The newest McMaster model of PBL includes a debriefing phase following every session during which learners have the opportunity to express feedback about the function of the team, themselves, and their peers. This debriefing phase leads to quality improvement of both self and team and is perhaps the most important 10 minutes of any PBL session. Within the Western Reserve2 Curriculum, facilitators coach the medical students through optimized debriefings using the small group debriefing pyramid (Fig. 9.3). Regardless of how long teams will continue working together, it is valuable to first focus on optimization of team function. Therefore faculty small group facilitators should coach their teams to focus initially on process. Once the team is functioning

effectively in terms of their collaboration toward learning goals and respectful interactions with each other, then the facilitator should coach them into revealing self-assessments around personal areas of strength and areas of selected growth for better supporting the effectiveness of the team's learning. The facilitator can remind medical students of the importance for physicians to be self-aware and good at self-assessment, which includes both areas of strength and needs for improvement. It may be useful to encourage teammates to take note of goals for improvement that their colleagues represent so that they are prepared for the next level of the small group debriefing pyramid. Once team members have expressed their own self-assessment, the group is typically ready to begin providing useful and constructive peer feedback to each other. This peer feedback should be specific, balanced, timely, and nonjudgmental.[35] Once the team has developed a firm foundation in terms of their process and peers have demonstrated their own fallibility, it becomes a much safer environment to carefully provide peer feedback that can be heard, received, and incorporated. Beginning too soon with peer feedback can lead to feelings of resentment and destabilization of the learning team. Although one might most reasonably assume that a facilitator would guide learners through the trajectory of their debriefing process, there is no reason that learners cannot take charge of this if provided with appropriate tools (see Fig. 9.3).

When effectively conducted, daily debriefing can have positive impacts on self-assessment and mindset. A learner may go beyond the recognition of his gaps in the realm of knowledge and may learn something about how he can adjust his own behavior to the benefit of the team. This kind of role adjustment is perhaps one of the greatest challenges for any of us but also represents a teamwork skill that is essential for the effective functioning of any team.

ONLINE LEARNING—THE MASTER ADAPTIVE LEARNER CLASSROOM OF THE FUTURE?

Although online learning classrooms are not currently used extensively in medical education, a number of online learning programs are increasingly being adopted—in both the formal and "parallel" curricula in which medical students are increasingly opting out of lectures in preference for online learning programs in many ways because these programs *do* employ a number of MAL-friendly characteristics.[22,36] Board preparation tools utilize known effective study strategies, such as knowledge retrieval practice and spaced repetitious learning, and can be calibrated to medical student's performance or learning goals.[37,38] Virtual patient programs are designed to assist medical students in elaborating on knowledge gained in clinical

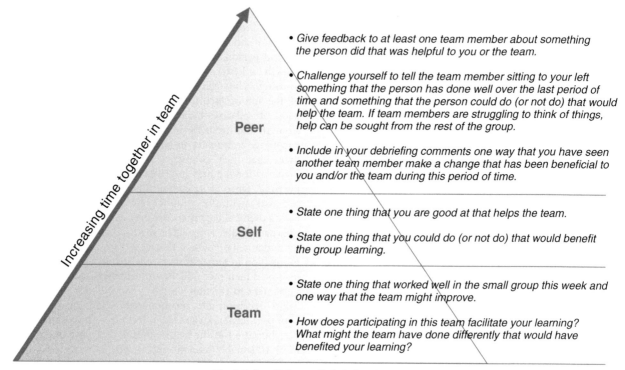

Fig. 9.3 Small Group Debriefing Pyramid

practice and, like caring for patients, promote interleaving and knowledge application within a safe learning environment.[39]

By its very nature, the online learning classroom can be constructed to provide many of the best features of in-person classroom learning for adaptive expertise. Online learning classrooms are being used effectively in nursing and other professional degree programs.[40] Often leveraging the expertise of e-learning designers, online faculty provide learners with a clear articulation of the learning outcomes to be achieved, construct the classroom experience to provide instructional sessions mapped to required learning materials, and supply progressive formative feedback, through dashboards and portfolios, that leverage pooled learning data to demonstrate an individual learners' progress toward the expected outcomes.[37,38] Programs are often paced to a given learner's learning or lifestyle needs and may provide equivalent content and conceptual learning along with some procedural learning at a much lower cost. Access to learning coaches who monitor and calibrate feedback and additional assignments, based on learner-specific performance gaps, is increasingly being employed.

BLENDING TECHNIQUES FOR OPTIMAL ALIGNMENT WITH MASTER ADAPTIVE LEARNING

Finally, we consider the fact that we have, for purposes of illustration, presented these classroom methods as separate and independent techniques. However, another perspective is to consider them a toolbox of techniques available to the creative educator. Blended courses may use focused lectures early in the week to efficiently deliver content needed to support TBL or PBL sessions at the end of the week. Online learning, through methods such as the flipped classroom, can be employed to support more valuable face-to-face learning activities such as collaborative problem solving. Another promising technique is the use of part-task cognitive trainers who allow deliberate practice to a precisely measured level of skill.[41-43] These techniques lean heavily on self-regulated learning, a core capacity of the MAL model. Given this burgeoning spectrum of available techniques, one of the most impactful applications of the MAL framework could be in guiding how to blend these often complementary techniques.

CONCLUSION

The common and popular teaching and learning methods considered in this chapter all have potential to foster the development of the master adaptive learner and can be adapted so medical students find themselves practicing skills that will support their development as master adaptive learners. As educators, we have a responsibility to consider how all of our classrooms can move medical students beyond lower-level knowledge acquisition and into development as master adaptive physicians prepared to care for patients in the changing health care landscape of the 21st century.

Vignette 1

Professor Adams is a junior faculty member who has been asked to take over the first-year pharmacology course for a large medical school class. He recently completed a faculty development program on active learning and is eager to implement these new methods and push his medical students to learn for expertise. The previous course director, who has been teaching the course for over 20 years, is known as a "great lecturer" by the medical student body. She is able to explain challenging concepts using a series of PowerPoint slides honed over time. While the course initially received high marks from medical students, over the years the evaluations have declined. Clinical faculty complain that medical students are unprepared to discuss therapeutic management on rounds, and medical students are turning to online tools for their content learning.

1. Professor Adams chooses to begin his work by observing his fellow colleagues teach their own courses. What should he be looking for?
2. What lecture hall techniques should Professor Adams consider to enhance medical student development of skills that will promote their growth as master adaptive learners?
3. What arguments can Professor Adams use with his basic-science colleagues to convince them it is a good investment of their time to help him transform the course and volunteer to facilitate problem-based learning or team-based learning groups?

Vignette 2

Dr. Patel is the curriculum dean at a medical school that is adopting a 3-year curriculum. To do so, she will need to ask all of the basic-science faculty to reduce their courses from 8 to 6 weeks with the aspiration of maintaining the same high level of core knowledge mastery. Furthermore, she would like to ensure that medical students gain a strong foundation of the basic-science core concepts needed for clinical practice and that they have the opportunity to hone their understanding multiple times over the preclinical phase.

1. What are the steps that Dr. Patel and her faculty should take to define the most important core concepts in the curriculum? How will they determine which core concepts should be revisited over time and in which courses?
2. Once the faculty have agreed upon the most important concepts, how should Dr. Patel work with them to refine and reduce the amount of content knowledge medical students need in order to understand these concepts?
3. Dr. Patel's medical students are eager to share the online study tools they have found most valuable. As key stakeholders, how should Dr. Patel engage them to ensure that the curricular goals of promoting adaptive expertise and transfer do not become secondary to the medical students' desire to do well on board examinations?

TAKE-HOME POINTS

1. Teachers should evaluate their classroom time and make intentional changes to foster development of the master adaptive learner. Even small changes may have a significant impact.
2. Classroom activities should be designed to make apparent the deeper conceptual understanding underlying the content and to facilitate appropriate clinical application.
3. Learning opportunities that stimulate curiosity, enhance motivation, and promote resilience facilitate engagement and reduce the drain on learner "batteries."
4. Faculty can be coaches, even in traditional classrooms.

QUESTIONS FOR FURTHER THOUGHT

1. What are the most important core concepts you teach? How do you ensure your colleagues in other courses leverage these concepts as well?
2. How do you encourage learners to set learning goals and self-assess their learning during your teaching sessions? What barriers prevent you from doing this more?

3. The excitement that medical students exude during their first days of medical school is palpable. How can you develop learning approaches that prevent the draining of your medical students' batteries (curiosity, motivation, growth mindset, resilience) over the year? How can you promote the recharging of the medical students' batteries?

ACKNOWLEDGMENTS

The authors would like to thank Nicole K. Roberts, PhD; Richard N. Van Eck, PhD; and Rosa Lee, MD for their contributions to this chapter.

ANNOTATED BIBLIOGRAPHY

1. Harden RM, Laidlaw JM. *Essential Skills for a Medical Teacher: An Introduction to Teaching and Learning in Medicine.* 2nd ed. Edinburgh, Scotland: Elsevier; 2017.
   This text is a practical curriculum planning and classroom guide for the medical educator.
2. Kulasegaram KM, Chaudhary Z, Woods N, Dore K, Neville A, Norman G. Contexts, concepts and cognition: principles for the transfer of basic science knowledge. *Med Educ.* 2017;51(2):184-195.
   This research article demonstrates the importance of conceptual structure in successful transfer.
3. Linsenmeyer M. Brief activities: questioning, brainstorming, think-pair-share, jigsaw, and clinical case discussions. In: Fornari A, Poznanski A, eds. *How-To Guide for Active Learning.* Huntington, WV: International Association of Medical Science Educators; 2015.
   This chapter provides multiple examples of approaches to make the lecture classroom more interactive and is framed within the context of a full active learning manual from the International Association of Medical Science Educators.
4. National Academies of Science, Engineering, and Medicine. *How People Learn II: Learners, Contexts, and Cultures.* Washington, DC: Author; 2018.
   This report, the second in a series of "How People Learn" consensus reports from the National Academies of Science, Engineering, and Medicine, focuses on new insights in learning science.
5. Streveler RA, Litzinger TA, Miller RL, Steif PS. Learning conceptual knowledge in the engineering sciences: overview and future research directions. *J Eng Educ.* 2008;97(3):279-294.
   This article from the engineering sciences provides a background in conceptual knowledge.

REFERENCES

1. National Academies of Science, Engineering, and Medicine. *How People Learn II: Learners, Contexts, and Cultures.* Washington, DC: Author; 2018.
2. Kulasegaram K, Min C, Ames K, Howey E, Neville A, Norman G. The effect of conceptual and contextual familiarity on transfer performance. *Adv Health Sci Educ Theory Pract.* 2012; 17(4):489-499.
3. Schmidt HG, Boshuizen HPA. On acquiring expertise in medicine. *Educ Psychol Rev.* 1993;5(3):205-221.
4. Bereiter C, Scardamalia M. *Surpassing Ourselves: An Inquiry into the Nature and Implications of Expertise.* Chicago and La Salle, IL: Open Court; 1993.
5. Streveler R, Litzinger T, Miller R, Steif P. Learning conceptual knowledge in engineering sciences: overview and future research directions. *J Eng Educ.* 2008;97(3):279-294.
6. Willingham D. Ask the cognitive scientist: is it true that some people just can't do math? *Am Educ.* 2009;33(4):14-39.
7. Wiggins G, McTighe J. *Understanding by Design.* 2nd ed. Alexandria, VA: Association for Supervision and Curriculum Development; 2005.
8. Norman G. Teaching basic science to optimize transfer. *Med Teach.* 2009;31(9):807-811.
9. Kulasegaram KM, Chaudhary Z, Woods N, Dore K, Neville A, Norman G. Contexts, concepts and cognition: principles for the transfer of basic science knowledge. *Med Educ.* 2017;51(2):184-195.
10. Mylopoulos M, Steenhof N, Kaushal A, Woods NN. Twelve tips for designing curricula that support the development of adaptive expertise. *Med Teach.* 2018;40(8):850-854.
11. Larsen DP, Butler AC, Roediger HL III. Test-enhanced learning in medical education. *Med Educ.* 2008;42(10):959-966.
12. Harden RM. What is a spiral curriculum? *Med Teach.* 1999; 21(2):141-143.
13. Bowen JL. Educational strategies to promote clinical diagnostic reasoning. *N Engl J Med.* 2006;355(21):2217-2225.
14. Batalden P, Leach D, Swing S, Dreyfus H, Dreyfus S. General competencies and accreditation in graduate medical education. *Health Aff (Millwood).* 2002;21(5):103-111.
15. Englander R, Cameron T, Ballard AJ, Dodge J, Bull J, Aschenbrener CA. Toward a common taxonomy of competency domains for the health professions and competencies for physicians. *Acad Med.* 2013;88(8):1088-1094.
16. Cutrer WB, Miller B, Pusic MV, et al. Fostering the development of master adaptive learners: a conceptual model to guide skill acquisition in medical education. *Acad Med.* 2017;92(1):70-75.
17. Michaelsen LK, Knight AB, Fink LD. *Team-Based Learning: A Transformative Use of Small Groups in College Teaching.* Westport, CT: Stylus Publishing; 2004.
18. Reimschisel T, Herring AL, Huang J, Minor TJ. A systematic review of the published literature on team-based learning in health professions education. *Med Teach.* 2017;39(12):1227-1237.

19. Barrows HS. Problem-based learning in medicine and beyond: a brief overview. *New Dir Teach Learn*. 1996:3-12. doi:10.1002/tl.37219966804.
20. Neville AJ, Norman GR. PBL in the undergraduate MD program at McMaster University: three iterations in three decades. *Acad Med*. 2007;82(4):370-374.
21. Dweck CS. *Mindset: The New Psychology of Success*. New York, NY: Ballantine Books; 2007.
22. Association of American Medical Colleges. *Medical School Year Two Questionnaire: 2017 All Schools Summary Report*. Washington, DC: Author; 2018.
23. Beichner R. *The Student-Centered Activities for Large Enrollment Undergraduate Programs (SCALE-UP) Project*. College Park, MD: American Association of Physics Teachers; 2007.
24. Prince M. Does active learning work? A review of the research. *J Eng Educ*. 2004;93(3):223-231.
25. Michael J. Where's the evidence that active learning works? *Adv Physiol Educ*. 2006;30(4):159-167.
26. Kober N. *Reaching Students: What Research Says About Effective Instruction in Undergraduate Science and Engineering*. Washington, DC: National Academies Press; 2015.
27. Springer L, Stanne MZ, Donovan SS. Effects of small-group learning on undergraduates in science, mathematics, engineering, and technology: a meta-analysis. *Rev Educ Res*. 1999;69(1):21-51.
28. Dochy F, Segers M, Van den Bossche P, Gijbels D. Effects of problem-based learning: a meta-analysis. *Learn Instruc*. 2003;13(5):533-568.
29. Freeman S, Eddy SL, McDonough M, et al. Active learning increases student performance in science, engineering, and mathematics. *Proc Natl Acad Sci U S A*. 2014;111(23):8410-8415.
30. Linsenmeyer M. Brief activities: questioning, brainstorming, think-pair-share, jigsaw, and clinical case discussions. In: Fornari A, Poznanski A, eds. *How-To Guide for Active Learning*. Huntington, WV: International Association of Medical Science Educators; 2015.
31. Angelo T, Cross K. *Classroom Assessment Techniques: A Handbook for College Teachers*. San Francisco, CA: John Wiley & Sons, Inc; 1993.
32. Harden RM, Laidlaw JM. *Essential Skills for a Medical Teacher: An Introduction to Teaching and Learning in Medicine*. 2nd ed. Edinburgh, Scotland: Elsevier; 2017.
33. O'Neil J, Croniger C. Critical appraisal worksheets for integration into an existing small-group problem-based learning curriculum. *MedEdPORTAL*. 2018;14:10682.
34. Straus SE, Glasziou P, Richardson WS, Haynes RB. *Evidence-Based Medicine: How to Practice and Teach EBM*. 5th ed. Edinburgh, Scotland: Elsevier; 2019.
35. Ende J. Feedback in clinical medical education. *JAMA*. 1983;250(6):777-781.
36. Le TT, Prober CG. A proposal for a shared medical school curricular ecosystem. *Acad Med*. 2018;93(8):1125-1128.
37. Menon A, Gaglani S, Haynes MR, Tackett S. Using "big data" to guide implementation of a web and mobile adaptive learning platform for medical students. *Med Teach*. 2017;39(9):975-980.
38. Berman N, Fall LH, Smith S, et al. Integration strategies for using virtual patients in clinical clerkships. *Acad Med*. 2009;84(7):942-949.
39. Berman NB, Durning SJ, Fischer MR, Huwendiek S, Triola MM. The role for virtual patients in the future of medical education. *Acad Med*. 2016;91(9):1217-1222.
40. Frazer C, Sullivan DH, Weatherspoon D, Hussey L. Faculty perceptions of online teaching effectiveness and indicators of quality. *Nurs Res Pract*. 2017;2017:9374189.
41. Ericsson KA. Deliberate practice and acquisition of expert performance: a general overview. *Acad Emerg Med*. 2008;15(11):988-994.
42. Lee MS, Pusic M, Carriere B, Dixon A, Stimec J, Boutis K. Building emergency medicine trainee competency in pediatric musculoskeletal radiograph interpretation: a multicenter prospective cohort study. *AEM Educ Train*. 2019;3(11):269-279.
43. Hatala R, Gutman J, Lineberry M, Triola M, Pusic M. How well is each learner learning? Validity investigation of a learning curve-based assessment approach for ECG interpretation. *Adv Health Sci Educ Theory Pract*. 2019;24(1):45-63.

10

How Will the Master Adaptive Learner Process Work at the Bedside?

Julie S. Byerley, MD, MPH, and Michelle M. Daniel, MD, MHPE

LEARNING OBJECTIVES

1. Create positive clinical learning environments to foster the master adaptive learner.
2. Describe how master adaptive learners can assess, adjust, plan, and learn at the patient's bedside in response to practice challenges.
3. Apply teaching strategies that promote self-monitoring, metacognition, reflection, and critical thinking during the clinical encounter.

CHAPTER OUTLINE

CHAPTER SUMMARY

Authentic clinical environments provide meaningful opportunities to foster the master adaptive learner. Establishing a positive learning environment is critical to success, but can be challenging to accomplish in chaotic workplace settings. Faculty and learners must be prepared to optimize the bedside experience with primacy for patient care while actively driving learning. Faculty can help learners identify teachable moments, triggered by a surprising presentation or clinical outcome, patient or panel data that demand attention, or sudden intuition that "something isn't right." Novel learning can also be found in the seemingly routine or everyday case.

This initiates the planning phase, wherein learners identify gaps in their knowledge and seek out resources to support their learning. Depending on the clinical setting (e.g., a fast-paced emergency department or a slower-paced rheumatology clinic), the next phases of learning, assessing, and adjusting may take place at varying speeds driven by both the needs of the learner and the urgency of providing excellent clinical care. Faculty must set clear expectations and inspire the learner. We should also use teaching strategies that promote self-monitoring, metacognition, reflection, and critical thinking. Well-established workplace learning theories, such as cognitive apprenticeship, can provide guidance to teaching-learning interactions.

Vignette 1

Three learners are rounding with their team on their surgery clerkship rotation. The team has just finished postoperative rounds. The attending of the day is known to ask tough questions. He first asks, "What are the most common causes of postoperative complications?" Alexia replies, "The 5 Ws—waves (electrocardiogram changes/myocardial infarct), wind (pneumonia), water (urinary tract infection), wound infection, and walking (venous thromboembolism). The attending nods, "Absolutely correct." He then asks, "What is the difference between Charcot's triad and Reynold's pentad?" Bob shyly offers, "The presence of shock and altered mental status, in addition to right upper quadrant pain, jaundice, and fever." The attending gruffly states, "Yes, and speak with more confidence next time. You seemed unsure." He then asks, "What is the diagnostic test of choice for acute cholecystitis with an equivocal ultrasound?" Cindy is put on the spot. She doesn't know. The attending suggests she "read more" and states that he expects all of them to perform their utmost best. Alexia leaves feeling validated that they are intrinsically "smart." Bob leaves worried, perseverating on his performance anxiety. Cindy is crushed and overwhelmed. There is so much to study in surgery, and she doesn't know where to begin.

1. How can the learning environment be improved for these three learners?
2. Alexia is encouraged to have a fixed mindset by receiving feedback that they are "smart." How can the learning environment be changed to encourage this learner?
3. How can the learning environment be altered to support learners Bob and Cindy?

Vignette 2

A second-year medical student, Debbie, is assigned to a mentor, Monisha, in a family medicine clinic as part of her clinical skills course (Doctoring). In class, Debbie is learning to take a very complete history and perform all the components of a physical exam according to lengthy checklists. On the first day in clinic, Monisha sends in Debbie to evaluate a patient and asks her to come back and give an oral presentation of the case. Debbie returns an hour later and provides a very detailed history. She was unsure what physical exam to perform for "generalized weakness," so she did a complete head-to-toe exam. Teacher and learner return to the room together, and Debbie

observes Monisha performing the encounter. She observes that her mentor appears to be "cutting corners" and is confused as to why Monisha doesn't perform the history and physical in the manner in which they were taught. Debbie tells her that "all the stuff" she is learning in the classroom doesn't appear to be needed "in real life."

1. How can Monisha convert this encounter into a teachable moment?
2. What strategies can Monisha use to foster master adaptive learning?
3. The size of Debbie's knowledge gap can feel overwhelming. How can Monisha coach the learner to set reasonable learning goals, employ effective learning strategies, continuously seek feedback, and implement change?
4. How can Monisha foster curiosity, motivation, resilience, and a growth mindset?

Vignette 3

Ms. Lyons, a 38-year-old woman with lupus, presents to the emergency department with marked facial, neck, and tongue swelling. This is the third time in 4 weeks she has had these symptoms. In relaying the story, the resident, John, notes that the patient has no history of atopy or allergic reactions, has no family history of angioedema, and is not on an ACE inhibitor. John rapidly diagnoses the patient with angioedema and initiates treatment with diphenhydramine, steroids, an H_2 blocker, and epinephrine. He prepares for advanced airway management and an ICU admission.

Later, the attending, Dr. Melissa Clark, asks John to reflect on the case. John clearly articulates three main causes of angioedema: allergic reaction, hereditary C1 esterase deficiency, and angioedema. He then asks, "But what else could this be? The patient has had two similar presentations, and there doesn't seem to be a clear reason why this patient develops angioedema." John has identified a gap in his knowledge, and Dr. Clark helps with shaping a clinical question. Ms. Lyons has lupus. Patients with lupus form multiple autoantibodies. Can a patient develop acquired C1 esterase deficiency through autoantibody production?

John engages in a literature search and critically appraises the findings. The next day, he emails Dr. Clark as well as the ICU team with his findings. Patients with lupus can form autoantibodies to C1 esterase. There is a special send-out test that can confirm the diagnosis. Dr. Clark praises the learner for his perseverance in asking the important "why" questions.

She encourages John to always seek to understand the "what," "why," and "how" of a case when the pieces don't add up. The resident's curiosity and the teacher's encouragement changed the course of this patient's treatment and may have saved her life.

1. What triggers should cause learners to switch from routine to adaptive expertise?
2. Describe the phases of master adaptive learning demonstrated in this case.
3. What strategies does Dr. Clark use to encourage master adaptive learning? What other strategies might be effective?

CREATING POSITIVE LEARNING ENVIRONMENTS

"The bedside" refers to the authentic clinical environment in which patients are being cared for by clinicians in inpatient and outpatient settings. Learners can participate concurrently in that clinical care delivery in an apprenticeship model for the purpose of their own education, but the primary intent at the bedside setting is always the care of the patient. Building on the pre–clerkship phase Master Adaptive Learner (MAL) skill development (see Chapter 9), master adaptive learning is at its most effective/relevant in an authentic clinical environment. There the master adaptive learner will find many opportunities to assess his understanding, adjust that understanding based on data and feedback, plan how to address an identified learning need, and, after new learning, reassess to continue to grow.

Addressing Potential Challenges

In the clinical setting the learner immediately identifies the pertinence of her need to know, thus the "real world" can be most inspiring. The greatest challenge in the clinical environment is, however, the very thing that makes it so inspiring: its authenticity and the primacy of patient care. Although learning can occur most dramatically in this setting, learning opportunities can also be missed without purposeful attention to the learning process. The clinical environment is unpredictable. The teacher does not control the learning material that emerges. Often the setting is fast paced and chaotic. Even when it is more controlled, patient issues and questions typically drive the material about which faculty and learners engage. Multiple levels of learners are often present, requiring teachers to meet different learners where they are in terms of skill and experience. There are even challenges in where and how teaching might physically occur in the clinical setting, which is usually designed with patient care, not education, in mind. Faculty have to adapt "on their feet" and must balance

multiple competing demands, including patient throughput and efficiency.[1]

Despite these challenges, faculty can come to understand that fostering the master adaptive learner is not necessarily time consuming, but, rather, can be aligned with the work of clinical care. To do that requires different strategies that we address in this chapter.

Engaging the Patient, Peers, and Other Health Professionals

Preparing the clinical environment for the shared goal of education paves the way for master adaptive learning success (see Chapter 11). Clinical care is typically delivered by teams, and multiple members of those teams participate in the teaching and learning process. Expectation setting and orientation to the clinical setting are essential for the master adaptive learner to thrive. Ideally, all those working in the clinical environment will understand the role and level of the learner training in that setting. The entire clinical staff, not just the precepting clinician, should be introduced to the learner and informed of the learner's role. Additionally, the learning environment is stronger if patients are informed of the concurrent educational mission in their care setting. Many institutions will label the educational mission to be applicable across the institution. In other settings, specific clinics might choose to inform patients through a variety of means, including signage, statements by the staff, an ongoing tradition of learner presence, or a combination of these. When all involved appreciate the dual (but prioritized) mission of (1) providing outstanding clinical care and (2) allowing the future workforce to learn simultaneously, the climate is established for dual mission success.

Establishing Safety and Support

Although an inclusive and collaborative team is essential, a single responsible educator must be identified as the learner's primary contact. This is a concrete demonstration of learner support and identifies a lead clinical instructor with whom the master adaptive learner will engage for inspiration, expectations, and feedback. This inspiration can be sparked by a framing conversation before the first patient is seen. In addition to setting specific expectations, the preceptor should clearly state the expectation that the master adaptive learner will be self-directed and approach learning with a growth mindset[2] (see Chapter 4). The educator could briefly outline the hope that in each clinical encounter the learner will first use metacognitive strategies to recognize his own understanding of the clinical situation, test that understanding by gathering data and feedback, and then establish his own learning need. The preceptor might describe that, in the authentic clinical setting, learning needs can be addressed through use of resources, such as literature review, clinical decision tools, or questioning of the patient or clinical team. Many learning needs can be tackled through the work of the day, but others will need to be noted for further exploration after tending to patient care, out of respect for the pace and priorities in the clinical environment.[3,4]

Once the expectations are clarified, the master adaptive learner must be invited to participate in the clinical care at a level appropriate for her experience and the patient's needs. The more a learner is allowed to actively participate, the more urgency and applicability is established for learning. Sometimes this is done in side-by-side work with the preceptor, but often, as the learners advance, a learner will engage with patients clinically before bringing her impressions and proposed plan to the preceptor. Early in a clinical rotation more scaffolding will be needed, while later learners will be able to identify gaps, set expectations, and operate more independently. The educator can use a coaching orientation, refining practice through frequent feedback and providing the minimal amount of support up front to allow for maximal independence and challenge (and, of course, risk taking and failure in the process).

Encouraging Questioning

Both to assess their own understanding and to fill gaps in knowledge and skills, master adaptive learners should be invited to ask questions at the bedside. To efficiently utilize the time of preceptors, to demonstrate the value of interprofessional teamwork, and to broaden clinical perspective, learners at the bedside must be encouraged to ask questions of the preceptor as well as other members of the team.

Techniques that clinician-educators can use to demonstrate interest in learner-generated questions are similar to techniques clinicians use to invite patients to express their own inquiries: patiently listening, providing supportive reflection, probing for a deeper rationale, and providing answers in terms the questioner can understand. In this way the educator teaches twice: through the substance of the question and in modeling optimal MAL clinician behavior.

- Patiently listening involves listening with all of the senses and a truly open mind to ensure that the educator is responding to what learners really want to know and enabling their personal growth. If the educator is uncertain about what the learner is asking, he should use inquiry to gain clarity. Too often, educators have their own ideas about a teaching pearl or lesson they wish to convey and they can "miss the mark" of what the learner actually needs.
- Providing supportive reflection can involve restating or rephrasing questions to ensure shared understanding

(e.g., "I want to ensure I fully understand your question so I can provide the best possible guidance for your learning. I am hearing you wonder about *xxx*. Did I summarize your question correctly?"). Supportive reflection can also involve affirmation of the value of a learner's question, to encourage future questions.
- Probing for a deeper rationale is important for understanding the genesis of a question, to get at the heart of true learning needs. This technique is central to the Socratic method for fostering critical thinking (e.g., "Why are you asking *xxx*?") Probing gets at the "what, why, or how" behind a query, providing explanations and clarifications that can be essential to optimal teaching-learning interactions.
- Providing answers in terms the questioner can understand involves targeting one's responses to the level of the learner. This is critical to avoid cognitive overload, which can impede learning.

Both learners and their preceptors should be encouraged to advance their questions to higher-order thinking. Precious time in the clinical environment is better utilized addressing application, analysis, and synthesis as compared to rote recitation of memorized facts. It can be particularly valuable to use "why," "how," and "what if" questions.[5] These stimulate learners to think deeply and mechanistically about what they are observing. Reflecting on Vignette 1, not only do the educator's responses discourage a growth mindset, but the questions the educator asked were low-order questions assessing simple recognition or memorization. Better questions invite the learner to apply his knowledge of possible postoperative complications to a particular patient being cared for, inviting the learner to suggest how a complication might present, for example.

When a learner expresses distress regarding the disconnect between what was taught in the slower-paced classroom experience as compared to the authentic clinical environment, as in Vignette 2, the educator intending to inspire adaptive learning can encourage self-assessment by probing for the learner's rationale behind her sentiment. Through sequential higher-order questioning, the learner is likely to come to her own recognition of her misunderstanding and make efforts to adjust.

In Vignette 3, the educator facilitates learning by simply asking the learner to reflect on the case. That simple step—forcing reflection—helps highlight a gap in learning and thereby drives the MAL cycle. The learner is stimulated to address a gap in understanding. He seeks out and critically appraises literature in the learning phase, receives feedback on his efforts, and, most importantly, individualizes the patient's care through the novel application of new knowledge. In the same case, as the clinician helps the learner shape a clinical question, the learner is supported in generating meaningful higher-order questions to drive that process.

PLANNING, LEARNING, ASSESSING, AND ADJUSTING IN RESPONSE TO PRACTICE CHALLENGES

Identifying Teachable Moments

Teachable moments abound in the clinical environment. Even the most mundane cases harbor teaching opportunities. Consider the young adult pack-per-day smoker who presents annually for a well visit. If the health professional waits for the patient to have a myocardial infarction from premature coronary artery disease, she has likely missed a lot of opportunities to teach about important topics such as smoking cessation. Teachable moments arise anytime an assumption turns out to be false or when something unexpected happens. Examples include spontaneous communication challenges, unusual physical examination findings, surprising results on diagnostic testing, or when disconnects are revealed in learner understanding. More serious struggles, failures, near misses, and poor outcomes can also be leveraged as teachable moments.[5]

Teachable moments, even the dramatic ones, can be missed without sign-posting,[6] done by a skilled educator or by the attentive master adaptive learner. One technique to ensure that teachable moments are recognized is activated observation. A preceptor can encourage activated observation by asking the learner to look for a surprise as she enters into a clinical encounter or by, immediately after an encounter, asking what the learner noted unexpectedly. Teachable moments should be used to launch the MAL cycle by encouraging the learner to adjust her understanding, in response to which she can plan, learn, assess, and then adjust again.

Engaging in Learning in Clinical Environments

The educator can prime the learner by stimulating learning concurrent with patient care and illustrating how to utilize learning resources. For example, the preceptor can ask the learner what his goals for the day are and how he will address those goals. Teachers, with more experience in the clinical environment, can assess learners' calibration and help them hone it to be realistic. For example, experienced clinicians can encourage medical students to read a textbook reference to learn the typical presentation, expected clinical details, and management choices regarding a patient expected in the operating room, and then utilize the precious operation time for the specific learning of live anatomy, surgical skill, and management of the unexpected in procedures.

Other ways to prepare the learner include sharing the next day's patient list and asking her to establish what she knows and what she may need to know (priming, goal setting). The learner should describe what her plan and approach for a patient examination will be prior to conducting it and why (metacognition). Then, she should conduct the examination under your supervision, asking probing questions, and intervening only when needed (challenge, risk, failure). The learner should self-evaluate her performance afterward, explaining where she had gaps, why you intervened, and what she will do moving forward to address gaps and enhance transfer.

Learners are typically most engaged when they are offered an appropriate amount of autonomy for their level of experience and skill. Beginning learners, for example, could be allowed to assess vital signs or take a history, while more senior learners should be allowed to initiate clinical care, as illustrated in Vignette 3. After the learner observes the teacher's history and physical, patient interviewing, and the like, the teacher should then ask him to explain what she did and why she did it, and establish gaps in his knowledge. The teacher should suggest that he develop a plan to remediate those gaps, implement it, and present his findings to her the next day.

In any of those situations, the teacher can motivate the MAL process by simply asking the learner, "Based on the data you gathered, what do you think is going on?" When the learner is forced to first propose her impression, rather than simply hearing the thoughts of others with more expertise, the learner is more engaged. When this is done in a safe, supportive learning environment, the master adaptive learner can advance to her potential.

Given that the major challenges to the MAL process at the bedside are the primacy of patient care and the pressure of limited time, it is unrealistic to expect learners to be able to articulate all questions that emerge or to be able to participate fully with autonomy in each encounter. Learning can be facilitated efficiently by thoughtful scheduling, spontaneous and variable direct observation of the learner, teaching with the patient or other professionals during the direct care delivery, prioritization of learning topics, and structured follow-up of learning topics outside of the clinical setting. Careful scheduling of patient time slots, to optimize the preceptors' pace of work while allowing the learner to have time with a fraction of patients, can be done ahead of time. Thinking through and clarifying the logistics of workflow, space utilization, and expected processes is worth the up-front investment of time.

Direct observation is an ideal method of preceptor assessment of the learner's clinical skill. This should be done by the preceptor as much as possible. This can be accomplished by bedside presentations both in the ambulatory setting and on family-centered rounds. Situations in which the learner and teacher are together with the patient optimize the recognition of the teachable moment and allow for the educator to teach the patient and the learner concurrently. Learners can also benefit from engaging with other members of the clinical team, such as pharmacists and nurses, at the bedside with the patient. Direct observation with clinical preceptors and other health professionals can be done during the entire clinical encounter, but observation of part of the visit is more common and perfectly appropriate because clinical care and learning are accomplished in concert. Daily brief observations with the medical student, selecting a 1- or 2-minute piece of a clinical encounter to be observed and followed by feedback, are realistic ways to watch learners progress over time. After direct observations, the preceptor should provide feedback: "In order to refine your practice, here's one thing you should keep doing, and here's one thing you should start doing/stop doing/do differently." Again, a key point of the MAL process in clinical environments is to teach the learner both the clinical approach and a learning approach.

Vignette 2 provides an example of a learner engaging in the clinical environment, likely without the proper clarification of expectations before beginning. Thoughtful expectation setting would have established that spending an hour in this setting without preceptor presence was not the desire of the teacher or the patient.

Self-Assessment and Feedback

The master adaptive learner must have time to reflect on his learning and to self-assess in order to establish learning goals. Learner self-assessment is refined with feedback from those who are more expert to create an informed self-assessment (see Chapter 6). Faculty should encourage self-assessment through questioning—simply asking, for example, "What do you think you need to learn now?", allowing the learner time to self-assess, and then reflecting on that self-assessment by delivering feedback.

Feedback is most effective when delivered promptly and privately or at least in a safe and supportive environment. Feedback, whether positive or negative, should always focus on behavior rather than provide a simple label of judgment. For example, in Vignette 1, the preceptor delivers feedback that is less than optimal in many ways. For the learner who answers correctly, the attending does not invite deeper understanding or investment but rather simply congratulates regurgitation of knowledge. Although this compliments the learner, it does not invite growth the way a follow-up probing question would. The second learner is embarrassed by the public feedback that calls out his lack of confidence, and the third learner is not invited to demonstrate her thinking when she cannot recall a factual answer.

In addition to asking better questions, this teaching encounter could have been improved by the preceptor providing feedback that challenges the next step of understanding for each of the learners. For example, the educator could have noted:

- "Alexia, it's great that you have memorized the 5 Ws. Be sure you think through each of them, prioritizing them for your patient. What do you think might be most likely for our patient?"
- "Bob, you are correct. Why did you seem unsure? It is okay for you to share what you think and let me help add to what you know."
- "Cindy, I see that you do not know this particular answer. That makes a good question for you to address today, then. See what you can learn on your own and then this afternoon tell me what you found."

Improvement-focused feedback that helps the learner shape the next step of his growth journey stimulates the MAL process.[7] Optimal feedback is based on concrete behavior that can be changed. The longitudinal relationship often created around bedside teaching allows feedback to be built upon over time. Preceptors should note improvements in effectiveness of behaviors in response to prior feedback and then provide additional feedback to drive incremental advancement. Bedside teachers experience developmental progression in giving effective feedback, and faculty development can influence this skill.[8]

Implementation of Learning

Learning at the bedside comes full circle and becomes self-reinforcing in the adjusting phase when what is learned can be implemented. This is illustrated in Vignette 3, in which the learner's mature question, shaped by forced reflection and supportive probing by the preceptor, leads to the learner digging deeper for the purpose of application immediately relevant in the care of the patient.

Thus, in bedside teaching, preceptor time is most effectively employed: (1) setting expectations that establish a supportive learning environment, (2) allowing engagement of learners in the clinical environment at the optimal autonomy for the learner experience, (3) directly observing the learner, (4) inviting self-assessment, (5) encouraging questioning, and (6) providing feedback to shape the MAL process.

Specific learner-centered educational techniques such as Wolpaw's SNAPPS model[9] can encourage learners to take a more active role in the educational experience. The teacher takes the role of facilitator rather than imparter of knowledge, having the learner "*SNAPPS*": *S*ummarize the history and findings, *N*arrow the differential to two to three possibilities, *A*nalyze the differential by comparing and contrasting diagnoses, *P*robe the preceptor with questions about areas of confusion, *Plan* diagnostic and management strategies for the working diagnosis and outline the next steps, and *Select* a case-related issue for deeper-dive learning.

TEACHING STRATEGIES TO PROMOTE SELF-MONITORING, METACOGNITION, REFLECTION, AND CRITICAL THINKING

Clinical teaching has been written about extensively in the medical education literature, yet there has been a relative lack of attention to teaching behaviors that can foster situated learning. Workplace-based learning likely requires different teaching strategies than non–workplace-based learning, particularly when it comes to fostering the master adaptive learner. Teaching strategies that can promote self-monitoring, metacognition, reflection, and critical thinking are crucial. One established theory of workplace-based instruction, cognitive apprenticeship, may provide a model for understanding how busy clinicians can inspire master adaptive learning while still prioritizing patient care.

Leveraging Theories of Workplace Learning

Cognitive apprenticeship was first described in the general education literature in 1989[10] and was later adapted in health professions education.[11,12] Cognitive apprenticeship

was designed to encourage experts to make their internal thought processes explicit for learners to observe, understand, and practice them. Cognitive apprenticeship describes six main teaching methods—modeling, coaching, scaffolding, articulation, reflection, and exploration—that can be applied to instruct a broad range of learner levels. Fig. 10.1 provides an overview of the steps in the cognitive apprenticeship model. Table 10.1 describes the different teaching methods and uses teaching vignettes to further clarify the model.

In Step 1 of the cognitive apprenticeship model (see Fig. 10.1), the focus is on facilitation by the preceptor. Faculty must help establish a supportive learning environment, then begin modeling behaviors while expressing their reasoning out loud. In this phase, faculty can help develop the master adaptive learner by encouraging questioning, particularly if there is a lack of clarity surrounding what the learner is observing. Thinking out loud by the faculty and questioning by the learner are critical elements that could have made the interaction in Vignette 2 very different. The faculty member might have stated, "In the classroom you learned all the tools in the clinician's toolbox. Now you must learn to select the right tools for the task at hand. My differential diagnosis for weakness includes anemia, hypothyroidism, and dehydration. Thus, on physical exam, I am looking for palmar or conjunctival

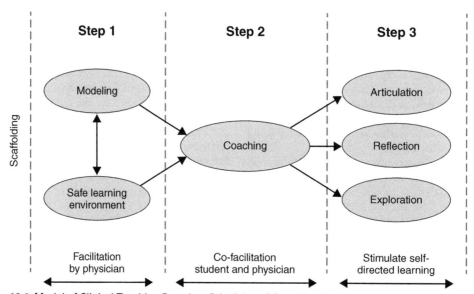

Fig. 10.1 Model of Clinical Teaching Based on Principles of Cognitive Apprenticeship. (From Stalmeijer R, Dolmans D, Snellen-Balendong H, van Santen-Hoeufft M, Wolfhagen I, Scherpbier A. Clinical teaching based on principles of cognitive apprenticeship: views of experienced clinical teachers. *Acad Med.* 2013; 88[6]:861-865.)

TABLE 10.1	Cognitive Apprenticeship Model With Teaching Vignettes.		
Teaching Method	Description	MAL Implications	Teaching Vignette
Modeling	Expert performs the task so that learner can observe. While performing the task, the expert externalizes the heuristics and control processes she uses in applying her basic conceptual and procedural knowledge (i.e., she thinks out loud).	While modeling, encourage questions to initiate MAL cycles. Model phases of the MAL model (e.g., describe how you critically appraise the literature and adjust your treatment plan based on what you find). This helps promote lifelong learning skills in the context of actual clinical practice.	The clinical teacher demonstrated different skills. During the demonstration the teacher explained the task, identifying aspects that are important for task performance and allowing me to ask questions. The teacher created opportunities for me to observe him. The teacher explained his processes (i.e., the sources he used for literature appraisal and how he used the findings to inform evidence-based practice).
Coaching	Expert observes learner during task performance—monitoring; offering hints, reminders, and immediate feedback; suggesting new tasks aimed at bringing the learner's performance closer to expert performance.	While coaching, facilitate aspects of the assessing phase: (1) hold up the mirror (e.g., describe what you observed) to allow for informed self-assessment, and (2) offer focused feedback for improvements. Also be sure to encourage curiosity, resilience, and a growth mindset.	The clinical teacher observed me on several occasions during my rotation in her department. After observing, the teacher described what she witnessed, so I could critique my performance. She then gave me specific, actionable feedback, which gave me a better idea of which aspects I could improve and how. She inspired me to get better by highlighting gaps in my performance that could have important impacts on patient safety.
Scaffolding	Expert diagnoses learner's current skill level and the availability of intermediate steps at the appropriate level of difficulty in carrying out the target activity. Expert provides support to learner for the parts of the task that the learner cannot yet manage. Support is gradually faded until the learner is on his own.	To provide scaffolding, analyze the learner's level, encouraging appropriate goal setting based on the desired learning outcome. Discuss learning strategies (e.g., the importance of engaging in spaced repetition or deliberate practice).	The clinical teacher was aware of my previous experience and offered sufficient opportunity for independent activities in line with my learning goals. The teacher helped when activities were difficult for me. The teacher taught me how to improve by discussing specific learning strategies, explaining the importance of repeated practice at intervals and guided practice with feedback. The teacher gradually reduced support so that I could become more independent.

Continued

TABLE 10.1   Cognitive Apprenticeship Model With Teaching Vignettes.—cont'd

Teaching Method	Description	MAL Implications	Teaching Vignette
Articulation	Expert stimulates learner to articulate her knowledge (or understanding, or both), reasoning, and problem-solving processes.	Articulation can be stimulated during the planning, learning, and adjusting phases of the MAL model. For example, the learner can be encouraged to discuss her questions or goals, describe her learning strategies to make them available to critique, and express how she plans to change her behaviors based on what she has learned.	The clinical teacher asked me to explain my actions/reasoning and helped me become aware of gaps in my knowledge and skills. The teacher questioned me regularly to increase my understanding and encouraged me to ask questions. He made me explain what I had learned and how I would make changes in my future practice.
Reflection	Expert stimulates learner to compare his problem-solving processes with those of an expert, another learner, or, ultimately, an internal cognitive model of expertise.	To encourage reflection, during the assessing phase, have the learner describe his perception of his strengths and weaknesses.	The clinical teacher encouraged me to become aware of my strengths and weaknesses and to consider what I could do to improve things.
Exploration	Expert stimulates learner to move to a mode of more independent problem-solving by setting general goals for the learner and then encourages her to focus on particular subgoals of interest to her, which will help her to overcome weaknesses and build on strengths.	Foster exploration during the planning phase by encouraging the learner to identify goals specific to her learning needs. During the adjusting phase, encourage the learner to consider not only how she will change practice at the individual level, but how she might apply what she has learned to health care systems (e.g., through population or policy applications).	The clinical teacher encouraged me to formulate learning objectives and pursue them. The teacher challenged me to keep learning new things, expanding my focus from the individual to broader issues in the health system.

Modified from Daniel M, Clyne B, Fowler R, et al. Cognitive apprenticeship: a roadmap to improve clinical teaching. *MedEdPORTAL*. 2015;11:10245. Available from: https://www.mededportal.org/publication/10245.

pallor, an enlarged thyroid gland, myxedema, and dry mucous membranes or poor skin turgor." If the learner felt confident asking questions in a welcoming learning environment, she could have asked: "Why did you perform maneuvers A, B, and C during the physical exam, but not X, Y, or Z?" Preceptors can also model several phases of the MAL model itself, especially planning (questioning and searching), learning (describing learning strategies and using critical appraisal of literature), and adjusting (by demonstrating individual or systems application of

new knowledge). This helps the learner relate the master adaptive learning process to lifelong skills.

In Step 2, the focus is on co-facilitation between the medical student and preceptor, with an emphasis on using coaching (see Chapter 12). Coaching can occur by utilizing frequent, brief (1- to 2-minute) observations and targeted feedback (i.e., identify one thing a learner should start doing, keep doing, or stop doing), or coaching can involve more prolonged engagement with more detailed feedback. During this phase, assessing (using external feedback and informed self-assessment) is emphasized, but all components of the MAL model can be coached. Faculty can play a critical role in helping learners refine questions to help set appropriate goals and accomplish change that will take them to the next level of learning. Faculty can also be very effective at "holding up the mirror," stating exactly what they observe about learner performance to highlight changes to be made in clinical care. The preceptor can further use techniques that tap into learner curiosity and motivation, using feedback that inspires change (i.e., she can help turn on or rev up a learner's batteries). For instance, a faculty member could state, "The selection of an ACE inhibitor to achieve blood pressure control in this patient with renal insufficiency could precipitate renal failure." This possible bad outcome can be highlighted to motivate the learner to further investigate the mechanisms of action of angiotensin-converting enzyme inhibitors, sparking his curiosity to ask "why" these drugs worsen renal failure.

In Step 3, the emphasis is on stimulating self-directed learning, a core skill for the master adaptive learner. First, more novice learners are encouraged to explain their reasoning. This articulation helps the preceptor better understand gaps in knowledge or skills, such that they can be highlighted to facilitate learners' goal setting. Then more advanced learners are encouraged to employ metacognitive strategies. Reflection encourages the learner to compare her own processes to those of an expert, to consider how her performance might be improved.[13] Reflection stimulates learners to think deeply about how they arrived at their conclusions. Facilitators may ask questions such as, "How did you arrive at that particular diagnosis? How do your underlying assumptions about adherence influence your perception of why this patient is not taking his medications?" Structured reflection, in which a learner provides supportive evidence for and against her leading hypothesis, as well as for and against her alternative hypotheses, has been shown to improve future diagnostic competence.[14] Exploration helps learners specify their own learning goals that build on their strengths and overcome their weaknesses. This is critical to adaptive expertise; otherwise, the learner runs the risk of making the same mistake over and over again. Individuals are hard-wired to build on their strengths, but it is harder for them to work on their weaknesses. Faculty can encourage exploration through recognizing what a learner does well, then helping identify growth areas. Once a learner identifies a gap and develops a strategy for learning and the interaction is complete, faculty should be sure to follow up next time, providing feedback on what was learned or celebrating new knowledge the learner brought to the team.

Across all steps of the model, scaffolding the experience with appropriate levels of support can ensure that learners remain in their zone of proximal development[15] (as discussed in Chapter 8). This is particularly critical to ensure that learners are not overwhelmed in authentic, whole-task, workplace-based environments. Faculty should rapidly assess a learner's current skill level by asking probing questions such as, "How many cases of *xxx* have you seen before? How many central lines have you placed, and how did the execution go?" This is particularly critical when the faculty member is meeting a learner for the first time and the two do not have an ongoing longitudinal relationship. Additional practical means of scaffolding in clinical settings may include such measures as: (1) priming the learning encounter by asking what the learner's goals for the day are, assessing her calibration, and helping her hone it; (2) carefully selecting patients who target the learner's level; (3) providing preemptive guidance concerning the questions to ask and examinations to perform (consider Vignettes 2 and 3) while ensuring adequate time for patient evaluations; and (4) granting access to electronic resources to supplement prior knowledge.

PRIORITIZING CLINICAL CARE WHILE CONCURRENTLY INSPIRING LEARNING

Cognitive apprenticeship was designed to enhance workplace-based instruction. Therefore its application is highly compatible with clinical practice to inspire the master adaptive learner. It does require faculty to carefully attend to externalizing their thought processes, and they must become practiced in using the techniques in the model. Starting small, by focusing on one teaching method at a time, will eventually ensure that the model becomes part of the teaching armamentarium to foster the master adaptive learner.

Eventually, faculty may come to see prioritizing clinical care and inspiring learning as synergistic processes, rather than mutually exclusive challenges. A curious, engaged learner who is appropriately primed to set realistic learning goals, seek out evidence, and implement changes in practice can become a value-added component of any health care team. Consider the resident in Vignette 3. This resident was stimulated to seek out new knowledge that impacted patient care. Imagine a future in which master adaptive learners are encouraged to make their learning an important part of (not an addition to) clinical care, with the potential to impact the experience for interprofessional teams, individual providers, patients, and learners alike.

CONCLUSION

The master adaptive learner can thrive in authentic clinical environments that are prepared to advance the concurrent missions of clinical care and education. The clinical material, applied in real time, forces the learner to assess, adjust, plan, learn, and then reassess. Accomplishing this efficiently, in a setting that prioritizes patient care and allows learners to add value, is essential. Clinical teachers can foster the MAL process by utilizing techniques that encourage self-monitoring, metacognition, reflection, and critical thinking during the clinical encounter. These techniques include establishing a safe and supportive learning environment that encourages questioning, setting expectations for learners, providing meaningful feedback, encouraging self-directed learner preparation and follow-up regarding content, and recognizing the teachable moments in both routine and surprising encounters. Engaging clinical teaching not only benefits master adaptive learners, but also inspires their clinician faculty and the patients whom both intend to serve.

TAKE-HOME POINTS

1. Teachers must work with learners to create a positive learning environment that fosters the growth of master adaptive learners at the bedside, establishing safety and support while encouraging questioning.
2. Teachers and learners can identify a vast array of teachable moments in the workplace that allow learners to engage in planning, learning, assessing, and adjusting in response to authentic practice challenges.
3. Teachers can develop strategies to foster the MAL process, using techniques drawn from theories of workplace learning that promote self-monitoring, metacognition, reflection, and critical thinking.

QUESTIONS FOR FURTHER THOUGHT

1. How can clinical settings be optimally designed to foster the growth of the master adaptive learner?
2. How can faculty better align with health care system leaders to concurrently optimize clinical care and education?
3. What one new teaching technique will you employ based on what you have learned about cognitive apprenticeship and fostering the master adaptive learner?

ANNOTATED BIBLIOGRAPHY

1. Lemaire JB, Wallace JE, Sargious PM, et al. How attending physician preceptors negotiate their complex work environment: a collective ethnography. *Acad Med.* 2017;92(12):1765-1773.
   The authors describe 100 hours of observation of 26 preceptors, noting competence, context, and conduct and citing relationships among those aspects of clinical teaching.
2. Ng B. The neuroscience of growth mindset and intrinsic motivation. *Brain Sci.* 2018;8(2):E20.
   In this review article, the author discusses the neuroscience underlying growth mindset and also intrinsic motivation, and discusses the relationship between the two. The author concludes that cultivating a growth mindset can build intrinsic motivation.
3. Eppich WJ, Hunt EA, Duval-Arnould JM, Siddall VJ, Cheng A. Structuring feedback and debriefing to achieve mastery learning goals. *Acad Med.* 2015;90:1501-1508.
   Though set in a simulation environment, the authors propose feedback techniques including "micro-debriefing" to encourage deliberate practice and performance improvement.
4. Wenrich MD, Jackson MB, Maestas RR, Wolfhagen IH, Scherpbier AJ. From cheerleader to coach: the developmental progression of bedside teachers in giving feedback to early learners. *Acad Med.* 2015;90(11 suppl):S91-S97.
   This qualitative study of faculty identified themes regarding their delivery of feedback in clinical settings, including cheerleading versus coaching, learner resilience, and balancing challenge and support.
5. Stalmeijer RE, Dolmans DH, Wolfhagen IH, Scherpbier AJ. Cognitive apprenticeship in clinical practice: can it stimulate learning in the opinion of students? *Adv Health Sci Educ Theory Pract.* 2009;14(4):535-546.
   This qualitative study of learners explored modeling, coaching, scaffolding, articulation, reflection, and exploration, the six teaching methods of cognitive apprenticeship in clinical teaching.

REFERENCES

1. Lemaire JB, Wallace JE, Sargious PM, et al. How attending physician preceptors negotiate their complex work environment: a collective ethnography. *Acad Med.* 2017;92(12):1765-1773.
2. Ng B. The neuroscience of growth mindset and intrinsic motivation. *Brain Sci.* 2018;8(2):E20.
3. Alguire PC, DeWitt DE, Pinsky LE, et al. *Teaching in Your Office: A Guide to Instructing Medical Students and Residents.* Philadelphia, PA: American College of Physicians; 2001.
4. Regan-Smith M, Young WW, Keller AM. An efficient and effective teaching model for ambulatory education. *Acad Med.* 2002;77(7):593-599.
5. Mylopoulos M, Steenhof N, Kaushal A, Woods NN. Twelve tips for designing curricula that support the development of adaptive expertise. *Med Teach.* 2018;40(8):850-854.

6. Turner T, Palazzi D, Ward M, Lorin M. *The Clinician-Educator's Handbook*. Houston, TX: Baylor College of Medicine; 2008.

7. Eppich WJ, Hunt EA, Duval-Arnould JM, Siddall VJ, Cheng A. Structuring feedback and debriefing to achieve mastery learning goals. *Acad Med*. 2015;90:1501-1508.

8. Wenrich MD, Jackson MB, Maestas RR, Wolfhagen IH, Scherpbier AJ. From cheerleader to coach: the developmental progression of bedside teachers in giving feedback to early learners. *Acad Med*. 2015;90(11):S91-S97.

9. Wolpaw TM, Wolpaw DR, Papp KK. SNAPPS: a learner-centered model for outpatient education. *Acad Med*. 2003;78(9):893-898.

10. Collins A, Brown JS, Newman SE. Cognitive apprenticeship: teaching the crafts of reading, writing, and mathematics. In: Resnick LB, ed. *Knowing, Learning, and Instruction: Essays in Honor of Robert Glaser*. Hillsdale, NJ: Lawrence Erlbaum Associates, Inc; 1989:453-494.

11. Stalmeijer RE, Dolmans DH, Wolfhagen IH, Scherpbier AJ. Cognitive apprenticeship in clinical practice: can it stimulate learning in the opinion of students? *Adv Health Sci Educ Theory Pract*. 2009;14(4):535-546.

12. Stalmeijer RE, Dolmans DH, Snellen-Balendong HA, van Santen-Hoeufft M, Wolfhagen IH, Scherpbier AJ. Clinical teaching based on principles of cognitive apprenticeship: views of experienced clinical teachers. *Acad Med*. 2013;88(6):861-865.

13. Mann K, Gordon J, MacLeod A. Reflection and reflective practice in health professions education: a systematic review. *Adv Health Sci Educ Theory Pract*. 2009;14(4):595-621.

14. Mamede S, Van Gog T, Sampaio AM, De Faria RM, Maria JP, Schmidt HG. How can students' diagnostic competence benefit most from practice with clinical cases? The effects of structured reflection on future diagnosis of the same and novel diseases. *Acad Med*. 2014;89(1):121-127.

15. Hedegaard M. The zone of proximal development as basis for instruction. In: Daniels H. *An Introduction to Vygotsky*. Abingdon, UK: Routledge; 2002:183-207.

11

How Does Master Adaptive Learning Interact With the Learning Environment?

Larry D. Gruppen, PhD; Michael Dekhtyar, MEd; and Nicole K. Roberts, PhD

LEARNING OBJECTIVES

1. Interpret complex learning environments to classify key components and dynamics that influence learning.
2. Use the Master Adaptive Learner model to identify and refine learner attributes and skills that enable them to adapt to diverse learning environments.
3. Evaluate your learning environment for characteristics that can foster (or hinder) the development and effectiveness of master adaptive learning.

CHAPTER OUTLINE

CHAPTER SUMMARY

As the diagram of the master adaptive learner in Chapter 1 illustrates, in the background of the various learning processes, learner characteristics, and learning outcomes is the learning environment (see Fig. 1.1). The diagram portrays the environment as part of the background, but it is important to recognize that the Master Adaptive Learning (MAL) process always takes place in context, a context that changes from situation to situation and varies from place to place. (Throughout this chapter, MAL refers to master adaptive learning, not master adaptive learners.) Although we can consider the MAL process in the abstract, any real-world application of the MAL model requires us to recognize the particular learning environment, an environment with features that make some aspects of master adaptive learning straightforward and other aspects very difficult.

Too often, the link between master adaptive learning and the learning environment is ignored, in part because the learning environment is contextual and, unless there is a problem with this context, we tend to ignore, screen out, and neglect it—like the background noise at a party that competes with the conversation you are having. Even when we focus on the learning environment, the situational nature of context makes each learning environment unique—unique individuals, unique institutions, unique learning activities—so it is often difficult to know what parallels one can draw between one learning environment and another.

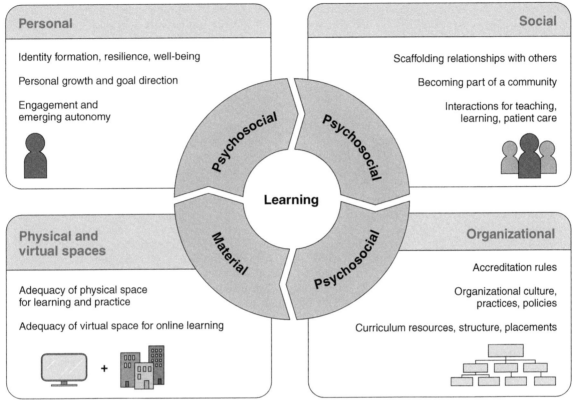

Fig. 11.1 A Conceptual Model of Learning Environments. (From Gruppen LD, Irby DM, Durning SJ, Maggio LA. Conceptualizing learning environments in the health professions. *Acad Med.* 2019;94:969-974.)

The learning environment interacts with the MAL process in complex ways. On the one hand, the MAL process may provide skills, resources, or habits that enable a learner to more effectively cope with a toxic learning environment and thrive in positive environments. On the other hand, there are some learning environment characteristics that may foster or hinder the operation of the MAL process. This chapter focuses on this two-way interaction between learning environment and learning, as described by the MAL model, by examining both theoretical relationships and practical applications.

LEARNING ENVIRONMENT

Key Components

Understanding how the learning environment interacts with the MAL process requires, first of all, a shared understanding of what we mean by "learning environment." The learning environment is a very complex construct. It is difficult to isolate the elements of the learning environment because, as reflected in the Middle French origins of the word "environment"[1] ("environ" or "around"), the learning environment is that which surrounds learning. However, unless the learning is defined, the "surrounds" cannot be specified; the environment is relative to the particular learning that we are interested in. This relativity means that almost anything can be considered part of the learning environment, to the extent that it influences learning. The wealth of possible components of learning environments cries out for some organizing framework to help make sense of it.

One framework (Fig. 11.1), developed for a consensus conference on the learning environment in the health professions, sponsored by the Josiah Macy Jr. Foundation,[2] incorporates theoretical features from living systems theory,[3] sociomateriality theory,[4,5] and prior models of the learning environment in the health professions.[6-9] It emphasizes that much of the learning environment is psychosocial in nature and can be considered at various levels of scale, ranging from the individual person to the organization. Personal characteristics that help define the learning environment include a learner's capacities, such as resilience, well-being, and professional identity, but also individual priorities and values, such as goals and level of engagement in learning.

Interactions among individuals produce the "social" level in the model, which describes how relationships can foster or hinder learning and the importance of learning and practice communities,[10,11] the learner-teacher interaction, the learner-learner interaction, and, in clinical settings, learner interactions with other health professionals, patients, and families. The "organizational" level highlights the impact of institutional and societal norms, regulatory structures, and culture.

Distinct from the psychosocial dimension is the material dimension, which represents the impact of physical spaces on learning[4] and the nature of virtual spaces for learning, such as course management systems, information systems, and data analytics.[12] The importance of the physical environment for education is illustrated by the extensive investment in new educational buildings[13] but also in routine concern for spaces that fit various methods of learning (lecture halls, small group rooms, clinical conference rooms, individual study spaces).

Dynamics That Influence Learning and Perceptions of the Environment

The learning environment model is useful for identifying and categorizing the numerous parts of a learning environment, but the model's key contribution is to draw attention to the interactions among these components and with the learning process and its outcomes. Recognizing and analyzing the direct impact of the various components and their interactions will encourage a deeper understanding of how the learning environment influences learning and how learning can define the learning environment.

Medical education can be characterized by two main types of learning environments: classroom and clinical (workplace). The classroom environment—which may be a lecture hall, a medium-sized traditional classroom, or a small group room—is often the site where students are introduced to foundational materials they will later be expected to apply to the clinical setting. Here, students might be encouraged to begin the process of developing their sense of community with a like-minded cohort of colleagues (a feature of a supportive learning environment). Schools that admit larger classes can develop smaller learning communities to foster the sense of belonging that encourages professional identity formation.[14] However, it is also possible to unintentionally create an environment where students compete for resources (high grades, attention from faculty), which can lead to a negative, stressful environment that may distort the process of physician identity formation.

The clinical environment, where students learn to engage in what will be their life's work, provides them opportunities for legitimate peripheral participation[10] and to finally see in person the lessons learned in the classroom. Although inherently exciting for learners, the clinical environment can also lead to stress, arising from heightened productivity demands on faculty, fragmented patient contact, complex team interactions, and constrained resources[15-20] (see Chapter 4). Through the social component of the learning environment, students learn how to interact with the environment by observing the ways established professions do so. Professionals who practice master adaptive learning can embrace challenges in their environments and demonstrate to learners how they identify gaps in practice, seek opportunities to learn more, and assess how well their solutions work in situ. This problem finding, addressing, solving, and testing can be applied in team-based settings with faculty and learners from all health professions, all of whom are a part of the learning environment. Although relationships may be a source of stress, they can also allow for a diversity of experience that can enhance, and indeed make possible, effective performance. Thus the hidden curriculum can serve for good or bad—with clinicians demonstrating either effective engagement or nonproductive reaction to situations that arise.

The Association of American Medical Colleges (AAMC), the Liaison Committee on Medical Education, and the Accreditation Council for Graduate Medical Education (ACGME) have raised national attention to the impact of the learning environment on patient safety and individual learners. Through the AAMC's Year Two Questionnaire and Graduation Questionnaire, the Independent Student Assessment, and the ACGME's Clinical Learning Environment Review (CLER) process, learners are encouraged to identify sources of mistreatment and potential breeches in patient safety. Organizations with master adaptive learners at the helm may use this identification as an inspiration to lead institutional learning, soliciting input from all levels of the organization. At the personal/individual level of the learning environment model, many schools struggle with student perceptions of the learning environment as engendering mistreatment or abuse. As schools strive to understand the dynamics of potential mistreatment at an institutional level, they may encounter the complexity of individual learner characteristics (expectations, priorities, prior experiences) and how these interact with characteristics of other individuals within the student body (social level of the model). In the assessing phase of the MAL model, leaders of an organization may find that the putative solution generated from their learning process is not perceived as expected, and they may have to adjust to accommodate a diversity of opinions. In general, there is no one-size-fits-all model to address these issues, because the milieu of each locale is different.[21] Thus it is important for institutions to demonstrate themselves to be learning organizations, open to feedback and conversation, and with an ongoing commitment to improvement.

Gaps in Measuring the Learning Environment

Measuring the learning environment in research and educational practice is a persistent problem. Virtually all tools developed to measure the learning environment depend on learner reports, usually of their subjective perceptions and beliefs.[8,22] Although this method may be valid for the personal level of the learning environment model, it is suspect as a measure of either the social or organizational levels of the psychosocial dimensions or of the material dimension.

Outside of learner self-report, it may be feasible to gather team- or group-level indicators of the learning environment, whether through aggregation of individual measures or through independent observer assessment of learning environment characteristics, or through unannounced simulated patients. At the organizational level, the learning environment may be best characterized by analysis of institutional culture—for example, document analysis, stakeholder interviews, institutional performance metrics, and analysis of learner outcomes, both cognitive, such as knowledge-based tests, and noncognitive, such as growth in professionalism—or analysis of other societal features, such as regulatory requirements, incentive structures, and goal definitions.

The ACGME CLER[23] process is a noteworthy initiative to systematically identify features of clinical learning environments. It seeks to identify basic characteristics of clinical work-learning environments (e.g., number of learners, inpatient-outpatient focus, number of programs) and relates them to various learning metrics and activities, such as interprofessional quality improvement projects, and team-based care. The CLER process is largely focused on the institutional level of the learning environment model, in contrast to a frequent focus on the personal and social levels in much of the research literature. Clearly, a broad perspective on the psychosocial aspects of the learning environment is needed for a fuller understanding of how learning environment and learning relate.

HOW THE LEARNING ENVIRONMENT CAN SUPPORT MASTER ADAPTIVE LEARNING

Both the learning environment and the MAL models focus on how the learning process is influenced by external factors (learning environment) and internal dynamics (master

adaptive learning). It is reasonable to expect that learning is optimized if there is a supportive learning environment in which the MAL process is facilitated to function effectively for all learners. The interaction of the MAL process and the learning environment is likely to be complex, and each can be seen as influencing the other. What follows are three examples of how the learning environment might be adjusted to support effective master adaptive learning. The next section gives examples of how the MAL process can be used to influence the learning environment.

Fostering Master Adaptive Learning Through a Culture of Inquiry and Curiosity

The MAL model suggests a number of learning environment interventions that could be explored in an effort to support master adaptive learning in students. One possibility would be to foster an overall organizational culture or environment that emphasizes and celebrates inquiry and curiosity.[24,25] Supportive learning environments must go beyond the narrow concern for factual knowledge and routine application to an emphasis on recognizing and accepting uncertainty and the need for individuals and the profession to pursue answers in ways that may be unproven and risky, and thus may indeed fail.[24,26] The organization's response to failure or mistakes can signal to the learner the degree to which an organization values improvement. Institutions are striving to move from a blame and punishment culture to one that acknowledges uncertainty, error, and transparency.[27] In some cases, schools have sought to augment the environment's emphasis on inquiry and curiosity by transforming it into an explicit part of the curriculum through scholarship tracks or research electives. This has the benefit of situating the learner in the Optimal Adaptability Corridor, as described in Chapters 3 and 16. In many other situations, this aspect of the larger organizational culture is more implicit and can promote many other activities besides education, such as quality improvement efforts, research infrastructure, promotion criteria, and recruitment priorities. In this sense, it is truly part of the environment in which learning takes place but is not solely focused on learning.

The relevance of this kind of learning environment for master adaptive learning may manifest in a number of ways. Observing faculty role models who pursue questions and knowledge gaps in the context of the MAL process will be a positive influence, as will the more general contribution of such a culture to the motivational aspects of master adaptive learning.

Role Modeling Master Adaptive Learning Behavior

It is ineffective for the institution to propagate the idea of the MAL process to its students if the students do not see this process used by faculty. Although it may be useful to develop a formal curriculum in which teachers share with learners their own strategies for addressing gaps and implementing the MAL process, fostering broad and lasting practice of master adaptive learning will benefit from its routine demonstration in diverse tasks, topics, and settings. For example, faculty may help students by not asking questions that reinforce existing knowledge, but instead asking questions that help students determine what is unknown. This type of question, referred to as a true question,[26] enables the faculty member to become a co-learner, so the faculty can role-model the MAL process as the learner is experiencing it. Master adaptive learning might also be fostered by faculty verbalizing their thought processes around deciding whether to change their practice in the face of new knowledge.[26]

Practicing Master Adaptive Learning in Learning Communities

Learning communities have become more prevalent and provide opportunity for learning about a variety of topics, including clinical skills, professionalism, leadership, and social determinants of health.[28] The MAL process could be integrated within these learning communities to help learners understand gaps in their knowledge and engage each other in asking true questions. These structured and regular sources of formative feedback may help learners further develop MAL skills by making these skills more public and subject to reflective analysis.

HOW MASTER ADAPTIVE LEARNING CAN SUPPORT THE LEARNING ENVIRONMENT

The prior examples demonstrated how the learning environment could be used to foster the MAL process, but the practice of master adaptive learning can also improve the effectiveness of the learning environment. If the MAL process enables learners to adapt to and learn in diverse situations, it could reduce the adverse effects of a negative learning environment and augment the benefits of a positive environment. In this way, the MAL process could protect learners against unhealthy learning environments and leverage the benefits of healthy ones.

Individual characteristics such as resilience, curiosity, motivation, and growth mindset in the MAL model (see Chapter 4) are factors that can moderate the impact of the learning environment. Learners with high levels of these characteristics will not only have greater success with master adaptive learning but also likely be more adaptable and better able to cope with adverse learning environments.

The self-direction and learner-centered skills and actions embedded in the MAL process may free the learner from overdependence on the learning environment and reduce the impact of negative environmental factors. The MAL process could serve to reduce any adverse impact of the learning environment by placing emphasis on the identification of gaps (whether originating from the learner or in the environment) that the learner takes responsibility for addressing (planning phase in the MAL model). Learning that will fill the gap will frequently reflect the resources and obstacles of the learning environment. Effective strategies for learning will tend to incorporate the methods and processes that adaptively overcome or circumvent learning environment deficiencies (learning phase).

The assessing phase, when the learner tries out the solution to her knowledge gap, is where the impact of the environment is likely to be most apparent. Learner-generated solutions may succeed or fail, but the MAL process depends on the learner's analysis and judgment of why her solution did or did not work. If the learner is able to distinguish the effects of an adverse learning environment from the inherent quality of her solution, she may be able to learn effectively in spite of a lack of feedback provided by the learning environment. In the face of a failed solution, the learner could use the MAL model to analyze where her solution may have failed. She could ask if her personal characteristics were at a point where she was ready to embrace a change in practice, if she was willing and open for appropriate coaching, and whether or not such was available. Thus practicing master adaptive learning enables the learner to use the information in the learning environment in an adaptive way to assess her own learning (see Chapter 16).

Learners can also examine their planning phase. Did they identify the proper opportunity for learning, access the proper resources, and implement the change effectively? And they could certainly look at the learning environment to see if they analyzed it appropriately to determine its readiness and willingness to agree to their change. Similarly, incorporating the new learning into practice (adjusting phase) is intimately linked to the environment and, once again, the learner who effectively applies the MAL process should be better able to sort out fundamental principles for implementation from the local and temporary considerations of a specific environment. For example, a learner may conclude that the change needed is an expanded dashboard of physician-specific patient outcome metrics. The adjustment phase of the MAL process could help him focus on the characteristics of the learning environment that might be facilitators or hindrances to making that adjustment.

A large-scale, programmatic adoption of master adaptive learning as a framework for teaching and learning could also alter the learning environment though a virtuous cycle. Implementing the MAL process could lead to changes in the educational system that are more supportive of master adaptive learning (e.g., relevant and timely assessment and feedback, learning resources, explicit analyses of learning implementation decisions, incentivizing mastery learning over rote learning). Thus practicing master adaptive learning will produce environmental changes that support master adaptive learning in a way that accelerates learning considerably (see Chapter 2).

The MAL framework may be used to help institutional stakeholders to identify and address gaps in their own learning environments. This would also involve stakeholders asking true questions of their organization's performance. In such a setting all stakeholders are co-learners aiming to understand what is unknown about their environment and working to improve it. However, as mentioned earlier, learning environment measures predominately focus on subjective learner perceptions and beliefs, which do not help institutions understand the quality of their physical and virtual social and organizational components. This reflects the need for program evaluation efforts on these levels that are specific to each institution's needs. Systematic and continuous program evaluations may help further sustain resulting interventions and increase the impact on the learning environment.

CONCLUSION

The MAL process always takes place in a context—the learning environment. The learning environment is complex and unique to each learning situation; however, it is useful to use a conceptual framework of the learning environment to guide educational planning and analysis. The model of the learning environment proposed in this chapter contains facets that reflect personal learner characteristics, social interactions, and institutional culture, along with physical spaces and virtual environments defined by information technology. These aspects of the learning environment interact with the MAL model in rich ways that enable learners and faculty to identify problems in the learning environment and develop interventions that can foster master adaptive learning. It also describes how the practice of master adaptive learning can, in turn, mitigate the impact of negative learning environments and leverage the benefits of healthy environments.

Vignette

Dr. Ima Lerner is now a new faculty member and Dean of Student Affairs at Utopia School of Medicine. The dean of the medical school consulted her,

worried there might be a problem between faculty and students. To orient herself to the school and the needs of the students, Dr. Lerner held meetings with the class representatives, student government members, and leaders of student clubs. All students expressed their passion for the school, but also their frustration in that they felt that most members of the pre-clerkship faculty were distant and unapproachable. Furthermore, the clinical faculty were intimidating and detached. Disturbed, Dr. Lerner then met with faculty members who led key courses and clerkship directors of core clerkships and found that they felt alienated from the students, as if the students did not appreciate their efforts. Further disturbed, Dr. Lerner consulted some colleagues with expertise in organizational development and change, who suggested that she gather resources focused on various mechanisms for convening groups of students and educators. She read about narrative medicine, visual literacy, and improv. She then convened a group of educators to consider the question: "What can we do to fully connect students and faculty, such that each is approachable to the other, and all are learning with and about each other?" She proposed that the group consider the three interventions she had read about. The group determined that they needed a month to consider the answer to this question and decided they would pilot an intervention within 2 months.

1. Would your environment support this type of organizational questioning? If not, which quadrant (see Fig. 11.1) of the learning environment is the biggest barrier? What aspects of that quadrant are challenging? If your environment does support this type of organizational questioning, where have you seen it take place? Which quadrant(s) were improved? What are the explicit goals of the change proposed?

2. How will learners employ the MAL process within the newly developed or improved-upon contexts you described? What are the roles and responsibilities for faculty and students to develop and sustain a learning environment within these contexts that promotes inquiry and curiosity? Within which quadrant(s) do improvements need to be made to facilitate further change processes?

3. How has Dr. Lerner employed the MAL cycle? Are there mechanisms in place within your own institution to encourage faculty to engage in the MAL process in their educational or clinical roles?

Vignette Continued

Dr. Lerner and her colleagues piloted a master's degree program in health systems science for students in the third and fourth year. While the students participated in traditional clerkships and electives, they also had coursework focused on teamwork, informatics, and patient safety. They met weekly with faculty to reflect on program content and their clinical experiences. Evaluation of this new opportunity piloted with the first class yielded mixed results. The learners were excited about the possibilities of health systems science. However, they also felt that the ideals discussed in the program were often inconsistent with their observations and experiences in clinical settings. In the subsequent AAMC Graduation Questionnaire, Dr. Lerner noted an incremental improvement in graduates' perceptions of their readiness for residency, but, coincidentally, there was also a large increase in their reports of mistreatment.

1. What should Dr. Lerner and her colleagues' next steps be upon realization of the mistreatment outcome? Which aspects of the MAL process may be hypothesized to have been affected by experiences of mistreatment? Which quadrant of the learning environment model should be further investigated? Which aspects of that quadrant, and how?

2. Likewise, what next steps should Dr. Lerner and her colleagues take in response to the positive results of increased preparation? Should they continue the program as is or should it be scaled up? What are appropriate strategies for scaling these types of educational interventions?

3. Upon the realization of these results, the dean of the medical school tasks Dr. Lerner to work with the Dean for Assessment and Evaluation on a system to understand the core of mistreatment issues at their institution. The dean also apprises them of a plan to begin a large-scale curricular change that integrates content and curricular experiences across all 4 years of medical school and wants the piloted program to be a central thread within the new curriculum. Lastly, the dean emphasizes his desire that they be prepared to address challenges in the integration process. What are next steps for Dr. Lerner and her colleagues?

TAKE-HOME POINTS

1. The learning environment is a pervasive influence on the MAL process, but its impact and effects are highly dependent on the nature and focus of the learning that is to take place.
2. The MAL process is facilitated by specific characteristics of the learning environment, including a supportive learner community, ready access to relevant learning resources, frequent and personalized feedback on performance, and an institutional culture that supports inquiry and innovation.
3. Learners who routinely practice master adaptive learning should be able to cope with a wider range of learning environments, particularly those that are adverse in various ways. By promoting a spirit of inquisitiveness, openness to feedback, and adaptation, learners can foster a virtuous cycle to promote healthy learning environments.

QUESTIONS FOR FURTHER THOUGHT

1. Every institution and program has its own learning environment. What aspects of your learning environment are supportive of, or create obstacles to, the practice of master adaptive learning?
2. What are viable interventions (large or small) that could improve your learning environment?

3. What is the interaction of your learning environment and work environment? Do the demands of the work environment promote or hinder master adaptive learning?

ANNOTATED BIBLIOGRAPHY

1. Colbert-Getz JM, Kim S, Goode VH, Shochet RB, Wright SM. Assessing medical students' and residents' perceptions of the learning environment: exploring validity evidence for the interpretation of scores from existing tools. *Acad Med.* 2014;89:1687-1693.

This recent review of learning environment measures provides a valuable analysis of validity evidence for each. This is an important contribution to improving the quality of the methods and tools used to assess aspects of the learning environment.

2. Gruppen L, Irby DM, Durning S, Maggio L. Interventions designed to improve the learning environment in the health

professions: a scoping review. In: *The Learning Environment in the Health Professions: A Consensus Conference Convened.* New York, NY: Josiah Macy Jr. Foundation; 2018.

This review of the health professions literature summarizes intentional and unintentional interventions to influence the learning environment in reference to a variety of learning outcomes.

3. Schönrock-Adema J, Bouwkamp-Timmer T, van Hell EA, Cohen-Schotanus J. Key elements in assessing the educational environment: where is the theory? *Adv Health Sci Educ Theory Pract.* 2012;17:727-742.

This review of measures of the learning environment also provides a conceptual framework for considering the particular focus of most of the commonly used instruments. It evaluates numerous instruments and classifies over 90% of the aggregated items into three categories: goal orientation, relationships, and organization/regulation.

REFERENCES

1. Merriam-Webster Dictionary. Meanings of environment. 2018. Available at: https://www.merriam-webster.com/dictionary/environment. Accessed June 4, 2018.
2. Gruppen L, Irby D, Durning S, Maggio L. Interventions designed to improve the learning environment in the health professions: a scoping review. In: *The Learning Environment in the Health Professions: A Consensus Conference Convened.* New York: Josiah Macy Jr. Foundation; 2018.
3. Miller JG. *Living Systems.* New York, NY: McGraw-Hill; 1978.
4. Oblinger D, Lippincott JK. Learning Spaces. *Brockport Bookshelf.* 2006;78. Available at: https://digitalcommons.brockport.edu/bookshelf/78. Accessed August 20, 2018.
5. Orlikowski WJ. Sociomaterial practices: exploring technology at work. *Organ Stud.* 2007;28(9):1435-1448.
6. Genn JM. AMEE Medical education guide no. 23 (Part 1): curriculum, environment, climate, quality and change in medical education—a unifying perspective. *Med Teach.* 2001;23(4):337-344.
7. Genn JM. AMEE medical education guide no. 23 (Part 2): curriculum, environment, climate, quality and change in medical education—a unifying perspective. *Med Teach.* 2001;23(5):445-454. doi:10.1080/01421590120075661.
8. Schönrock-Adema J, Bouwkamp-Timmer T, van Hell EA, Cohen-Schotanus J. Key elements in assessing the educational environment: where is the theory? *Adv Health Sci Educ Theory Pract.* 2012;17(5):727-742. doi:10.1007/s10459-011-9346-8.
9. Gruppen LD, Rytting ME, Marti KC. The educational environment. In: Dent JA, Harden RM, Hunt D, eds. *A Practical Guide for Medical Teachers.* 5th ed. Edinburgh: Elsevier; 2017:376-383.
10. Lave J, Wenger E. *Situated Learning: Legitimate Peripheral Participation.* New York, NY: Cambridge University Press; 1991.
11. Wenger E, Trayner-Wenger B. Communities of practice: a brief introduction. https://wenger-trayner.com/introduction-to-communities-of-practice/.
12. Ellaway RH, Pusic MV, Galbraith RM, Cameron T. Developing the role of big data and analytics in health professional education. *Med Teach.* 2014;36(3):216-222. doi:10.3109/0142159X.2014.874553.
13. Association of American Medical Colleges. New Buildings. 2018. Available at: https://www.aamc.org/members/gip/private/149582/newbuildings.html. Accessed January 20, 2018.
14. Osterberg L, Goldstein E, Hatem D, Moynahan K, Shochet R. Back to the future: what learning communities offer to medical education. *J Med Educ Curric Dev.* 2016;3:S39420. doi:10.4137/JMECD.S39420.
15. Tackett S, Wright S, Lubin R, Li J, Pan H. International study of medical school learning environments and their relationship with student well-being and empathy. *Med Educ.* 2017;51(3):280-289. doi:10.1111/medu.13120.
16. Lee N, Appelbaum N, Amendola M, Dodson K, Kaplan B. Improving resident well-being and clinical learning environment through academic initiatives. *J Surg Res.* 2017;215:6-11. doi:10.1016/j.jss.2017.02.054.
17. Jennings ML, Slavin SJ. Resident wellness matters: optimizing resident education and wellness through the learning environment. *Acad Med.* 2015;90(9):1246-1250. doi:10.1097/ACM.0000000000000842.
18. Lachance S, Latulippe JF, Valiquette L, et al. Perceived effects of the 16-hour workday restriction on surgical specialties: Quebec's experience. *J Surg Educ.* 2014;71(5):707-715. doi:10.1016/j.jsurg.2014.01.008.
19. Dahlin M, Fjell J, Runeson B. Factors at medical school and work related to exhaustion among physicians in their first postgraduate year. *Nord J Psychiatry.* 2010;64(6):402-408. doi:10.3109/08039481003759219.
20. Cross V, Hicks C, Parle J, Field S. Perceptions of the learning environment in higher specialist training of doctors: implications for recruitment and retention. *Med Educ.* 2006;40(2):121-128. doi:10.1111/j.1365-2929.2005.02382.x.
21. Skochelak SE, Stansfield RB, Dunham L, et al. Medical student perceptions of the learning environment at the end of the first year: a 28-medical school collaborative. *Acad Med.* 2016;91(9):1257-1262. doi:10.1097/ACM.0000000000001137.
22. Colbert-Getz JM, Kim S, Goode VH, Shochet RB, Wright SM. Assessing medical students' and residents' perceptions of the learning environment: exploring validity evidence for the interpretation of scores from existing tools. *Acad Med.* 2014;89:1687-1693. doi:10.1097/ACM.0000000000000433.
23. Accreditation Council for Graduate Medical Education. Clinical Learning Environment Review (CLER). 2019. Available at: http://www.acgme.org/What-We-Do/Initiatives/Clinical-Learning-Environment-Review-CLER. Accessed March 8, 2019.
24. Cutrer WB, Atkinson HG, Friedman E, et al. Exploring the characteristics and context that allow Master Adaptive Learners to thrive. *Med Teach.* 2018;40(8):791-796. doi:10.1080/0142159X.2018.1484560.
25. Dyche L, Epstein RM. Curiosity and medical education. *Med Educ.* 2011;45(7):663-668. doi:10.1111/j.1365-2923.2011.03944.x.

26. Cooke M, Ironside PM, Ogrinc GS. Mainstreaming quality and safety: a reformulation of quality and safety education for health professions students. *BMJ Qual Saf.* 2011;20 (suppl 1):i79-i82. doi:10.1136/bmjqs.2010.046516.

27. Kachalia A, Kaufman SR, Boothman R, et al. Liability claims and costs before and after implementation of a medical error disclosure program. *Ann Intern Med.* 2010;153(4): 213-221. doi:10.7326/0003-4819-153-4-201008170-00002.

28. Smith S, Shochet R, Keeley M, Fleming A, Moynahan K. The growth of learning communities in undergraduate medical education. *Acad Med.* 2014;89(6):928-933. doi:10.1097/ ACM.0000000000000239.

How Can I Best Support Master Adaptive Learners Using Coaching?

Nicole M. Deiorio, MD, and Amy Miller Juve, MEd, EdD

LEARNING OBJECTIVES

1. Define coaching, differentiating it from advising, mentoring, and other traditional faculty roles.
2. Describe how coaching supports the Master Adaptive Learner model.
3. List competencies and toolkit items of successful coaches.

CHAPTER OUTLINE

CHAPTER SUMMARY

In this chapter, academic coaching is highlighted as a way to augment the development of a master adaptive learner (MAL). We review the definition of coaching and summarize the theoretical frameworks supporting it. Coaching for the different stages of the MAL process is discussed, including logistical considerations.

INTRODUCTION

Vignette 1

Amir is a first-year medical student who is beginning his first clinical experience in a preceptorship in the family medicine clinic. Wanting to be prepared, he turns to a strategy he has used successfully in his undergraduate career: talking to a trusted adviser. He schedules an appointment with his family physician, with the agenda of receiving advice on how to be successful in this clinical experience.

1. What information is Amir likely to receive from this encounter?
2. What are the benefits and potential pitfalls to this approach?

In Vignette 1, Amir reaches for a common, traditional resource in the world of medical education: the physician adviser. A tried-and-true model, advising can be relied upon to provide the learner with expert answers to the learner's questions. This model, however, can overly weight the expertise of the adviser in solving the learning challenges and can minimize the power of the learner's own experiences and self-reflection in creating and executing learning goals. Although mentors, another traditional physician role, do often have in-depth, personal knowledge of their learners, the mentorship model typically assumes a more intimate relationship in which the mentor feels personal responsibility and, in turn, fulfillment when the protégé succeeds. Often, a more objective look and framework are needed to help learners develop the skills needed to be a master adaptive learner (MAL) (Fig. 12.1).

Applying coaching to medical education can take advantage of its well-known utility in the higher education, business, and sports worlds and implement it in the unique environment of undergraduate medical education (UME), graduate medical education (GME), and continuing medical education (CME).[1,2]

Atul Gawande, MD, MPH, described the value of coaching via direct observation in improving his surgical skills and complication rates—a natural leap from sports to the physical sphere of surgical performance.[3] In addition to improving technical skills, coaching also shows promise in the acquisition of cognitive knowledge, attitudes, and behaviors.[4,5]

The framework of coaching differs from that of advising or mentoring in that it assumes the learner is the expert in understanding what she needs to improve. A coach can draw out this expertise with thoughtful questioning and guided reflection in the protected setting of a trusted longitudinal relationship.[6]

Similar to the educational alliance described in the feedback literature,[7] coaching can foster a supportive relationship that also provides an objective framework to distill external feedback in a way the learner is more likely to trust and incorporate. A coach can also provide external accountability and a structured but safe space for goal setting. We know that the human capacity for self-assessment is, at baseline, unreliable.[8] Ideally, coaching should be used to help learners improve their ability to self-assess by modeling a matter-of-fact approach to eliciting, internalizing, and acting on feedback regarding the inevitable gaps or next steps in skill and knowledge acquisition—a skill that will be practiced lifelong during one's medical career (see Chapter 6).[9,10]

In this chapter, we define the goal of coaching as being to, "support a developmental process whereby an individual learner meets regularly over time with a coach to create goals, identify strategies to manage existing and potential challenges, improve academic performance, and further professional identity development toward reaching the learner's highest potential."[11]

When used in this manner, coaching has the power to positively influence each of the gears in the MAL process (see Fig. 1.1).

General Coaching Skills and Competencies

Whereas advisers and mentors rely on personal experience to provide guidance to the learner, coaches need to demonstrate specific skills that may require formal training. Depending on the structure of the coaching meetings, skills that could facilitate the different gears of the MAL model process might include facilitating appreciative inquiry and self-reflection, motivational interviewing, health and wellness coaching, and a knowledge of the program's resources and legal guidelines. The coaches may need to receive coaching themselves.

COACHING FOR THE PLANNING PHASE

Vignette 2

Sonia is in the first term of her first preceptorship. In contrast to Amir, she has had more than the average amount of clinical experience prior to entering medical school, having worked as a scribe in an emergency department for 2 years. Her school has a required coaching program, but Sonia is having trouble feeling invested in the program, because by all accounts she

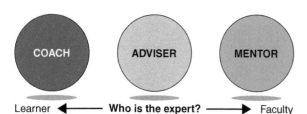

Fig. 12.1 Identification of Expertise, Depending on the Relationship. (From Deiorio NM, Hammoud MM. Coaching in medical education; 2017. https://www.ama-assn.org/education/accelerating-change-medical-education/coaching-medical-education-faculty-handbook. Accessed February 11, 2019.)

is performing above the expected level. Most of the data in her academic portfolio consist of numeric scores based on multiple-choice knowledge examinations. She wonders if her time is better spent in enrichment experiences that could improve her eventual residency application. Sonia's coach would like to engage her in the coaching process, since she believes Sonia has the potential to be an outstanding physician, but struggles to find topics for goal setting due to the multiple-choice exam-based nature of the early medical school years.

1. What assumptions and preconceived ideas might Sonia be bringing into the coaching relationship?
2. What domains might be valuable for Sonia to set goals in?
3. What resources and techniques could Sonia's coach use to add value to their initial coaching sessions?

Information the Coach Needs for the Planning Phase

Because the planning phase usually occurs in the first meeting between coach and learner, it is important to build the framework for a strong relationship in this step by agreeing on and aligning expectations. In this phase, the coach will first need an understanding of what the learner values in his education and professional development, the coaching program, and a coach. A mutually agreed-upon coaching contract that also clarifies the nonnegotiable components of the program can add value

to this step. Additional methods for relationship building include asking about the learner's pursuits outside of school, such as hobbies and interests; coming to meetings on time and prepared to coach the learner; and following up on topics and goals discussed at previous meetings.

Operationally, an academic coach will ideally have full access to a learner's record in order to ensure that the learner is targeting appropriate areas for improvement. Advising relationships can fall prey to the situation in which a learner (intentionally or not) withholds key, possibly unfavorable, pieces of assessment data, because the learner is responsible for guiding the content of the sessions. Because coaching is designed to stimulate and support appropriate self-reflection and improve self-assessment, the relationship benefits from the coach having a full range of assessment, performance, and formative and summative feedback data at her disposal. This should not detract from the concept of having the learner drive the meetings, however. Normative data, used sparingly and intentionally, can be a powerful motivator for some learners, although this may be overwhelming for others. Care should be taken to keep the focus on improving as a physician, as opposed to earning certain scores or grades or giving global comparisons against peers or national averages. In the event the learner is performing well, the coach should also have access to assessment tools, such as institutional clerkship assessments or national rubrics such as milestones, to stimulate discussion and goal creation around skills and knowledge needed to become a more advanced learner (Fig. 12.2).

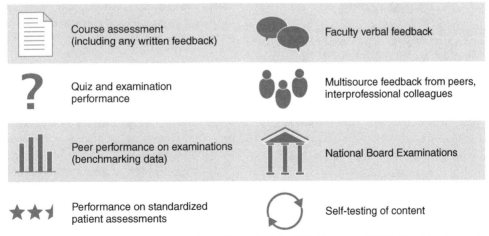

Sources of Feedback to Consider:

Course assessment (including any written feedback)

Faculty verbal feedback

Quiz and examination performance

Multisource feedback from peers, interprofessional colleagues

Peer performance on examinations (benchmarking data)

National Board Examinations

Performance on standardized patient assessments

Self-testing of content

Fig. 12.2 **Sources of Feedback to Consider.** (From Deiorio NM, Hammoud MM. Coaching in medical education; 2017. https://www.ama-assn.org/education/accelerating-change-medical-education/coaching-medical-education-faculty-handbook. Accessed February 11, 2019.)

Coach's Role and Needed Competencies in the Planning Phase

The first step in the planning phase is for the "aha" moment to occur, wherein a learner identifies a gap in knowledge or performance and is motivated to address this gap. Here, the coach plays a powerful role in prompting the learner's questioning and aiding the learner in identifying gaps, selecting opportunities for learning, and searching for resources. Self-reflection can favorably influence goal creation in medical education,[12] and proper attention needs to be paid to reflection if thoughtful decisions are going to be made.[13] Reflective practice is one way to approach the stimulation of questioning and create meaning from experiences. Although reflection can occur before, during, or after experiences (and may therefore have relevance to all the gears in the MAL cycle), this practice might resonate best with a beginning master adaptive learner. For example, a learner performs below average in a core clerkship yet has a long-term goal of matching into a highly competitive specialty. The coach might help the learner reflect on her choice of specialties or future clerkship performance. The Gibbs model of reflection breaks down the act of reflection into six steps: description, feelings, evaluation, analysis, conclusions, and action plan.[14] Having facility in these frameworks can be a key component of coach training (Fig. 12.3).

Goal setting is a critical action in the planning phase of the MAL cycle and is a rich topic of potential discussion for the coaching meetings. Goals of beginning learners, in particular, tend to be broad, vague, and impossible to attain, but can be expected to improve with coaching. Coaches should guide learners to create goals that are specifically linked to the identified "aha" moment. A coach can shepherd this process by reminding the learner to come prepared to discuss a moment in which he felt perplexed or uncertain.[13] Through thoughtful questioning, the coach can help the learner explore *why* he felt perplexed or uncertain (e.g., perhaps he did not know how to examine a knee before seeing a patient with knee pain) and then guide him to use tools such as ISMART[15] to create goals to address the identified gap. The ISMART acronym prompts the learner to articulate a goal that is Important, Specific, Measurable, offers Accountability, is Realistic, and contains a Timeline. A rubric for learners to self-assess their ISMART goal(s) is also available, and the coach should encourage her learner to "grade" his ISMART goal after it is developed.[15] Another tool that can be used for goal creation is the Wish-Outcome-Obstacle-Plan (WOOP) strategy.[16] In this framework, the learner is prompted to focus on visualization (the Outcome) and anticipate and plan for a way to overcome the obstacle(s) to their vision. Unlike ISMART, WOOP does not have an assessment rubric; however, it has been shown to be a more effective method for setting and achieving goals than utilizing an unguided goal-setting process. WOOP incorporates the imagination of a desired future state that overlaps with another theoretical model, that of appreciative inquiry. Appreciative inquiry uses a strengths-based approach to engage a learner in identifying her strengths and postulating how those strengths can be used to achieve a desired outcome.

Prioritization is a crucial skill for helping individuals select and plan an opportunity for learning.[17] It can be overwhelming for a learner to focus on too many learning goals.[18] Prioritization needs to occur during several steps of the MAL process, but, since the learning phase could be the most time consuming, coaches can ensure that proper attention is paid to prioritization of goals in the planning phase. Learners should pick one to two goals on which to focus. There are several models the learner can use to help prioritize tasks. Popular tools include the Eisenhower Decision Matrix (Fig. 12.4) and the ABC analysis. Using the Eisenhower model, the coach should help the learner decipher between urgent versus not urgent and important versus not important goals.

The goals are categorized and placed into a table to help illuminate what should be done first. Subsequently, learners further group tasks into three ABC categories. Category A includes tasks that are urgent and important, Category B includes tasks that are important yet not urgent, and category C includes tasks that are unimportant but can be urgent or not urgent. Tasks in category A should be completed first. Using these or other prioritization strategies can help

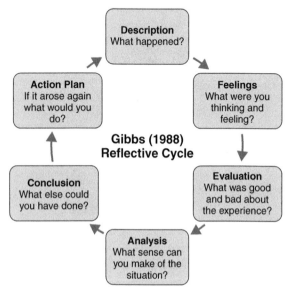

Fig. 12.3 Gibbs' Reflective Cycle. (From Gibbs G. *Learning by Doing: A Guide to Teaching and Learning Methods.* Oxford, UK: Oxford Polytechnic Further Education Unit; 1988.)

	Urgent	Not urgent
Important	DO-Tasks that are both important and urgent	SCHEDULE-Tasks that are important but not urgent
Not important	DELEGATE-Tasks that are not important and urgent	ELIMINATE-Tasks that are not important and not urgent

Fig. 12.4 Eisenhower Decision Matrix Sample Table. (From Toolshero. Eisenhower decision matrix; 2017. https://www.toolshero.com/time-management/eisenhower-matrix/. Accessed February 11, 2019.)

learners better understand where to focus their time and resources. Coaches may be physicians also, adding a layer of credibility to the prioritization discussion.

In considering the part of the planning phase in which resources are identified, coaches do not need to serve as content experts, nor do they need to be expert in where to direct learners for more information. Their role is to assist learners to find the answers. While tempting, serving as a content expert can lead to a coach slipping into an advisory role. Rather, a coach needs to activate the learner, through thoughtful questioning, into identifying the correct sources for additional knowledge, training, or support.

PITFALLS TO AVOID AND STRATEGIES TO USE FOR COACHING THROUGH THE PLANNING PHASE

Pitfall	Strategy
Assuming the learner understands coaching, has buy-in, and shares your expectations.	Create a structured protected space for planning to occur so the learner understands that this work is important and expected. Provide consequences when a learner is not prepared, such as asking him to reschedule.
Providing answers to all of the learner's questions without giving her the chance to explore her own problem-solving abilities though reflective practice.	Use validated techniques such as reflective inquiry and practice. Be overt with your guidance in coaching meetings and provide credibility and structure for the adaptive learning process.
Defining goals for the learner.	Apply a framework, such as the ISMART rubric or WOOP, to encourage a learner to better hone his goals.[15,16] Act as an accountability partner and be sure to follow up on goal progression at each meeting or key deadlines.
Allowing the learner to set vague, overly large, or unrealistic goals.	Ask the learner what goals she has defined for herself and ask her what data she used to identify the need for the identified goal.
Allowing e-mails or casual meetings to count as coaching meetings.	Coaches may consider holding intermittent group meetings with their learners. Especially in the planning phase, group discussion can demystify the coaching process, decrease imposter syndrome, and send the message that all learners have gaps—a gap should not be considered a marker of a weak physician or physician-in-training.

COACHING FOR THE LEARNING PHASE

Vignette 3

Ken is a second-year medical student deep into coursework and preceptorship experiences and is getting ready to take the USMLE Step 1. Over the past several meetings with Ken, you have noticed that his excitement about being in medical school has dwindled and he seems less motivated to study and less engaged in his coursework. You know this is a tough point in the curriculum for most students, and the dark winter months can be tough on student motivation.

1. Is Ken experiencing a learning strategy issue? What other issues may be affecting the learning stage?
2. What question(s) do you ask Ken to ensure that he knows the appropriate resources to access to help him with his concerns and potential performance issues?
3. How do you gauge whether or not Ken is proficient at self-reflection so that he may identify and create goals around any identified academic performance or wellness concerns?
4. What techniques do you coach Ken to consider in order to address potential time management and wellness issues?

In the learning phase of the MAL model, the coach may be more "hands-off" than in the planning phase. The learner will rely on the skills he has gained through the coaching process to integrate new understanding into previously held knowledge, beliefs, or attitudes. He will revisit and deconstruct the "aha" moment identified in the planning phase in order to attend to his gaps in knowledge and learning needs.

Information the Coach Needs in the Learning Phase

Before the learner enters this phase, the coach should ensure that the learner is able to access the resources needed both to learn and to support her learning. In addition to educational resources, a full spectrum of services are needed in order to aid a learner's professional growth and academic performance.[19] Ensuring that the learner knows about and has access to available resources will allow her to recognize that she can problem-solve and address her learning needs with little direction or guidance from her coach, instead of asking the coach for help. In this phase most of all, the coach must guard against slipping into the "expert adviser" role and teaching, instead of coaching, the learner. Also pivotal in the learning phase are academic

resources, such as portfolios or academic data; contact information for clerkship directors or preceptors, professional or peer tutors, and learning specialists; and tools for self-assessment. Resources also include those that support social and emotional development, such as the counseling center, cultural or religious communities, a center for equity and inclusion, and activities that promote physical fitness. Finally, resources such as financial advising, career advising, the student affairs dean, and the ombudsman are needed to promote the transition into medical school and the profession of medicine. Although coaches need not be content experts in support areas, they must know that such resources exist to be able to guide goal-setting conversations toward these areas when necessary.

Once support is in place, ensuring that the learner knows about and can access resources is an important next step in supporting the master adaptive learner through the learning phase and into the assessment phase. To do this, the coach should carefully review the learner portfolio and learning data to confirm that the learner is identifying the most pertinent knowledge gaps. In the form of guiding questions, the coach should review learner-created goals and action plans for completeness.

Coach's Role and Needed Competencies for the Learning Phase

Strategies such as knowledge retrieval practice, spaced repetition learning, calibration, elaboration, and concept interleaving are known to be some of the most effective strategies for deep and durable learning. However, learners tend to rely on quicker, much less effective learning strategies such as re-reading, cramming, or highlighting to achieve their learning goals.[17] Such strategies may have been effective for the learner in the past, but the rigors of medical training and the need to integrate knowledge into practice can often necessitate a retraining in study skills. Coaches can provide foundational skills to help learners select the most effective strategy for their intended learning goals by helping them gain reflective skills, develop the skills needed to participate in "learningful" conversations,[20] and become increasingly self-regulated in their learning.

As previously noted, learners need to engage in the reflective process in order to make thoughtful decisions about their learning.[13] Coaches can help learners develop their reflective prowess by encouraging journaling or talking through an experience with their coach or peers using Gibbs' model of reflection as noted earlier,[14] which can aid in both the learning and the assessment phases.

Another skill coaches can help learners develop is the ability to participate in learningful conversations with others in their learning environment. Learningful conversations provide a mechanism to stimulate learning by

PITFALLS TO AVOID AND STRATEGIES TO USE FOR COACHING THROUGH THE LEARNING PHASE

Pitfall	Strategy
Not following up with the learner to check on the progress of her goals and learning.	Encourage your learner to schedule frequent check-ins with you. In person is preferable but via e-mail or phone is also acceptable. Ask the learner about the progress of her identified goals and, if the learner is struggling to meet a goal, ask her to identify her plan to get back on track.
Not ensuring the learner has support in place to help him achieve a goal.	Ask the learner to identify what support services he will use to achieve his goals. Having him list relevant support services will allow you the opportunity to suggest services he may have overlooked, such as the librarian, a learning specialist, or the counseling center.
Assuming the learner knows the best learning strategy to meet her identified learning needs.	Be a sounding board as the learner attempts different learning strategies that are proven more effective in developing deeper understanding. It is easy for learners to fall back to ineffective, easy-to-complete strategies such as re-reading.
Taking it upon oneself to diagnose a learning disability or mental health issue such as anxiety or depression in the learner.	Be alert for special situations such as learning disabilities or mental health support needs. It is important to remember that a coach is not the health care provider for her learner. A coach is responsible for referring her learner to appropriate resources such as counselors or someone trained to assess for a learning disability.

empowering learners to engage in meaningful knowledge acquisition with preceptors, peers, and others. Learningful conversations are a balance between inquiry and self-advocacy[20] wherein the learner reflects upon his own thinking, beliefs, and evidence before responding to feedback. To develop the capacity to engage in learningful conversations, coaches can provide feedback on reflections in order to ensure they are meaningful rather than superficial. They can also ask learners to identify supporting facts (data from their learning portfolio, literature etc.) for their beliefs or actions. By doing this, learners explore their actions and beliefs against objective data.

Finally, encouraging learners to increase their propensity to engage in self-regulated learning is key for helping learners develop through the learning phase. Self-regulated learners create better learning habits such as choosing and applying strategies to improve their academic outcomes,[21] and monitoring and assessing their performance.[21,22] Furthermore, self-regulated learners have been found to ask more questions and to seek out advice or support when needed.[22,23] Coaches can help learners develop self-regulation skills by ensuring that they use ISMART or other tools to identify and articulate goals. Coaching learners on how to use these tools early in their transition to medical school will help underscore how they support efficient and effective learning rather than being a burdensome distraction from studying. Coaches can also encourage learners to try new approaches to achieve a different learning outcome, such as trying spaced repetition learning to achieve a higher grade on their next examination. Providing the scaffolding needed for learners to try new learning strategies allows them to gain independence while working toward achieving their goals.

COACHING FOR THE ASSESSING PHASE

Vignette 4

Kim is a third-year medical student. She is an average student academically but is heavily engaged in student government and participates in national organizations, including serving as the national vice president of the Association of American Medical Colleges' Organization of Student Representatives. She has identified that, in order to match into her specialty choice of emergency medicine, she needs to focus much more heavily on her grades. She has created several ISMART goals related to academic achievement and leadership but has met only her leadership goals to date. She is very concerned she might not match into her desired specialty and is looking to you for advice and mentorship. You have received several e-mails stating, "Tell me what to do, and I'll do it." You respond back using coaching strategies, asking thoughtful questions. You can tell Kim is getting frustrated because you are not providing "any advice or answers." You suggest a meeting to review her concerns.

1. How do you address Kim's apparent frustrations with the coaching process?
2. What strategies do you coach Kim to consider for prioritization of tasks?
3. How do you ensure that Kim is self-assessing correctly in order to appropriately identify and address her learning needs and ISMART goals?

Information the Coach Needs for the Assessing Phase

In the assessing phase, the coach serves as a trusted partner who helps the learner assess objective performance data. In order to do this, the coach and the learner need to have an established relationship in which the learner trusts the guidance and judgment of the coach. The concept of an educational alliance[7] emphasizes the importance of unity of goals, agreement of goals, and the bond in creating an environment in which feedback is likely to be truly heard and incorporated.

The coach and learner will rely on external feedback and data such as examination scores, grades, and feedback from preceptors and other health care professionals to appropriately assess the learner. Having access to this information in an online portfolio or dashboard will be beneficial for ensuring that all data are considered in the assessment of performance. If the coaching relationship begins at the planning phase, then by the time a learner enters the assessment phase, the coach should have a good understanding as to the learner's ability to self-reflect, an important component of assessment. Physicians struggle with accurate self-assessment.[8,24] It has been found that learners who are less competent are less able to accurately self-assess than their more competent peers (see Chapter 6).[25] Knowing if the learner is using informed self-assessment effectively will help a coach understand where he needs to focus his coaching efforts.

Coach's Role and Needed Competencies in the Assessing Phase

As in prior phases, a coach should encourage habitual self-reflection using all available assessment data.[26] Self-reflection is a process by which the learner reviews a specific experience or a constellation of experiences in order to instill meaning or learn insights that will inform future practice.[13] A coach can help learners incorporate feedback by recounting times in which they have reflected upon their practice, including conveying their "aha" moment, recognized gaps in knowledge or instances in which they want to take their performance to the next level, their

action plan or ISMART goal, and any related outcomes. The coach will specifically want to identify any assessment data they used in reflecting upon their practice. Another way in which a coach can encourage habitual reflection is to verbally walk through Gibbs' reflective cycle with the learner during each check-in meeting (see Fig. 12.3). It is important for the coach to prompt the learner prior to meeting in order for the learner to arrive prepared to discuss a recent "aha" moment. This will allow the reflection to be a meaningful activity rather than just an activity needed to "check a box."

A good self-assessment is one that is informed by data (see Chapter 6). Unlike self-reflection, self-assessment uses implicit or explicit standards to help guide the learner in identifying gaps in knowledge or learning.[27] It is a critical skill that is needed in order for the master adaptive learner to progress to the adjusting phase. Unguided self-assessment has been shown to be inaccurate[28]; therefore the process should be one in which the learner looks outward for feedback and objective assessment data in order to guide his findings. The coach can support the practice of good self-assessment by asking the learner to identify the data he used to inform his assessment. If the coach believes the data set is incomplete or inaccurately assessed, she should carefully guide the learner to additional assessment data using thoughtful and targeted questions such as "What feedback did you receive on how you performed when taking a history?" or "What was your last in-training exam score?" A coach can also help the learner develop a checklist of data points to review before he performs his next self-assessment. Data could include longitudinal competency achievement, examination scores, reflections, peer assessments, verbal and written feedback, and, if relevant, patient outcome data.

Medical education is a time of learning, discovery, and development of new skills, with a steep learning curve to becoming a physician. To that end, and similar to the prioritization that takes place during the planning phase, coaches should help their learners prioritize their self-reflection and self-assessment findings in order to help them identify activities that will aid them in reaching their goals. The coach can also help the learner assess the value of the identified activities. For example, in revisiting the learner in Vignette 4, we can see that perhaps Kim does not need to volunteer for additional committees or projects and needs to focus on other tasks, such as joining a study group, that will ultimately help her reach her desired goal of matching into emergency medicine, if the coach can guide the learner in objectively using her performance data to categorize herself as currently a strong, average, or weak applicant to an emergency medicine residency.

Finally, perhaps the most valuable role coaches can serve is that of an objective, trusted interpreter of assessment

PITFALLS TO AVOID AND STRATEGIES TO USE FOR COACHING THROUGH THE ASSESSING PHASE

Pitfall	Strategy
Failing to prepare prior to meeting with the learner.	Review all assessment data on performance dashboards or learner portfolios. These tools will help you gain insight into not only how your learner is doing academically but also whether or not he is properly self-assessing and self-reflecting.
Downplaying or not addressing the importance of asking for and obtaining performance feedback.	Guide learners toward asking for feedback by giving examples of when you have asked for feedback. You can also ask your learner to jot down a list of who she feels would be able to provide her with the best snapshot of her performance. Coach the learner in how to ask that person for feedback by role playing. Then, when you meet again, check in to find out how the encounter went and ask what insights the learner gained.
Missing the opportunity to normalize the feedback process.	Be a model for receiving feedback. Help learners understand that feedback is not criticism. Feedback is a data point that can be used to change and improve performance. Tell stories about when you last received feedback and how you used it to change your practice. After all, assessment is a lifelong practice that physicians need to embrace in order to achieve the very best outcomes for their patients.
Assume that all coaching must occur in individual meetings to be most successful.	Facilitate peer meetings to normalize self-reflection, self-assessment, and the process of receiving feedback. Having learners engage with each other and share how they have engaged in these key practices will help them understand that everyone participates in this important step.

data.[17] By serving in this role, they can help the learner frame assessment data as positive and a required component of providing competent patient care. We know that informed self-assessment will help guide each physician's future practice and is required by most licensing bodies as part of maintaining credentials or certification. Developing a rapport with a learner, wherein the learner knows the coach has her best interest in mind, is key in helping the learner trust the coach's guided interpretation of assessment data.

COACHING FOR THE ADJUSTING PHASE

Vignette 5

Stefan is by all accounts a high-performing fourth-year student. He is easily able to navigate the varied clinical environments through which he rotates, but does acknowledge he can become privately frustrated when an approach or treatment he learns from a preceptor in one environment is not always viewed as the correct approach in his next rotation, even if he is speaking from an evidence-based position. He asks you for help in sorting out whether he should focus his energies on learning the "right" answer for each system until he has completed his training and can decide on his own style of doing things, or whether he is in a

position now to try to effect change in less-well-functioning systems.

1. What questions could the coach ask to help Stefan decide how address his frustrations?
2. What resources could the coach give Stefan to help him navigate decisions on how and when to effect change?

Information the Coach Needs for the Adjusting Phase

The adjusting phase represents the final step of the MAL cycle. Having tried out new knowledge and skills, the learner can now incorporate these into habitual practice. The coach can be impactful during this phase as well. Learners, particularly early learners, can have trouble assessing the scope of change needed in practice[17]: is an individual accommodation called for, or should the learner work toward transformative, system-wide efforts? Early learners may want to focus on individual practice change first. Learners may be overly ambitious or idealistic in predicting the amount of external change they should influence, yet we would not want to discourage them from bringing a progressive growth mindset to potentially stale practice patterns. The coach, with likely more seasoned experience in the health care system, can offer credibility and direction in this part of the process. Although care

PITFALLS TO AVOID AND STRATEGIES TO USE FOR COACHING THROUGH THE ADJUSTING PHASE

Pitfall	Strategy
Acting in a system or content expert role, giving advice and filling in knowledge gaps of learners.	When assisting with goal setting in the adjusting phase, the coach may offer credibility in steering the conversation in a realistic direction, but should avoid taking over the conversation as the clinical or system expert.
Relying on quantitative data in the portfolio or dashboard as the only type of assessment data.	Coaches can remember that there may be relevant assessment data to be mined for conversations in this stage as well, such as interpersonal and leadership skills feedback. Qualitative comments may better illustrate a trend the learner might be resisting and be more credible or impactful.
Missing the opportunity to coach the learner to explore barriers to system-wide changes, if identified, or inappropriately squelching his idealism.	If a learner identifies a system-wide change that is needed, ask the learner what barriers he may face when trying to make the change. Who else is impacted? What buy-in do they need to get before attempting their change?
Assuming the learner (especially novice learners) can differentiate between an individual-level change and a system-level change.	Ask the learner thoughtful questions about who/what the change would affect.

should be taken so that the coach's role does not shift into focusing on herself as the expert, a coach with clinical experience can assist the learner in recognizing the importance of focusing on the correct level of change: individual, departmental, organizational, and the like (see Chapter 16).

The Accreditation Council for Graduate Medical Education's Practice-Based Learning and Improvement and Systems-Based Practice competencies and specialty milestones highlight the expectation that GME learners learn to improve the system in which they practice care.[29] Coaches can appraise themselves of and assist the learner in setting goals related to local system efforts and direct them to resources that may already exist for GME learners.[30-32]

Assessment data around leadership skills, initiative, and teamwork may also be used to guide conversations around plans to create broader change. Even if the anticipated change in practice patterns will only be at the individual level, guided reflection on understanding oneself can lead to more substantive efforts to creating habits and new workflows, potentially influencing eventual system-wide changes.

Coach's Role and Needed Competencies in the Adjusting Phase

As in the learning phase, the coach must resist teaching the learner herself and will need to be mindful of staying in the coaching role. This threat exists since the gap between the learner and the coach regarding the health care system is likely the widest at this point. The coach should focus her coaching on asking questions, rather than telling the learner about the health care system. Questions such as "Do you know why it is important to maintain proper chart notes?" after an identified charting deficiency or "Tell me what happens when a patient safety concern is reported?" can help the coach guide the acquisition of knowledge as opposed to imparting knowledge. Keeping the conversation focused on interpreting data and goal setting can help the coach avoid slipping into giving advice or direction.

ASSESSMENT AND EVALUATION OF COACHING

Once a program has implemented coaching to develop master adaptive learners, faculty involved will find it helpful to explore the assessment and evaluation of the coaching practice. How do we know that coaching is working to promote master adaptive learning? What metrics do we use to measure coaching success? To date, few instruments exist to measure coaching. Ideally, assessment and evaluation will occur of the learner, the coach, the relationship between the coach and learner, and the coaching program to provide evidence of effectiveness. As described earlier, it is likely that coaching will be more impactful in certain gears of the MAL model than others, and effective evaluation will allow programs to deploy resources strategically toward those parts of the MAL cycle. For now, widely available instruments can be adopted to measure certain activities within coaching, such as those measuring the coach-learner relationship,[11] depth of learner reflection,[33] the quality of goals,[34] and others. Such data can then help convince stakeholders of the value of the coaching process.

Final Vignette: Amir, Sonia, Ken, Kim, and Stefan

At graduation, the students reflect on their medical education to date. They have gained an understanding of the lifelong commitment they have made to keep up their skills and knowledge as physicians. Yet, rather than being overwhelmed, through coaching they feel they have gained the tools to fold self-monitoring, reflection, and goal-setting skills into their practice as they enter residency training and beyond. While hopeful that their residency programs offer a coaching program, they know these activities will be a permanent habit for them.

1. How will their coaching needs change, if at all, as they become GME learners?

2. How might coaching become more challenging yet also richer when applied in the GME sphere?

Although in this chapter we have addressed the individual phases of the MAL model and tied coaching strategies to each phase, the goal of a coaching program should be to train learners to perform these cycles on their own, holistically, and continuously. With a foundational experience in coaching, learners will hopefully understand the value that coaching can provide throughout their careers, but will also ideally improve their own self-assessment and self-monitoring skills so that they can independently work on their quest of becoming master adaptive learners.

CONCLUSION

Coaching has the potential to support all of the phases of master adaptive learner development. Coaching can incorporate many different theoretical frameworks, each of which may have benefit to different learners. Coaching requires specific training, yet, done well, it will uniquely allow learners to create their own educational goals and path.

TAKE-HOME POINTS

1. Coaching, via its unique framework of support that differs from advising, can enhance the process of each of the phases of the master adaptive learner framework.
2. Particular aspects of coaching that can benefit learners are providing a structure to do this work, encouraging reflective practice, and adding accountability for learners.
3. It is important that coaches rely on thoughtful questioning, as opposed to advice giving or mentoring, to help develop the learner through the various phases of adaptive learning.
4. It is vital that coaches have access to all learner assessment data in order to help learners develop skills that will lead them through each phase (or gear) of the MAL process.
5. Tools are available that can help assess the effectiveness of various aspects of coaching.

QUESTIONS FOR FURTHER THOUGHT

1. Can coaching serve as the only external support a master adaptive learner needs? What other roles might be necessary?
2. In what gears of the MAL model might coaching be the most useful for the development of the master adaptive learner in the program you work in?
3. How can we know when coaching has been successful?
4. What assessments or tools can the coach use to understand how well the learners are developing skills to become master adaptive learners, such as ISMART goals and self-reflection?
5. What are some things coaches should avoid when engaging the learner (think back to the differences among coach, adviser, and mentor)?

ANNOTATED BIBLIOGRAPHY

1. Davis DA, Mazmanian PE, Fordis M, Van Harrison R, Thorpe KE, Perrier L. Accuracy of physician self-assessment compared with observed measures of competence: a systematic review. *JAMA*. 2006;296(9):1094-1102.

This literature review reveals that practicing physicians have limited self-assessment skills in a variety of domains.
2. Deiorio NM, Hammoud MM. Coaching in medical education; 2017. https://www.ama-assn.org/education/accelerating-change-medical-education/coaching-medical-education-faculty-handbook. Accessed February 11, 2019.

In this handbook, the authors provide operational aspects for coaching utilizing best practices and consensus from experts in the field of academic coaching.

3. Gibbs G. *Learning by Doing: A Guide to Teaching and Learning Methods*. Oxford, UK: Oxford Polytechnic Further Education Unit; 1988.

This seminal work describes how learners can use reflective practice to link theory and practice to enhance and support their learning.

4. Gifford KA, Fall LH. Doctor coach: a deliberate practice approach to teaching and learning clinical skills. *Acad Med*. 2014;89(2):272-276.

The paper presents a framework that organizes coaching and deliberate practice concepts.

5. Wolff M, Stojan J, Cranford J, et al. The impact of informed self-assessment on the development of medical students' learning goals. *Med Teach*. 2018;40(3):296-301.

In this original research, the investigators show that when self-assessment influences learning goals, the goals are more likely to be reached.

REFERENCES

1. Griffiths KE. Personal coaching: a model for effective learning. *J Learn Des*. 2005;1(2):55-65.
2. Hamlin RG, Ellinger AD. Toward a profession of coaching? A definitional examination of "coaching," "organization development," and "human resource development." *Int J Evid Based Coach Mentor*. 2009;7:13-38.
3. Gawande A. Personal best. *New Yorker*. 2011;3:44-53.
4. Gifford KA, Fall LH. Doctor coach: a deliberate practice approach to teaching and learning clinical skills. *Acad Med*. 2014; 89(2):272-276.
5. Gazelle G, Liebschutz JM, Riess H. Physician burnout: coaching a way out. *J Gen Intern Med*. 2015;30(4):508-513.
6. D'Abate CP, Eddy ER, Tannenbaum SI. What's in a name? A literature-based approach to understanding mentoring, coaching, and other constructs that describe developmental interactions. *Hum Res Dev Rev*. 2003;2(4):360-384.
7. Telio S, Ajjawi R, Regehr G. The "educational alliance" as a framework for reconceptualizing feedback in medical education. *Acad Med*. 2015;90(5):609-614.
8. Eva KW, Cunnington JP, Reiter HI, Keane DR, Norman GR. How can I know what I don't know? Poor self assessment in a well-defined domain. *Adv Health Sci Educ Theory Pract*. 2004;9(3):211-224.
9. Cavalcanti RB, Detsky AS. The education and training of future physicians: why coaches can't be judges. *JAMA*. 2011; 306(9):993-994.
10. Hauer KE, Lucey CR. Core clerkship grading: the illusion of objectivity. *Acad Med*. 2018;94(4):469-472.
11. Deiorio NM, Carney PA, Kahl LE, Bonura EM, Juve AM. Coaching: a new model for academic and career achievement. *Med Educ Online*. 2016;21(1):33480.
12. Wolff M, Stojan J, Cranford J, et al. The impact of informed self-assessment on the development of medical students' learning goals. *Med Teach*. 2018;40(3):296-301.
13. Schön DA. *The Reflective Practitioner. How Professionals Think in Action*. New York, NY: Basic Books; 1983.
14. Gibbs G. *Learning by Doing: A Guide to Teaching and Learning Methods*. Oxford, UK: Oxford Polytechnic Further Education Unit; 1988.
15. Lockspeiser T, Schmitter P, Lane J, Hanson J, Rosenberg A. A validated rubric for scoring learning goals. *MedEdPORTAL*. 2013;9:9369.
16. Saddawi-Konefka D, Baker K, Guarino A, et al. Changing resident physician studying behaviors: a randomized, comparative effectiveness trial of goal setting versus use of WOOP. *J Grad Med Educ*. 2017;9(4):451-457.
17. Cutrer WB, Miller B, Pusic MV, et al. Fostering the development of master adaptive learners: a conceptual model to guide skill acquisition in medical education. *Acad Med*. 2017;92(1):70-75.
18. Vygotsky LS. *Mind in Society: The Development of Higher Psychological Processes*. Cambridge, MA: Harvard University Press; 1980.
19. Paul G, Hinman G, Dottl S, Passon J. Academic development: a survey of academic difficulties experienced by medical students and support services provided. *Teach Learn Med*. 2009;21(3):254-260.
20. Senge PM. *The Fifth Discipline: The Art & Practice of the Learning Organization*. New York: Doubleday/Currency; 1990.
21. Harris KR, Graham S, Mason LH, Saddler B. Developing self-regulated writers. *Theory Pract*. 2002;41(2):110-115.
22. de Bruin AB, Thiede KW, Camp G, Redford J. Generating keywords improves metacomprehension and self-regulation in elementary and middle school children. *J Exp Child Psychol*. 2011;109(3):294-310.
23. Clarebout G, Horz H, Schnotz W, Elen J. The relation between self-regulation and the embedding of support in learning environments. *Educ Technol Res Dev*. 2010;58(5):573-587.
24. Davis DA, Mazmanian PE, Fordis M, Van Harrison R, Thorpe KE, Perrier L. Accuracy of physician self-assessment compared with observed measures of competence: a systematic review. *JAMA*. 2006;296(9):1094-1102.
25. Violato C, Lockyer J. Self and peer assessment of pediatricians, psychiatrists and medicine specialists: implications for self-directed learning. *Adv Health Sci Educ*. 2006;11(3): 235-244.
26. Cutrer WB, Atkinson HG, Friedman E, et al. Exploring the characteristics and context that allow Master Adaptive Learners to thrive. *Med Teach*. 2018;40(8):791-796.
27. Epstein RM. Reflection, perception and the acquisition of wisdom. *Med Educ*. 2008;42(11):1048-1050.
28. Eva KW, Regehr G. "I'll never play professional football" and other fallacies of self-assessment. *J Contin Educ Health Prof*. 2008;28(1):14-19.
29. Accreditation Council for Graduate Medical Education. *ACGME Common Program Requirements*. Available at: https://www.acgme.org/Portals/0/PFAssets/ProgramRequirements/CPRs_2017-07-01.pdf.

30. Myers JS, Nash DB. Graduate medical education's new focus on resident engagement in quality and safety: will it transform the culture of teaching hospitals? *Acad Med.* 2014;89(10):1328-1330.
31. Wolpaw J, Schwengel D, Hensley N, et al. Engaging the front line: tapping into hospital-wide quality and safety initiatives. *J Cardiothorac Vasc Anesth.* 2018;32(1):522-533.
32. Blanchard RD, Pierce-Boggs K, Visintainer PF, Hinchey KT. Integrating quality improvement with graduate medical education: lessons learned from the AIAMC national initiatives. *Am J Med Qual.* 2016;31(3):240-245.
33. Wald HS, Borkan JM, Taylor JS, Anthony D, Reis SP. Fostering and evaluating reflective capacity in medical education: developing the REFLECT rubric for assessing reflective writing. *Acad Med.* 2012;87(1):41-50.
34. Lockspeiser TM, Li ST, Burke AE, et al. In pursuit of meaningful use of learning goals in residency: a qualitative study of pediatric residents. *Acad Med.* 2016;91(6):839-846.

Can the Master Adaptive Learner Process Help the Struggling Learner?

Lynnea M. Mills, MD, and Patricia S. O'Sullivan, EdD

LEARNING OBJECTIVES

1. Describe steps in diagnosing why a learner has struggles in learning in health professions education.
2. Analyze when an individual's challenges constitute typical learner struggles versus when an individual

is "a struggling learner," requiring extra support and resources, often in the form of remediation.
3. Apply the Master Adaptive Learner model to learners with struggles and "struggling learners."

CHAPTER OUTLINE

CHAPTER SUMMARY

Medical training is hard. All learners are expected to encounter content and tasks that feel challenging to master. These are struggles that are typical of a learner who is progressing at an appropriate pace, and there are specific ways to help support these individuals. Other learners, however, face challenges significant enough that they have fallen off the typical trajectory and require additional mentoring, resources, and remediation; these individuals are often referred to in the literature as "struggling learners." Here we describe background on remediation and then turn to the Master Adaptive Learner (MAL) perspective in remediation,

which we suggest requires additional skills around recognition and management of the emotion attendant to the remediation process. Two MAL characteristics often invoked in the remediation process are growth mindset and resilience; here we offer practical tips to spot learners struggling with these characteristics, as well as ways to address them in remediation settings. All phases of the MAL model can present challenges for struggling learners; we pay special attention in this chapter to the planning, assessing, and adjusting phases for demonstrating the utility of the framework. This chapter is not intended to be a how-to guide for remediation or a comprehensive review of key information on the remediation process; rather, it is meant to give the interested reader a sense of how the remediation process can be viewed through the lens of the MAL model. To achieve that end, we have included references to the literature where appropriate and draw on our own experiences and expertise (signposted in the text, e.g., with "we recommend") in offering ideas and approaches.

STRUGGLES WITH LEARNING

Medical training is rightfully rigorous, and all learners are expected to struggle at various points with learning content, mastering skills, managing stress, and more. Successful learners use techniques to learn from and overcome these challenges and continue moving forward on the expected trajectory in their professional development. Just as the MAL model can guide learners as they first approach their learning, it can also help them react appropriately at times when their learning is not proceeding as they wish.

Planning Phase Struggles

> **Vignette 1**
>
> Suzie is a third-year student on her pediatrics clerkship. She is excited to begin her inpatient rotation at Children's Hospital because she thinks she wants to be a pediatrician. As she begins her clinical work, however, she realizes that she is encountering a great deal of content with which she is unfamiliar, and she quickly becomes overwhelmed each day with all of the things she doesn't know. She dutifully keeps a list of unanswered questions in her notebook, but can't seem to find the time to investigate answers to her questions.

Suzie is encountering a fairly normal struggle for a new clinical student. Suzie's difficulty in finding time to engage in her desired learning indicates she has a problem in the planning stage, which involves identifying a gap, selecting a learning opportunity, and searching for resources. She sets goals but has trouble finding time to work toward them because of challenges in prioritizing tasks in her day and prioritizing particular learning points. There are some clues that a learner may be struggling in the planning phase:

- Learner appears disorganized.
- Learner has (or reports) trouble with time management.
- Learner has unrealistic expectations for himself about what he can accomplish (e.g., when asked for learning goals, says he wants to learn "everything").
- Learner consistently has trouble meeting deadlines or makes commitments and then complains of not having enough time.

- Learner is surprised by her own inability to achieve desired tasks due to feeling a task was manageable and then discovering it was harder than expected.

These clues may appear to be fairly egregious deficits, but they often represent very normal processes in professional growth, such as in Suzie's case.

Vignette 1 Continued

Suzie's attending, Koki, checks in with her a few days into the rotation, and Suzie reveals she is struggling to find enough time to do the reading she wants to do to feel knowledgeable about each of her patient's illnesses. Koki discovers Suzie did well in her preclinical courses and is unsure why this is so tough for her. With more questioning, Koki learns Suzie is feeling flustered and "pulled in too many directions" while on the wards. She is never quite sure where to focus her attention. Koki also discovers how many different resources Suzie is trying to use for her learning. Koki tells Suzie he thinks she's having a common struggle in the planning phase of learning. He helps her make a list of and prioritize her learning tasks, as well as assigning specific amounts of allowable time for each task. He helps Suzie identify one specific resource to focus on when she does her reading. The following week, Suzie reports she has had increased time to do outside reading and feels less frazzled.

Suzie's challenge is one that can easily be managed by her direct clinical supervisor; in fact, all educators expect they will need to guide learners for whom the material is hard. To help address challenges with the planning phase, the supervisor should first assess the learner's metacognitive skills by asking the learner to reflect on her planning strategies and by inquiring about the learner's prior performance history in other settings with complex tasks. Some learners have strong metacognitive abilities but may just feel overwhelmed by new learning settings. In these cases, simply pointing out where the issue lies may be sufficient to help learners create self-directed approaches that lead to improvement without further intervention required. Learners with less metacognitive skill likely require more specific guidance on how to address these issues. They can turn to resources in the lay press on time management, organization, and prioritization. Some experts have modified similar resources for use by medical professionals,[1] including developing to-do lists that prioritize each task based on multiple factors (who else can accomplish it, how urgent it is, how important it is), and setting aside a specific amount of time each day for to-do list tasks.

Many learners are trying to do too much and therefore end up doing nothing. We recommend setting a very realistic goal of a small time commitment and a specific amount of ground to cover (one topic) so that it can feel more accomplishable. Our usual advice for learners who "don't have enough time to read" is to set aside 10 uninterrupted minutes each night to read on one topic—whichever feels most urgent from the topics that arose that day—using an accessible resource, which may or may not be primary literature. Developing ISMART (Inspired, Specific, Measurable, Accountability, Realistic, and Timeline) goals, as described in Chapter 12, helps learners structure their approach so as to accomplish goals and promote lifelong learning.

In general, the corrective process for planning phase challenges is the same as for challenges with any phase of the MAL model:

1. Assess the learner's metacognitive skill and the learner's current approach to that phase of the cycle.
2. Elicit the learner's self-assessment of what is working and what is not, then offer your external perspective by indicating areas of strength and areas for improvement (thereby creating a more informed self-assessment; see Chapter 6 for details).
3. Ask the learner to make connections between a specific behavior (e.g., using too many resources) and an outcome (e.g., feeling frazzled); point this link out to the learner if it is not apparent. This can include learning from functional processes that are working and dysfunctional processes that are not.
4. Elicit a plan from the learner on how to change a behavior in order to improve the outcome (e.g., via ISMART goal). Create accountability by making a plan to follow up at a specific time in the future.
5. Follow up with the learner to ask for her self-assessment of progress and offer your own perspective. Scaffold the learner's goal setting as often as needed.

Note that when learners make plans for addressing deficits, creating their own plans, rather than just being told what to do, is valuable (see Chapter 12). There is a balance here, though: if a learner creates a plan that ends up being completely unsuccessful, he will feel frustrated. It is important for the supervisor to weigh in on how realistic a given plan is and to do some coaching to help make sure that the plan is likely to lead to some degree of success. If the learner's plan is not the optimal solution, though, this is okay, because he may learn something valuable from the process, and reflecting on what was imperfect about the approach will likely enhance his skills in the future.

It is worth taking a moment to discuss the diagnostic process, because some planning phase challenges might not be as clear-cut as Suzie's. The MAL model can be useful for diagnosing the nature of a given learner's problem. For example, a learner who delivers clear presentations on morning rounds but has trouble answering questions "on the fly" may be struggling with planning, due to a lack of ability to strategize about how to increase her knowledge base around each case. This learner is only able to demonstrate skill when reporting on information already discussed with the team or known to be part of the case. However, the same challenge could be due to a problem with the learning phase, such as if the learner is reading appropriate sources but not getting material to "stick." Or this problem could be with the assessing phase: the learner may be underconfident or not getting enough feedback about expectations for answering impromptu questions. And, of course, the problem could be due to personal issues (lack of sleep, anxiety, etc.). The challenge in diagnosing the issue may be compounded by the fact that, especially in team settings, some team members may purposely or inadvertently compensate in ways that minimize appearance of deficits in learners (e.g., by feeding them differential diagnoses and plans). Figuring out exactly where in the MAL model a learner is struggling can be challenging, and some learners may have deficits in multiple phases. To help continue to delineate the differences, we will now turn to the identification of struggles with other phases.

Learning Phase Struggles

Vignette 2

Teo is a second-year obstetrics and gynecology resident who really wants to do well in residency and, specifically, on his current labor and delivery rotation. He tries to spend time each night reading and rereading systematically through the textbooks recommended by his adviser. He underlines and highlights as he goes, but never seems to remember what he has read.

Teo's struggle is also common: he is having difficulty with the learning phase of the MAL model. Teo continues to use the same learning strategies, even though they are not successful for him. This is a typical challenge for learners at many stages of training. There are some clues that a learner may be struggling in the learning phase:

- Learner has a subpar knowledge base in the context of
  - appearing motivated.
  - appearing well organized.
- Learner appears fatigued (the learning phase is very hard in the setting of fatigue because it is easy to fall back on previously developed learning strategies when exhausted).

- Learner reports being "a bad test-taker."
- Learner reports challenges making sense of different available learning resources.

With well-developed metacognitive skills (see Chapter 5), Teo could recognize his difficulties and potentially reset his approach by talking with peers, consulting the literature, or getting advice from more experienced clinicians on successful approaches to improving medical knowledge. Alternatively, if Teo is unable to see the issue and needs more hands-on help, any adviser or coach who notices the issue could point it out to Teo and help him strategize better approaches. For learners struggling on standardized assessments in a classroom-based setting, this challenge will be made clear by low performance. In some settings, though, this challenge may not be obvious to the learner or supervisors. For example, a learner on a busy clinical service might produce reasoning described by prior providers in the patient's chart, and the fact that the learner does not have a deep understanding of the issue may not be apparent. This highlights the importance of clinical supervisors checking in on learners to reveal challenges that may be less visible. This often takes the form of questions to probe a learner's understanding in a nonthreatening way (see Chapter 11). Longitudinal coaching programs may also help meet this need by providing learners with coaches who know them well and can address challenging skill areas.[2]

To address challenges with the learning phase, we can look to the literature around improving medical knowledge. Most of that literature draws from learning theory and practical applications of adult learning processes. Learning and study practices that are effective and likely to improve learners' knowledge base include spacing out their practice or study on a given topic; reorganizing information, such as in charts or outlines; self-testing with flash cards or question banks[3]; and interleaving content on different topics when studying.[4] We often point learners toward several of these methods and ask them to start with the one that seems most feasible for them. Specifically, Teo's strategy of highlighting has been shown to be a relatively ineffective strategy.

Assessing Phase Struggles

Vignette 3

Aisha is a busy junior faculty member who works as an outpatient general internist. A month ago, she realized her diabetic patients' core measures were not as well controlled as she had hoped, and she has since reviewed the literature to verify that she is up-to-date on all the current recommendations regarding diabetes management. After this, she doesn't know where to turn to identify what's going wrong.

Aisha's challenge here is with the assessing phase, which involves testing out her new learning, including self-assessment. She recognized her problem and has created a plan but does not have the ability to see where the barriers are or to modify her approach to meet the needs of the situation. There are some clues that a learner may be struggling in the assessing phase:

- Learner demonstrates an adequate knowledge base but outcomes are not as good as expected.
- Learner can describe expected outcomes and appropriate strategies to achieve them, but has trouble operationalizing these strategies. This can sometimes look like a logistical challenge.
- Learner's self-assessment does not match supervisor's or peer's assessment.

To manage challenges with this phase, learners need help with their informed self-assessments (see Chapter 6). Self-directed learners may be able to find this guidance on their own, by talking with peers or turning to the literature, but others will need it more explicitly spelled out by supervisors. In that case, a recommended strategy would be to ask the learner to take one exemplar case and walk, step by step, through his approach to managing it. The supervisor can then ask questions to prompt reflection at key time points and help the learner uncover missed or inappropriate steps.

Adjusting Phase Struggles

Vignette 3 Continued

Aisha invests time and energy in reviewing all of her patients' charts and talking with colleagues. She realizes that she does not have a system for ensuring patients get their labs checked as often as needed to stay on top of their progress in managing their diabetes. She reviews the literature for the best methods of adhering to necessary timelines for diabetes management and decides her practice should create a system in which the medical assistants keep track of diabetic patients' labs and send alerts to the clinicians when new labs are due. She feels like it should be effective and has buy-in from the other physicians about the idea, but she is stuck when figuring out how to implement the new program in her clinic. Her frustration has led her to consider giving up on the idea.

Aisha's problem now is with the fourth phase in the MAL model: the adjusting phase, which involves incorporating new learning into one's routine or practice. Specifically, she is struggling with change management (individual vs. system implementation). Although she had identified individual changes, the systems changes are more difficult. This is an example of how the MAL model can allow a broader perspective than traditional remediation models. There are some clues that a learner may be struggling in the adjusting phase:

- Learner has trouble deciding how to apply learning to new situations that arise.
- Learner has trouble seeing big-picture issues and approaches (can't "see the forest for the trees").
- Learner has realistic goals and plans but has difficulty implementing them.
- Learner is unsure how to navigate systems-level concerns.
- Learner is unaware of the roles of other people in the setting (often especially true for new members of a team).
- Learner cannot list stakeholders in given processes or anticipate ways in which they will be impacted by changes.

A colleague with a background in systems work could help Aisha, or she could potentially find sufficient information on systems implementation from books and online resources to help her figure out how to get her project off the ground. More broadly, challenges with the adjustment phase benefit from being broken down into small chunks and considered reflectively. For Aisha, it would be helpful to sit down with other stakeholders (the medical assistants, as well as other clinic staff) to create lists of potential barriers to implementation, as well as resources available. Investigating the extent that each barrier contributes to the issue can help Aisha prioritize aspects of the plan to roll out first and can help her see areas where she may need to go back to the beginning phase to seek out new information/learning to help her understand the systems landscape better. After going through this process, Aisha might realize, for example, that her practice's medical assistants do not have enough time to take on this role, but the practice manager may be able to teach Aisha how to set up alerts in the electronic health record so she can track these lab dates herself.

Bringing It All Together

All of the previous vignettes portray learners struggling with common aspects of learning to become successful clinicians. In each of these cases, the learner may just need a supervisor to look at the issue and discuss it with the learner (e.g., discussing how to choose the right resource for outside learning). From there, the learner may be able to discern appropriate strategies to correct the issue without further guidance, provided the learner does have the metacognitive abilities of a master adaptive learner. Educators can help support learners in these processes by shedding light on specific areas of struggle, and can teach learners the entire MAL model so that they may continue to use it for self-directed learning and to overcome learning challenges. These learners often will not need additional support structures in order to succeed.

"STRUGGLING LEARNERS"

All learners struggle, many in the ways described in the previous section. Some learners, however, struggle more, to the point that they fall off the normal developmental curve as their deficits become more significant compared to their peers or to their school's or program's expectations. These individuals are often referred to as "struggling learners." "Struggling learners" need and deserve institutional efforts to remediate their deficits. Though remediation does not have one agreed-upon definition in the literature, for our purposes here, we will use the concept of an extracurricular skill-building process. A learner who needs remediation is one we expect will not achieve desired competency within the usual educational structures and needs additional work and guidance outside or alongside the standard curriculum.[5,6] This process usually entails intensive coaching from a skilled faculty member. It can be extremely time consuming and resource intensive,[6] but it is our obligation as educators to both the learner and her patients.

Background on Remediation

No one knows exactly how many learners have remediation-level struggles in health professions education—estimates from larger studies often indicate about 3%,[7-9] ranging up to about 15% according to Frellsen and colleagues,[10] or even a third,[11] of all learners—but it is clear that learners at all levels undergo remediation[12] for deficits in a broad range of areas.[13] The work of Guerrasio and colleagues[13] (Fig. 13.1) showed variability in the types of deficits most prevalent at different stages of training, but learners at all levels struggle with knowledge, interpersonal skills, professionalism, and more.

In this chapter, we focus on trainees, but faculty can and do require remediation. Additionally, we have found in our own work that this is not a problem localized to "struggling" institutions or programs; institutions of all sizes, calibers, and reputations have learners who require remediation.

There are no formal criteria or agreed-upon guidelines for determining when an individual with struggles becomes a "struggling individual" and requires remediation. Many experts frame these issues in the context of competencies,[6,14] and learners who do not achieve expected

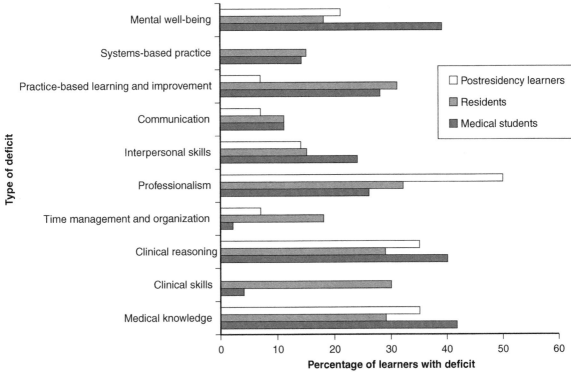

Fig. 13.1 Percentage of 151 learners with each type of deficit by level of training, University of Colorado School of Medicine remediation program, 2006-2012. Although trends emerged among the learners, the only statistically significant finding was that mental well-being difficulties were more common in medical students (P = .03). Most learners had more than 1 of the 10 deficiencies studied. (Reprinted with permission from Guerrasio J, Garrity MJ, Aagaard EM. Learner deficits and academic outcomes of medical students, residents, fellows, and attending physicians referred to a remediation program, 2006-2012. *Acad Med.* 2014;89[2]:352-358.)

competencies in the traditional time frame are considered to be in need of additional attention and remediation. Learners who do not pass standardized examinations or clinical rotations clearly need extra support in the form of remediation. Outside of these formal assessment processes, learners may be identified as needing remediation based on singular events so egregious as to warrant immediate attention or based on patterns of deficits across clinical settings that are noticed by supervisors. Multiple studies have revealed that relying solely on supervisors' numerical ratings, or even narrative descriptions, in summative evaluations of learners may be insufficient to detect problems. Verbal conversations between education leadership and direct supervisors are most likely to lead to identification of struggling learners.[15-17] This suggests that many struggling learners are coming to attention late.

Though there is no easy set of criteria to guide educators on when to direct learners to remediation processes, our advice is to err on the side of referring learners for remediation whenever there is a question as to whether it could be warranted. This is especially the case if remediation programs are low-stakes and formative. This approach of "catching" more struggling learners earlier on benefits both them and patients in the long run. Ideally, all learners would receive whatever coaching they need in their authentic learning environments without needing to be referred to additional resources, but, in our current system, working with "struggling learners" requires additional skills. The approaches to the work with these learners, especially the metacognitive components, may be different. Therefore determining whether a learner is "struggling" or is a "struggling learner" is not just an academic exercise.

Vignette 4

Joel, a third-year medical student who did well in all his pre-clerkship coursework, is referred for remediation coaching because he failed his objective structured clinical examination (OSCE) prior to beginning clinical rotations. Review of his scores and video recordings reveals that Joel missed obvious diagnoses in multiple cases cutting across different specialties, preferring to focus on esoteric and rare diagnoses. Joel is a "struggling learner."

1. Who is best situated to help Joel, given the broad-ranging effects of his challenge?
2. What skills does the coach need to have?
3. What should be this coach's approach to working with Joel?

Although there is good evidence that learners can develop their own goals and remediation plans[18] and are sometimes successful carrying out remediation work independently,[19] we believe remediation work is best done with support from a trained faculty member, whom we refer to here as a remediation coach. All remediation coaches need some degree of expertise in the area in which they are remediating. In Vignette 4, Joel is lacking in clinical reasoning, and his remediation coach should be someone whose clinical reasoning skills are well honed, ideally with pedagogical knowledge in this area as well. Although these are skills of effective teachers in general, remediation requires an additional skill set beyond this. In the remediation setting, the content knowledge is important but takes a backseat to specific skills in this context. Kalet and Zabar described key competencies that remediation coaches must demonstrate before beginning the work.[20] An abbreviated, noncomprehensive list is included here; we have organized them into our own categories:

Knowledge and application to remediation

- Articulate how current learning theories apply to routine medical teaching and assessment practice as well as remediation.
- Discuss the underlying assumptions of various assessment strategies and common misunderstandings.
- Discuss the impact of bias and prejudice on achievement.
- Explore personal perspectives, attitudes, and beliefs that inhibit identification of learners who struggle.
- Define clinical competence in a behaviorally specific and measurable manner.

Remediation programming skills

- Demonstrate taking an educational history from a trainee, including addressing clues suggesting the

presence of a verbal or nonverbal learning disability or attention deficit disorder.
- Construct with learner useful individualized remediation plans with proper accountability, based on critical review of the objective and subjective assessment data for an individual learner.
- Identify and design authentic complex tasks in which trainees can demonstrate competence.

Relational skills

- Demonstrate exceptional metacognitive skill and awareness.
- Give effective reinforcing feedback as well as direct and difficult-to-receive constructive feedback.

Many of these coaching competencies add value in general coaching settings, but they are truly crucial in remediation. As noted, we group these skill sets into three categories:

1. Knowledge and application to remediation—knowing about assessment, bias, and remediation background information
2. Remediation programming skills—ability to develop a learner-centered approach to targeting specific deficits
3. Relational skills—engaging and giving appropriate feedback to the learner, drawing out information and making appropriate diagnoses on that basis, and being aware and reflective throughout the process

The first category requires that remediation coaches be well versed in the curriculum's goals and the expected standards for learner achievement. This is ideally someone with extensive experience working with learners at this level (for purposes of understanding typical development). The remediation coach also needs to understand the epidemiologic data described earlier, as well as the fact that some learners' assessments reflect systemic issues and bias.[21-25] The second category involves remediation coaches being aware of and facile with techniques to address specific types of deficits, such as medical knowledge or organization. Some of these are addressed later, but describing all of them is beyond the scope of this chapter. For further reading, we recommend the textbooks by Guerrasio[6] and Kalet and Chou.[26]

The third category deserves to be parsed more specifically, because the relational component of the remediation process is probably the most important and the most challenging. This skill set is often described outside the health professions education literature as emotional intelligence; here we refer to this domain as relational skills. Although the ability to build strong relationships with learners is useful in a general educator or supervisor, it is not required. Many learners learn just fine in the context of cordial, formal, and fairly superficial relationships with supervisors, but the remediation context is different.

Many learners develop significant deficits as a result of mental health issues, substance use, large personal life stressors, and the like. Though faculty who work as remediation coaches for medical learners are not expected to provide mental health services, skillfully drawing out any potential contributions of mental health issues to poor performance is usually the first step in remediation. Learners in these situations likely cannot begin their remediation work until these issues have been at least partially addressed, which involves referral to experts outside the remediation program.

Even for learners for whom such stressors are not present, the mere fact of being singled out for one's substandard performance is likely to bring significant stress and emotional challenge, including such negative emotions as shame, denial, and fear. Moreover, the need to engage in additional remedial work, on top of an already daunting regular workload, can feel extremely cognitively and psychologically burdensome. To be able to recognize the presence of any relevant emotional/psychological issues and to support learners in dealing with the emotional stress of the remediation process requires remediation coaches to have special skills in developing rapport and trusting relationships with learners, as well as in giving challenging feedback in a supportive manner. Recall from Chapter 6 on cognitive processes that feedback is best accepted when it is concordant with the learner's self-assessment, even if it is critical feedback. As described in that chapter, interpretation of feedback depends on both the content and the quality of the source of feedback. When the content feels hard to receive—when it is discordant with the learner's self-assessment—internalization of the feedback will require an increase in the quality of the source of the feedback. We recommend a strong relationship as the single best way to increase the perceived quality of the feedback giver.

For remediation to work, learners must feel the remediation coaches are "in their corner." Furthermore, because of the need to address institutional standards and deadlines, the remediation process is sometimes quite time limited, meaning this strong relationship must be built quickly. Remediating learners corroborate the importance of these relationship skills in their remediation coaches, emphasizing honesty, high standards, and skill with facilitation as being key to a remediation coach's success.[27] Remediation programs that neglect the psychosocial, mental health, and emotional aspects of failure and remediation are less successful for learners.[28] This work is challenging and may not be realistic to expect of all educators who supervise learners. Many institutions have developed stand-alone, referral-based remediation programs in which faculty remediation coaches are specially selected and trained; resources offer guidance on developing programs for this purpose.[6,29,30]

This conversation raises an important question: how is a remediation coach different from a (general) coach? As described in Chapter 12, a coach is a trusted individual who helps guide a learner to develop his own plan for learning and improvement and serves to help the learner interpret outside information. Here we have purposely used the term *remediation coach* to be clear that people in this role must possess all the same skills as outlined in Chapter 12, but they must have additional skills. Remediation coaches need the same relationship-building skills as coaches but will need to be able to work with stronger emotion, on shorter time frames, and with learners with more deficits. They need increased ability to identify learners' learning edges (also known as the zone of proximal development, described in Chapter 8). Remediation coaches need the same ability as other coaches to guide learners' reflections and self-assessments but also need to feel comfortable being more directive when learners' metacognitive abilities are insufficiently developed (e.g., pointing out deficits learners cannot see). Remediation coaches must be exceptionally comfortable delivering bad news in a supportive way and must be realistic and honest about their learners' performance. In our experience, long-term coaches often "root for" their learners and may feel challenged seeing their deficits. While good general coaches can model MAL skills well, remediation coaches need increased focus on their own MAL skills, especially metacognition, in order to guide learners with significant deficits. Additionally, unlike for the general coach, the remediation coach's work cannot be primarily driven by the learner's goals but must achieve a delicate balance between learner goals and institutional requirements for academic progress. Finally, they must possess outstanding ability to "read" a variety of learners. Some people call this intuition, but it is not an ingrained quality; rather, it is an important capacity that can be developed with deliberate practice. Misinterpreting a learner's cue can have a detrimental effect on the relationship or the learner's progress because of the high-stakes nature of remediation.

Once we have identified and trained appropriate remediation coaches and addressed barriers presented by mental health issues, personal life stressors, and the like, we may turn to the MAL model to frame our remediation work. Every MAL characteristic and phase may be implicated in a struggling learner's challenge, but here we emphasize selected characteristics and phases that are especially likely to be involved in remediation cases.

General Remediation Approaches and the Master Adaptive Learner Framework in the Context of Remediation

The literature on addressing specific deficits is too broad to recount here, though there are some overarching themes that can help guide all remediation plans. Hauer and co-workers grouped the common components of remediation plans into three key domains: deliberate practice, feedback, and self-assessment.[12] These can be further elaborated via the lens of the MAL model. Although we do not know of specific papers that frame the remediation process in terms of the MAL model, the general literature on remediation maps well onto this model.

CHALLENGES WITH MASTER ADAPTIVE LEARNER CHARACTERISTICS

Learners may struggle with all of the characteristics described in Chapter 4 (curiosity, motivation, growth mindset, and resilience). Here we focus on two characteristics that are particularly relevant to remediation: growth mindset and resilience.

Vignette 5

Two students fail their general surgery clerkship due to challenges with clinical reasoning and are required to repeat it. Mario, while embarrassed, reports that he wants to get "as much help as possible" and is eager to receive lots of constructive feedback to help him succeed on his repeat rotation. Olivia, on the other hand, expresses that she failed only because her evaluators were "out to get me" and "didn't look for my real skills." Mario's high likelihood for success during the repeat rotation, relative to Olivia's, seems obvious to the faculty involved, because of his growth mindset.

1. How can the remediation coaches help Olivia recognize the value of working to improve her skills?
2. How much work can be done with Olivia on her clinical reasoning with her mindset in its current state?
3. What should be the first step in remediation?

Growth Mindset

Although there is some evidence of the impact of mindset-targeted interventions on student performance,[31] recent research calls into question the effect of the growth mindset on academic achievement.[32] Though the growth mindset has been explored in the education literature for decades, its

link to long-term learner outcomes remains unclear. Many health professions learners succeed without a growth mindset. We find that in remediation, however, a growth mindset may be of differentially more importance. Learners who do not have a growth mindset *can* successfully remediate deficits in their mindset, but this is not ideal. Take, for example, a learner who is referred for remediation of poor communication skills on a standardized examination. She feels the test is unfair and that she does not truly have problems, but she is willing to "jump through the hoop" of the remediation process because it is required. She does successfully improve her skills on subsequent assessments. However, this is certainly not the best approach. First, it is unclear if learners without a growth mindset are seeing intrinsic value in the improvement process or are doing it solely for external validation. Indeed, it is quite possible that Olivia might have seen those skills as for use only during examinations and abandoned them the rest of the time. Second, a fixed mindset makes the remediation process harder because learners are less likely to recognize their deficits (needing the remediation coach to spend extra time pointing out issues, to make up for the lack of insight) and less ready to jump into activities to build skills. The learner buy-in certainly facilitates remediation processes and is much more likely to occur when the learner possesses a growth mindset regarding the task at hand.

In Vignette 5, Olivia's deficit (clinical reasoning) is a far-reaching issue that may be unrelated to her problems with mindset. But her response to her need for remediation is likely evidence of lack of a growth mindset and affects the remediation process. There are some clues that a learner may not have a growth mindset in a given situation:

- Learner is defensive about his deficits.
- Learner is resigned ("I'll just never be good at this").
- Learner verbalizes generalizations about characteristics or is not behaviorally anchored in observations of others ("Gio is a good communicator," rather than, "Gio really put that patient at ease with his calm tone" or "Nisha is so smart," rather than, "Nisha studies a lot and it shows").
- Learner prefers to continue skill-building in areas where she is already strong, rather than addressing weaker areas.

The summary of these clues is that the learner does not believe he can learn and grow in certain areas, potentially because of an assumption that his capacity is fixed. Defensive learners, especially, are often stuck in a fixed mindset. They may interpret constructive feedback as commentary on their intrinsic skills or competency and see this as a sign that they are not believed to be capable of meeting standards. For some learners, constructive feedback or other comments on performance are not viewed as efforts to help them improve behaviors and actions, but instead as negative comments on them as people. This may manifest as a defensive response to the information.

Defensiveness, as well as the other comments and behaviors described, reveals a lack of insight about one's capacity to learn and improve. Some experts argue that capacity to change in clinical practice is based on a combination of motivation and insight, and that absence of insight can cause some deficits to be irremediable.[33] Certainly, insight and attitude—and metacognition more broadly—have profound and far-reaching effects on the remediation process. Winston and colleagues described learner feedback on critical aspects of remediation programs. The majority centered on the programs' focus on enhancing metacognitive and affective skills: "changes in ways of thinking and studying," "development as flexible, reflective learners," and "emphasis on attitude and motivation."[27]

So, what can we do about mindset problems in remediation? Clearly a fixed mindset makes remediation work more challenging. Ideally, we would help guide learners toward a growth mindset. In Vignette 5, Olivia may be too defensive or stressed to be able to internalize efforts to help her shift her mindset. For that reason, implementing the overt techniques described in Chapter 4 to enhance the growth mindset (e.g., teaching about neuroplasticity) may be unsuccessful and possibly even backfire if they serve to alienate Olivia. A better approach may be to focus on the relationship—having her remediation coach demonstrate genuine interest in Olivia as a person and validate her feelings of frustration while coaching her through the skills practice—and allow Olivia to develop trust and respect for the remediation coach, which may well seep over into the skill and the remediation itself. The real-life "Olivia" from this example actually found the repeat assessment experience much more fun and engaging after doing this remediation work. She reached out to her remediation coach with excitement regarding her final evaluations; this may indicate that seeing the benefits of the process helped Olivia recognize in retrospect the value of a commitment to seeking help and improving one's skills—and, by extension, a growth mindset—to her long-term success. In this way, the growth mindset may be something that the remediation process can develop, even if it is not tackled head-on in the process.

Practical tips for working with struggling learners who have trouble with a fixed mindset include the following:

- Focus on the relationship.
- Attend to affective components of the learner's communications; validate feelings of frustration, anger, etc.
- Do not mention mindset up front; unlike in other domains of remediation in which naming the challenge and linking it to phases in the framework may help the learner via metacognition, naming a fixed mindset can feel threatening if the learner is not ready to hear it.

- Maintain high standards.
- Especially early on, guide the learner to see specific, demonstrable outcomes of improving the skill (e.g., improved patient outcomes), as she may not have sufficient internal motivation for the task.
- Utilize the modeling behaviors described in Chapter 4.
  - First, normalize the process of wanting to improve and asking for help doing so:
    - Consider offering personal stories that demonstrate how you as a remediation coach have improved your own skills. ("I used to have such a hard time hearing heart murmurs—I never identified a single one correctly when I was a student, but I really worked at it and got some coaching, and now I catch subtle murmurs all the time, which feels great.")
    - Consider introducing stories of other successful individuals who seek out help. (We often encourage learners to read Atul Gawande's 2011 *New Yorker* piece on coaching[34] as mentioned in Chapter 12.)
  - Second, praise effort and hard work, as well as improvement and progress, not specific outcomes. ("This is fantastic—your differential diagnosis there was so much broader than the last one you did" versus "You got the answer right!")
- When noting deficits, tie behaviors to observed responses and invite reflection. ("When you smiled while delivering the diagnosis, I saw the patient withdraw. What did you notice in that moment? Why do you think she reacted that way?")
- Tie constructive feedback to specific, actionable behaviors. ("When you introduce yourself and shake the patient's hand, make sure you are making eye contact.")
- Remember that learners will not have the same mindset in all situations; be on the lookout for areas where the learner has a growth mindset, then highlight and play those up for the learner.
- Be realistic; this work will often move more slowly than remediation work with learners with a growth mindset. Taking on too big of a challenge can reaffirm the learner's fixed mindset if he fails to achieve the goals.

Resilience

A lack of resilience may be implicated in two distinct ways in remediation cases. Either a lack of resilience may have caused the learner to have difficulty pushing through on challenging tasks and therefore demonstrating competence, leading to the need for remediation (a cause of the deficit), or lack of resilience may make it challenging for learners to invest in the work required to remediate other deficits (a barrier to addressing the deficit). The former issue is often related to mental health and other psychological concerns, including lack of meaning in one's work, overwhelming personal obligations, and the like. Cultivating resilience in these settings is important, though outside the scope of this chapter.

For learners who have other deficits but lack the resilience to engage fully in the necessary steps to remediate the deficit, the remediation process is likely to feel extremely burdensome, even if they see the value of working to improve their skills. Many remediating learners have experienced repeated disappointments in their academic careers and have become habituated to feel frustrated and let down by attempts to address the issues. We frequently encounter learners who are not surprised by their referral for remediation (unlike their fixed mindset compatriots) but lack the energy or drive to engage in the work. There are some clues that problems with resilience may be interfering with a learner's remediation:

- Learner seems disengaged or distant.
- Learner does not seem to derive enjoyment or other positive emotions from successes.
- Learner appears fatigued or describes juggling numerous obligations.

The best approach to working with learners in this situation is, again, to emphasize the relationship with the remediation coach and address the emotional challenges. Supporting resilience in the challenging setting of remediation work is best accomplished via a comfortable, enthusiastic relationship in which the learner strongly feels the remediation coach is unconditionally there to support him, and in which that remediation coach encourages reflection and personal awareness during each step of the process. One valuable approach for this work is the appreciative coaching model, in which the coach focuses on learners' strengths to help address deficits.[35] In the appreciative coaching model, rather than emphasizing what is going wrong, the coach asks the learner to describe her strengths and then envision the ideal scenario. The two then work to map out proactive strategies to leverage the learner's strengths to close the gap between reality and ideal. The approach fits perfectly with the resiliency remediation situation. This does not mean the remediation coach does not give honest, constructive feedback (always important in the remediation process), but rather that the emphasis is on starting from a place of strength, rather than weakness (avoiding the "deficit model").

Note that this work is also hard for remediation coaches. Promoting resilience for them requires a good sense of community with other remediation coaches, as well as faculty development targeting the common challenges and highlights of the experience. Because of the confidentiality usually inherent to the process, remediation coaches are often not recognized for their hard work, and it can feel like a thankless job; institutional efforts to recognize, appreciate, and validate remediation coaches' work will help promote resilience for them.

Practical tips for working with struggling learners who lack resilience include the following:

- Make the relationship between remediation coach and learner the top priority.
- Emphasize reflection after each task.
- Start from places of strength and build upward (appreciative coaching model).
- Attend to and validate emotion; do not gloss over it or try to distract the learner from it.
- Address fatigue and emotional exhaustion first, then continue addressing them throughout the remediation process. Learners may need a time out from their program or curriculum to address burnout before they can proceed.
- Constantly seek out systemic factors contributing to lack of resilience; sometimes changing a clinical schedule or team can dramatically impact a learner's readiness to engage.

Comparing the Relationship in Growth Mindset Versus Resilience Challenge Situations

In both the growth mindset and the resilience situations described, the learner–remediation coach relationship is the foundation on which to build successful work, but the type of relationship and the skills the remediation coach employs will likely be different for different scenarios. For learners with a fixed mindset, for example, the relationship needs to feel especially nonthreatening. Many learners who do not have a growth mindset will feel they do not need help. Confronting them with their need can be off-putting and disruptive to the relationship. This often means that the remediation coach needs to introduce constructive feedback more slowly, in a more measured way, and that reflective (metacognitive) conversations may need to be subtler and occur later. Learners with a fixed mindset who are upset about undergoing remediation may have adversarial feelings toward the process or the institutional leadership that deemed them as "failing." The goal for the remediation coach here is to get on the learner's team in that perceived conflict. This does not mean throwing the leadership under the bus or questioning the validity of the assessment's outcome—that would be counterproductive and confusing for the learner—but it does mean aligning with the learner from the start. This is accomplished by focusing on the shared goals and tabling efforts to help learners be more reflective. With Olivia, for example, the remediation coach might say, "It sounds like there are lots of things that have contributed to you not getting the grade you want. The goal we both have now is for you to get a better grade the second time around. So, let's talk about how we can achieve that." Any efforts to help the learner see her own role in her struggles (reflection) may be poorly received in the beginning of the process. Investigating the learner's backstory early in the relationship may make the learner feel accused, like some part of his background is being blamed for the performance issue; therefore, we also recommend holding off on exploring much personal background until the learner has gotten a chance to start working in a concrete way toward his goal (passing the institution's assessment) and feels more trusting of the remediation coach. Finally, because they do not recognize their need for improvement, learners with mindset challenges are most likely to be willing to engage in the process if the remediation coach is someone perceived by the learner as an expert in the domain being addressed, since someone who is not clearly expert in that area will have "nothing to teach me."

Learners struggling with resilience, however, need a different kind of relationship. Here, there is no need to wait to push for reflection or to hold off on exploring personal stories and contributions to performance. There is also no requirement to dole out constructive feedback more cautiously. In fact, the nonresilient learner often appreciates a very open, honest relationship with the remediation coach, which can feel like a necessary support, as long as the remediation coach is cautious not to push the learner too far or deliver feedback the learner is not ready for, given her lack of emotional reserve. Remediation faculty are not (usually) therapists, nor do they usually have special training in wellness, but their emphasis in working with these learners should be to get to know and support the whole person, not just the challenge at hand (Table 13.1).

CHALLENGES WITH MAL PHASES

Learners may struggle with any phase of the MAL model. Here we highlight challenges with the planning phase and the learning phase. Learners also may struggle with the assessing and adjusting phases, but we do not describe a specific approach to remediation of those challenges here because it is largely the same as the process described previously for the learner with a "typical struggle," just potentially lengthier and more intensive.

Planning

Planning is frequently a challenging phase for learners requiring remediation. Especially at times of transition to new tasks or new levels of responsibility, learners can feel overwhelmed and may have a hard time mapping the gap between their performance and the competency standard and then selecting areas for learning. Furthermore, being

TABLE 13.1 Optimal Remediation Relationships for Learners Struggling With Growth Mindset and Resilience Issues.		
	Lack of Growth Mindset	**Lack of Resilience**
Optimal remediation coach characteristics to achieve learner buy-in	Remediation coach is perceived as expert in the domain being addressed	Remediation coach is perceived as warm, relatable, understanding
Time to explore and address issues related to mental health, substance use, significant stressors	Immediately	Immediately
Time to explore personal backstory and prior experiences	Not until relationship has formed	Early and often
Initial focus of the work	Focused, targetable skills	Emotions
Nature of feedback	Begin with targeted, behaviorally anchored reinforcing feedback and ease into constructive feedback more slowly	Supportive and open throughout, building from strengths, but watching out for emotional overload
Encouragement of metacognition	Not until learner starts to see skill improvement (and therefore recognizes value in the work)	Early and often
Metaphor for relationship	Alignment; team	Support network

noted to be struggling leads to increased stress that can prove paralyzing in the process of appropriate planning.

Earlier in this chapter, we outlined clues that a learner may be struggling with the planning phase in a "typical" way. Those same clues will also apply in a setting with a learner who is struggling more significantly.

Many learners who struggle in this phase probably have insight but are unable to use it to get back on track because they are overwhelmed by stress. The key to managing this challenge is again to emphasize a comfortable, trusting relationship that feels low-stakes and, to the extent possible, formative for the learner. Once the stress is minimized, the learner can shift that cognitive bandwidth to more appropriate planning strategies, provided the insight is present. For learners who lack metacognition in this realm and are unable to plan even when stress is largely reduced, it may be worth spending some time thinking about direct or indirect approaches to mindset or motivation (see Chapter 4). Tackling challenges with planning in a remediation setting may be less straightforward than in a "typical struggle" scenario, because the learner may be working with strongly ingrained maladaptive strategies. Doing a careful and thorough assessment of the learner's usual approach and then creating small "chunks" of work, slowly progressing over time, will often help these learners develop new habits; trying to make large shifts at once is likely to be overwhelming to the learner and unsuccessful.

Practical tips for remediating planning phase issues include the following:
- Use the process to model planning for the learner.
  - Perform a thorough review of the learner's organizational techniques/structures, including observing the learner utilizing them in real time if possible.
  - Set detailed schedules for your work together and the learner's other tasks.
  - Ask the learner to keep a record of plans and follow-through (e.g., "use Bates to review abdominal exam for 10 minutes tonight" → "I did this!") so as to build connections and metacognition around successful strategies.
  - "Chunk" tasks into very small pieces and set realistic expectations (probably lower than you would initially think).
- Allow self-direction within guardrails.
  - Ask the learner to weigh in on preferred options (i.e., of organizational schemes) that will work with his learning preferences, but do not provide too many choices; limit to two or three.
  - Conduct frequent (okay to be brief; we sometimes use e-mail) check-ins on the learner's accomplishment of tasks or subtasks; with improvement, space these out slowly.

Learning

The learning phase is a challenge for many learners, but in the remediation context it often manifests as a significant pattern of "inability to put the pieces together" or to transfer knowledge. Most learners, by the time they have reached this point in their education, have taken so many tests that "book knowledge" is less challenging to come by than the ability to learn how to apply information and process it.

A common learning phase problem in remediation settings is challenges with clinical reasoning. Medical student Joel in Vignette 4 struggled with his differential diagnoses and constantly landed on "zebras." This is a problem with illness scripts because Joel does not have appropriate illness scripts that include prioritization of the most likely etiologies of common syndromes.

Modifying their thinking to enable learners to reason more appropriately and apply knowledge across varied contexts requires use of thoughtful, guided exercises to work through one's approach to a case aloud, with purposeful reflection at the end (e.g., "What is your problem representation now that we have talked through this case? What other kinds of cases would this apply to?") This process can be painstaking and slow, but learners can gain increasing autonomy managing their own remediation work as their metacognitive skills improve with practice. Unlike remediation of other deficits (communication, physical examination, etc.), actual practice in authentic workplace settings might not be the most efficient way to remediate clinical reasoning deficits; classroom- or office-based step-by-step discussions of learners' evolving thinking around a case can be the best way to target this deficit. The key is to get the learner to dive into the thinking, over and over. Coaches should make sure that they revisit the same concepts (with minor variations) multiple times, because this promotes retention and transfer of knowledge. The process of using drills to test learners on their skills promotes learning via the testing effect, is much more effective than continued studying,[36] and enhances retention through retrieval.[37,38]

Practical tips for remediating learning phase issues include the following:
- Spend less time exploring the reasons for the struggles (learners often have no idea) and spend more time with skill building. Clinical reasoning drills are helpful.
- Revisit concepts several times.
- Use advance organizers, analogies, and the like that promote development of connections. Avoid mnemonics that can lead to memorization without understanding or application.
- Assign homework to practice skills at home and bring in records of the work.

CONCLUSION

The MAL model can be useful in helping gauge a learner's challenges and developing an approach to addressing them. Trying to determine the combination of phases and characteristics at play in any given deficit will be key to helping the learner. Although some learners may have challenges that cannot easily be organized into the MAL phases, this approach represents a good starting point for work with struggling learners.

How will we know if we are successful? Unfortunately, remediation is a newcomer to the empirical research world (work spanning only a few decades); the relative infrequency of the issue, as well as the need for privacy, also contribute to a paucity of data surrounding outcomes. We do know that many education leaders are not confident in the success of their remediation approaches[12,24] and that improvements are not necessarily sustained,[7] though remediation efforts may decrease attrition rates.[39] One study examined learners' outcomes in internal medicine residency after needing remediation during their internal medicine clerkship in medical school; the majority of these learners did not have issues noted in internship, but the remediated learners were significantly more likely to have problems than their nonremediated peers.[40] There is definitely room for improvement. A benefit of using the MAL model to try to fill this gap is that it simultaneously tackles two issues—identifying the learner's area of struggle and emphasizing metacognitive aspects of the learning process—both of which are key to remediation's success. The time investment is significant, but the efforts feel worthwhile when the learner's improvement is obvious.

TAKE-HOME POINTS

1. All learners will struggle to learn content and skills relevant to their professions; these struggles are normal, and the feedback required to help these learners attain proficiency is an expected part of medical training. Some learners, however, veer farther off course and require additional assistance. These individuals are termed "struggling learners."
2. The MAL model can be applied to both typical struggles and "struggling learners," but identifying which is at play in a given situation is valuable because this can guide the approach and the mobilization of appropriate resources. The best resource for a "struggling learner" is a remediation coach with enhanced coaching skills and special skills in relationship building.
3. "Struggling learners" can have challenges with any of the characteristics or stages of the MAL model. Ones that are especially common are issues related to mindset and resilience, as well as challenges with planning, assessing, and adjusting.

QUESTIONS FOR FURTHER THOUGHT

1. When was the last time you worked with a learner who was struggling, you felt, to master the content you were teaching? Was it a typical struggle or further outside the norm? Where in the MAL model do you think the learner had the greatest challenge? How would you approach the situation again if you could go back in time?
2. How can institutions leverage MAL principles to design institutional frameworks for supporting struggling learners?

ANNOTATED BIBLIOGRAPHY

1. Guerrasio J, Garrity MJ, Aagaard EM. Learner deficits and academic outcomes of medical students, residents, fellows, and attending physicians referred to a remediation program, 2006-2012. *Acad Med.* 2014;89(2):352-358.
   This is possibly the most comprehensive published review of a remediation program and gives insightful information about who the learners are, what they struggled with, and how they did with remediation; note that this is just one institution's experience, but many aspects may be generalizable.
2. Hauer KE, Ciccone A, Henzel TR, et al. Remediation of the deficiencies of physicians across the continuum from medical school to practice: a thematic review of the literature. *Acad Med.* 2009;84(12):1822-1832.
   This paper reviewed published literature on remediation and developed frameworks for thinking about approaches to the work; several pieces of research have been published since this review, but it remains a great resource for understanding the field broadly.
3. Kalet A, Chou C, eds. *Remediation in Medical Education: A Mid-Course Correction.* New York, NY: Springer; 2014.
   This book describes numerous aspects of remediation, ranging from skill development in coaches to designing structures to support remediation work to developing plans to remediate specific deficits; it is our go-to resource when

someone needs guidance on how to work with a struggling learner.

4. Patel RS, Tarrant C, Bonas S, Shaw RL. Medical students' personal experience of high-stakes failure: case studies using interpretative phenomenological analysis. *BMC Med Educ*. 2015;15:86.

This is one of a handful of papers investigating the learner's perspective on failure and the remediation process, and one of the most recent.

REFERENCES

1. Christie S, Green M. How to improve your time management skills. *BMJ*. 2012;344:e1156.
2. Lovell B. What do we know about coaching in medical education? A literature review. *Med Educ*. 2018;52:376-390.
3. Cutting MF, Saks NS. Twelve tips for utilizing principles of learning to support medical education. *Med Teach*. 2012;34(1):20-24.
4. Gooding HC, Mann K, Armstrong E. Twelve tips for applying the science of learning to health professions education. *Med Teach*. 2017;39(1):26-31.
5. Ellaway RH, Chou CL, Kalet AL. Situating remediation: accommodating success and failure in medical education systems. *Acad Med*. 2018;93(3):391-398.
6. Guerrasio J. *Remediation of the Struggling Medical Learner*. 2nd ed. Irwin, PA: Association for Hospital Medical Education; 2018.
7. Pell G, Fuller R, Homer M, Roberts T. Is short-term remediation after OSCE failure sustained? A retrospective analysis of the longitudinal attainment of underperforming students in OSCE assessments. *Med Teach*. 2012;34(2):146-150.
8. Zbieranowski I, Takahashi SG, Verma S, Spadafora SM. Remediation of residents in difficulty: a retrospective 10-year review of the experience of a postgraduate board of examiners. *Acad Med*. 2013;88(1):111-116.
9. Guerrasio J, Brooks E, Rumack CM, Christensen A, Aagaard EM. Association of characteristics, deficits, and outcomes of residents placed on probation at one institution, 2002-2012. *Acad Med*. 2016;91(3):382-387.
10. Frellsen SL, Baker EA, Papp KK, Durning SJ. Medical school policies regarding struggling medical students during the internal medicine clerkships: results of a national survey. *Acad Med*. 2008;83(9):876-881.
11. Kinnear B, Bensman R, Held J, O'Toole J, Schauer D, Warm E. Critical deficiency ratings in milestone assessment: a review and case study. *Acad Med*. 2017;92(6):820-826.
12. Hauer KE, Ciccone A, Henzel TR, et al. Remediation of the deficiencies of physicians across the continuum from medical school to practice: a thematic review of the literature. *Acad Med*. 2009;84(12):1822-1832.
13. Guerrasio J, Garrity MJ, Aagaard EM. Learner deficits and academic outcomes of medical students, residents, fellows, and attending physicians referred to a remediation program, 2006-2012. *Acad Med*. 2014;89(2):352-358.
14. Kalet A, Pusic M. Defining and assessing competence. In: Kalet A, Chou C, eds. *Remediation in Medical Education: A Mid-Course Correction*. New York, NY: Springer; 2014.
15. Hemmer PA, Pangaro L. The effectiveness of formal evaluation sessions during clinical clerkships in better identifying students with marginal funds of knowledge. *Acad Med*. 1997;72(7):641-643.
16. Hemmer PA, Hawkins R, Jackson JL, Pangaro LN. Assessing how well three evaluation methods detect deficiencies in medical students' professionalism in two settings of an internal medicine clerkship. *Acad Med*. 2000;75(2):167-173.
17. Schwind CJ, Williams RG, Boehler ML, Dunnington GL. Do individual attendings' post-rotation performance ratings detect residents' clinical performance deficiencies? *Acad Med*. 2004;79(5):453-457.
18. Bierer SB, Dannefer EF, Tetzlaff JE. Time to loosen the apron strings: cohort-based evaluation of a learner-driven remediation model at one medical school. *J Gen Intern Med*. 2015;30(9):1339-1343.
19. White CB, Ross PT, Gruppen LD. Remediating students' failed OSCE performances at one school: the effects of self-assessment, reflection, and feedback. *Acad Med*. 2009;84(5):651-654.
20. Kalet A, Zabar S. Preparing to conduct remediation. In: Kalet A, Chou C, eds. *Remediation in Medical Education: A Mid-Course Correction*. New York, NY: Springer; 2014.
21. Kelly S, Dennick R. Evidence of gender bias in true-false-abstain medical examinations. *BMC Med Educ*. 2009;9:32.
22. Woolf K, Potts HW, McManus IC. Ethnicity and academic performance in UK trained doctors and medical students: systematic review and meta-analysis. *BMJ*. 2011;342:d901.
23. Yeates P, O'Neill P, Mann K, Byrne G, Eva K. Bias in assessing trainees' clinical competence: the influence of assessors' recent experiences of other performances on present assessment scores. *Lancet*. 2014;383(Special Issue):S113.
24. Hauer KE, Lucey CR. Core clerkship grading: the illusion of objectivity. *Acad Med*. 2019;94(4):469-472. Aug. doi:10.1097/ACM.0000000000002413.
25. Teherani A, Hauer KE, Fernandez A, King Jr TE, Lucey C. How small differences in assessed clinical performance amplify to large differences in grades and awards: a cascade with serious consequences for students underrepresented in medicine. *Acad Med*. 2018;93(9):1286-1292.
26. Kalet A, Chou C, eds. *Remediation in Medical Education: A Mid-Course Correction*. New York, NY: Springer; 2014.
27. Winston KA, Van Der Vleuten CP, Scherpbier AJ. At-risk medical students: implications of students' voice for the theory and practice of remediation. *Med Educ*. 2010;44(10):1038-1047.
28. Patel RS, Tarrant C, Bonas S, Shaw RL. Medical students' personal experience of high-stakes failure: case studies using interpretative phenomenological analysis. *BMC Med Educ*. 2015;15:86.
29. Kalet A, Tewksbury L, Ogilvie JB, Yingling S. An example of a remediation program. In: Kalet A, Chou C, eds. *Remediation in Medical Education: A Mid-Course Correction*. New York, NY: Springer; 2014.

30. Kalet A, Guerrasio J, Chou C. Twelve tips for developing and maintaining a remediation program in medical education. *Med Teach*. 2016;38(8):787-792.

31. Blackwell LS, Trzesniewski KH, Dweck CS. Implicit theories of intelligence predict achievement across an adolescent transition: a longitudinal study and an intervention. *Child Dev*. 2007;78(1):246-263.

32. Sisk VF, Burgoyne AP, Sun J, Butler JL, Macnamara BN. To what extent and under which circumstances are growth mind-sets important to academic achievement? Two meta-analyses. *Psychol Sci*. 2018;29(4):549-571.

33. Hays RB, Jolly BC, Caldon LJ, et al. Is insight important? Measuring capacity to change performance. *Med Educ*. 2002;36(10):965-971.

34. Gawande A. Personal best. *New Yorker*. 2011;3:44-53.

35. Kemp White M, Barnett P. A five step model for appreciative coaching: a positive process for remediation. In: Kalet A, Chou C, eds. *Remediation in Medical Education: A Mid-Course Correction*. New York, NY: Springer; 2014.

36. Larsen DP, Butler AC, Roediger HL III. Repeated testing improves long-term retention relative to repeated study: a randomised controlled trial. *Med Educ*. 2009;43(12):1174-1181.

37. Roediger HL III, Butler AC. The critical role of retrieval practice in long-term retention. *Trends Cogn Sci*. 2011;15(1):20-27.

38. Kornell N, Hays MJ, Bjork RA. Unsuccessful retrieval attempts enhance subsequent learning. *J Exp Psychol Learn Mem Cogn*. 2009;35(6):989-998.

39. Schwed AC, Lee SL, Salcedo ES, et al. Association of general surgery resident remediation and program director attitudes with resident attrition. *JAMA Surg*. 2017;152(12):1134-1140.

40. Lavin B, Pangaro L. Internship ratings as a validity outcome measure for an evaluation system to identify inadequate clerkship performance. *Acad Med*. 1998;73(9):998-1002.

How Can the Master Adaptive Learner Model Advance Leadership Development?

Maya M. Hammoud, MD, MBA; Susan M. Cox, MD; and Katherine R. Zurales, MD, MBA

LEARNING OBJECTIVES

1. Describe the importance of leadership development for physicians.
2. Apply the Master Adaptive Learner model as a framework for leadership development in learners.
3. Summarize the intersection of leadership skills with those of the master adaptive learner.

CHAPTER OUTLINE

CHAPTER SUMMARY

In this chapter, we review leadership skills for physicians and present the Master Adaptive Learner (MAL) model as a framework for leadership development. We discuss the different phases of the MAL model with their application to leadership development. In addition, we present a summary of how the skills of being a leader overlap with the skills of being a master adaptive learner.

INTRODUCTION

"Leadership and learning are indispensable to each other."[1]

This line was central in a speech to be given in late 1963 by former President John F. Kennedy. Though the speech went undelivered, his strong leadership through pivotal times in the United States' history exhibited the interconnected nature of leadership and learning. In her recent book *Leadership: In Turbulent Times,* Doris Kearns Goodwin chronicled this critical connection for other important presidents as well: Abraham Lincoln, Theodore Roosevelt, Franklin Delano Roosevelt, and Lyndon B. Johnson.[2] As Goodwin demonstrated, continuous deep learning played a central part in the development of their leadership abilities.

In this chapter, we first examine the importance of leadership development for future physicians and review key skills necessary for effective leadership. We then explore how the Master Adaptive Learner (MAL) model makes an excellent framework for leadership development. Finally, we conclude with a discussion of the intersection between leadership development and the MAL model.

WHY IS LEADERSHIP IMPORTANT FOR MEDICAL STUDENTS, RESIDENTS, AND PHYSICIANS?

Medical school graduates are entering a dynamic health care system that requires them to lead in multiple ways. Patient care necessitates not only that they are able to apply clinical expertise, but that they can collaborate with, coordinate, and influence interdisciplinary teams. Beginning to address the complex, fragmented health care system requires physicians to serve as change agents, using their voices and experience to improve care delivery, affordability, and quality (see Chapter 15). Finally, physicians are inherently looked to as models of leadership. They set the tone for the team, model expectations of behavior, and contribute significantly to the culture of the clinical environment.[3] Despite evidence showing that high-quality physician leadership improves patient and health care system outcomes, physicians are often not prepared to lead due to a lack of formal training in medical school and residency.[4] As a result, leadership development is beginning to be recognized as an important component of undergraduate medical education,[5] with application of the MAL model supporting and enhancing this development.

To meet the growing needs of the health care system, learners must be equipped with leadership skills, qualities, and behaviors that can be used in any setting, regardless of their rank or title. Numerous leadership theories have been recognized over time, such as charismatic, transformational, transactional, servant leadership, and more.[6] Although some individuals choose a predominant theory to guide their actions, others believe a great leader is one who chooses the best approach for the desired goals. Regardless of the theory or approach an individual chooses to follow, there are similarities in skills that are common across many of these theories.

Therefore the next section focuses on those general leadership skills that intersect multiple theories in order to guide learners in building a foundation for great leadership.

WHAT DOES EFFECTIVE LEADERSHIP LOOK LIKE?

In "Why Doctors Need Leadership Training" published in *Harvard Business Review,* Rubenstein and colleagues identified two key competencies that are critical for future physicians: interpersonal literacy (an understanding of personal relationships) and systems literacy (an understanding of the health care system).[4] Leaders with interpersonal literacy have a high degree of emotional intelligence, empower high-performing teams, and communicate effectively. Leaders with systems literacy leverage their knowledge of the health care system to create change. Although described separately here, the skills required to attain both interpersonal and systems literacy often overlap and ultimately enhance one another. In this section, we highlight some of the key attributes of effective leaders within each literacy. Medical educators can assist learners in applying the MAL model to each of the following literacies to help learners build foundational leadership skills throughout undergraduate medical education.

Interpersonal Literacy
Emotional Intelligence

The most effective leaders are self-aware. They embrace the MAL process by taking the time to reflect, self-assess, and adjust their actions and behaviors based on internal and external feedback. They have a high degree of emotional intelligence—the ability to recognize and manage their own emotions as well as the emotions of a group. The four domains of emotional intelligence include self-awareness, self-management, social awareness, and relationship management.[7,8] The most effective leaders hone expertise in these domains to model the behavior they seek to bring out in others. They realize that, before they can lead others, they must first be able to look within and adapt their own understanding, attitudes, and actions. The most effective leaders strive to constantly learn from both successes and failures in order to improve their own performance and ultimately that of the team. Finally, they have a strong sense of purpose, utilize goal setting to achieve that purpose, and consistently reflect on progress toward those goals.

Teamwork

Effective leaders recognize that followership is equally as important as leadership for optimal performance.[9] Therefore they strive to serve as team players, or followers, who also inspire passion, purpose, and high-quality performance among team members.[9] Learners naturally fall into a followership role as members of a larger team during training; nonetheless, they have the ability to influence the team. Thus training is an optimal time to use the MAL process to hone teamwork skills.

At a high level, teamwork consists of collaborating with others and cooperating to reach a shared goal. Effective leaders serving as team players trust their team members, embrace constructive conflict, and go the extra mile to help others.[10] They are actively engaged and frequently lead by example, supporting their teammates through daily tasks, but also take the initiative to step up during challenging times. Setting their focus on team building, they work to create a sense of connection and belonging within their teams to cultivate loyalty and trust. Effective leaders realize that empowered teams—teams made up of individuals who take initiative, confidently suggest bold ideas, and balance individual demands with needs of the team—are more productive and proactive.[10] To empower their teams, leaders collaborate with their teammates to set stretch goals. They encourage the team to utilize their strengths to reach them. The most effective leaders coach and develop others, and their significant investment in people often results in superior outcomes.[11]

Communication

Successfully achieving a mission requires coordinating multiple people in ambiguous, constantly changing environments. To do so, the most effective leaders communicate frequently and openly, utilizing the MAL process to adapt their communication style to varying situations and audiences. Regular, open communication fosters trust within the team, inviting innovative ideas and opening the door for feedback.[9] Effective leaders articulate bold visions with clear objectives and expectations, ensuring that all team members are aligned and know their mission. They also serve as coaches, providing frequent check-ins on performance and regularly communicating both positive reinforcement and constructive feedback in an open, objective manner.[10] They are willing to engage in critical, sometimes difficult conversations. When conflicts arise, they resolve them quickly, directly, and fairly to increase cooperation.[11] Active listening and understanding the needs of their audience is critical in helping leaders tailor their communication to enhance its effectiveness. Ultimately, just as critical for effective leadership is a willingness to listen and receive feedback.

Systems Literacy

The health care system today is fragmented, composed of multiple stakeholders with complex, sometimes conflicting incentives. Changing this system to improve health outcomes and manage costs requires leaders who have a strong understanding of the industry landscape and who are able to take a high-level view of the system. These leaders can identify and critically appraise problems. Within an understanding of systems-level structures and drivers, they use the MAL process to identify gaps, develop solutions, and ultimately serve as change agents.[4] They are prepared with change management skills, including the ability to engage a variety of stakeholders, articulate a vision and direction, and take action steps to implement that vision. These change management skills are critical to effectively navigating the adjusting phase of the MAL process that makes positive tangible changes based on the preceding learning. In addition, they are well versed in quality and safety processes, such as lean management, process improvement, and impact analysis.[12] Strong systems literacy is central to effective leaders' ability to leverage these skill sets and create change.

In the following section, we discuss how the MAL model can be applied to the development of leadership qualities and skills.

MASTER ADAPTIVE LEARNER MODEL AS A FRAMEWORK FOR LEADERSHIP DEVELOPMENT

Vignette

Hannah is a fourth-year medical student on her internal medicine subinternship. She is assigned to a team that is composed of the following: attending, resident, intern, third-year medical student, nurse, caseworker, and PharmD student. Anticipating being an intern in a few months, she is stepping into a leadership role to manage two patients (a 60-year-old man with congestive heart failure and a 72-year-old woman with poorly controlled diabetes). For her last subinternship, she felt she had a hard time "decoding" what the attending and her senior resident wanted from her. In talking to her coach, they identified that at times she struggles with emotional intelligence.

She sets two goals for herself. First, she would like to lead by working collaboratively with the interdisciplinary team caring for their patients. Second, she would like to receive feedback on how she is performing on perceiving emotions.

1. What leadership skills and qualities will Hannah need to reach her goals for the subinternship?

2. How can Hannah use the Master Adaptive Learner model to reach her goals and improve her leadership capabilities?

"The 21st century physician leader must be equipped with a new toolkit of skills for the leadership agility necessary for them to respond proactively to rapidly changing environments."[13] Unfortunately, there is incongruity between leadership development as it exists and the skills leaders actually need. This mismatch is enormous and widening.[14] Using the MAL model to develop leadership skills will help learners identify the right gaps that need development early on, particularly beginning before or during medical school.[12] Stoller highlighted factors underscoring the need to systematically develop physician leaders, including addressing the unhelpful perception that physicians are more likely to value autonomy versus collaboration.[15] The health care system is a challenging environment that makes it difficult to lead, and education programs may not pay adequate attention to training learners on leadership competencies. Being master adaptive learners will help future physicians identify and develop the leadership skills and traits needed to navigate those complex systems because many of the features of good leaders resonate with the MAL framework (Table 14.1).

In the following sections, we present a plan for using the MAL model to foster long-lasting individual leadership development that results in leadership agility. Additionally, we explore how Hannah can use this model to improve her leadership capabilities with a focus self-awareness.

Planning Phase: Diagnosis of Leadership (In)competencies

One approach to applying the MAL model to leadership development might occur during the planning phase. The learner—ideally with the support of a coach—describes what makes a great leader. Next, the learner develops a list of traits, characteristics, and skills that define a great leader. Traits such as honesty, vision, integrity, exceptional communication, empathy, attentive listening, fairness, impartiality, courage, responsiveness, and accountability are just a few to consider. Then the learner identifies a gap that may be present in her own leadership core characteristics.

There are many resources and tools to help the learner with self-assessment, such as the Myers Briggs Personality Inventory (https://www.myersbriggs.org/my-mbti-personality-type/take-the-mbti-instrument/), the Big 5 Personality test, StrengthsFinder, the HIGH 5 Test (https://high5test.com/), and 16 Personalities (https://www.16personalities.com/free-personality-test). There is also a self-assessment tool for core values (https://www.whatsnext.com/life-values-self-assessment-test/). It is important to remember that self-assessment can be flawed and that multisource feedback such as a 360-degree review might provide a more informed self-assessment (see Chapter 6).

The learner should review and reflect on her core characteristics and values. Then she should create a personal vision statement considering her prioritized core characteristics and values. This will help her to set her goals. This step is essential for entering the learning cycle. In Hannah's case, she has difficulty with self-awareness and, in particular, perceiving emotions. Her personal vision statement is to be a thoughtful and effective leader. She recognizes the gap in her self-awareness and that this is an area she wants to focus on in order to become an effective leader.

Phase of MAL Process	**MAL Process for Learning and Developing Leadership**	**Leadership Characteristics That Enhance MAL Development**
Planning	• Identifies the qualities of a good leader • Identifies a gap—learn about your deficiencies as a leader • Creates a personal leadership development plan	• Motivated to identify a gap • Sensitive to signals in the environment • Creates a clear vision • Sets realistic goals
Learning	• Engages with learning leadership literature, including leadership styles and skills	• Committed to self- and team improvement • Committed to adult learning pedagogy • Committed to lifelong learning
Assessing	• Practices new skills to improve leadership attributes	• Committed to feedback agility • Appreciation of teams' perspective • Desire to create high-functioning teams
Adjusting	• Adjusts and adapts styles based on feedback	• Engages in continuous performance improvement • Understands health care system • Seeks to apply learning to broader system

TABLE 14.1 Complementary Characteristics of Leaders and Master Adaptive Learners (MALs).

Goal setting is key for leadership development just as it is a key activity for the master adaptive learner. Leaders find goal setting to be important to build confidence and demonstrate competence to their team members. Leaders also use goals to assign ownership and direction to the team. Goals should be specific in order to create a means to deliberately focus leadership development. Goals should also be measurable and realistic as well as attainable. Just about any goal is attainable when steps are planned wisely and a realistic time frame is established.

Recognizing what conditions would have to exist to accomplish leadership goals is also important. Leadership goals should be skills and literacies the learner is willing and able to work toward—things the learner believes can be accomplished and wants to accomplish. Goals should be grounded within a specific time frame.

Vignette Continued

Now that Hannah has a better understanding of her leadership gaps, she sets a goal to improve her self-awareness during her fourth year. She identifies a recent *Harvard Business Review* article that focuses on the 12 elements of emotional intelligence (Fig. 14.1). She is invested in developing her emotional self-awareness and looks for other resources to help. Her coach directs her to TalentSmart, a consulting firm that offers numerous online assessment tools for individuals that can pinpoint strategies to increase emotional intelligence.

Learning Phase: Leadership Can Be Grown

The learning phase for leadership development may include formal training as well as experiential learning. There are complex leadership skills that need to become the fabric of one's identity to become sustainable. Action learning linked to real issues provides a significant context for learning. The choice of the learning experiences is guided by an attempt to decrease the self-identified leadership gaps and increase the defined leadership competence to reinforce the use and importance of the core values.

Many organizations offer leadership development programs that vary in content, time commitment, and delivery methods. There are online and face-to-face programs. Other programs use a case-based format and work with challenging case studies. Others use role modeling and experiential activities as the major pedagogy. The most effective leadership development programs build on vital lessons related to how adults learn best, with an emphasis on reflection, interaction, and application of concepts in real situations. Frequent assessment and feedback are also key.

Although there are many physician leadership development programs[16] that are associated with significantly improved self-assessed knowledge and expertise, these may be less useful for medical student learners. Very few programs address personal growth and self-awareness, which are key features of the MAL model. Other noteworthy resource examples for physician leadership development include the Harvard Business School Leadership modules on self-awareness,[17] building self-awareness with help from your team,[18] and the *Harvard Business Review*'s five ways to become more self-aware: psychometric testing, meditation,

Self-awareness	Self-management	Social awareness	Relationship management
Emotional self-awareness	Emotional self-control	Empathy	Influence
			Coach and mentor
	Adaptability		Conflict management
	Achievement orientation	Organizational awareness	Teamwork
	Positive outlook		Inspirational leadership

Fig. 14.1 **Emotional Intelligence Domains and Competencies.** (Reprinted by permission from Goleman D, Boyatzis RE. Emotional intelligence has 12 elements. Which do you need to work on? *Harvard Business Rev.* 2017;February 6. Copyright ©2017 by Harvard Business Publishing; all rights reserved.)

documenting plans and priorities, seeking feedback at work, and asking friends for direct observation and feedback.[19]

Vignette Continued

After setting leadership goals in the planning phase, Hannah shifts to the learning phase. She aims to find resources to help her accomplish her goals. Hannah reads about the four self-awareness archetypes (Fig. 14.2), and she decides to focus her attention on requesting observational feedback. She requests feedback and follow-up on her progress to achieving self-awareness.

Assessing Phase: Did It Work?

In the assessing phase, the learner applies the newly learned skills in the workplace, practicing the leadership traits that were identified as a gap, asking for feedback and practicing again. Because leadership skills can be difficult to evaluate with written examinations or formalized assessments, applying the assessing phase to leadership development can require a slightly different approach. One effective method for evaluating leadership development is seeking out real-time observation and subsequent feedback from a diverse group of colleagues and teammates. The learner can do this by asking a trusted colleague to observe her leadership behaviors and let her know how she comes across to others. The learner is pursuing candid, critical, and objective perspectives. Another strategy is to ask the colleague to point out when she is behaving in a way the learner already knows she wants to change. Healthy, constructive, formalized feedback allows the learner to clearly see her strengths and weaknesses. Feedback is also a mechanism whereby the learner can see if there is evidence that she is learning.

It is important to note that just introspection and self-reflection alone will not lead to an improvement in the learner's self-awareness. The learner needs to take the next step to iterate and apply any insights gained in the adjusting phase of the MAL model.

Vignette Continued

Eager about the prospect of reaching her leadership goals, Hannah attempts to apply the lessons she learned about self-awareness during her subinternship. Using clear communication, she articulates her objectives to her teammates and asks them to provide candid feedback. At the end of each day, she humbly and openly asks what went well, what did not, and if there were emotional clues she missed. During the adjusting phase, Hannah will apply what she has learned from the results of her teammates' day-to-day observational feedback and feedback from the 360-degree peer review.

	Low external self-awareness	High external self-awareness
High internal self-awareness	**INTROSPECTORS** They're clear on who they are but don't challenge their own views or search for blind spots by getting feedback from others. This can harm their relationships and limit their success.	**AWARE** They know who they are, what they want to accomplish, and seek out and value others' opinions. This is where leaders begin to fully realize the true benefits of self-awareness.
Low internal self-awareness	**SEEKERS** They don't yet know who they are, what they stand for, or how their teams see them. As a result, they might feel stuck or frustrated with their performance and relationships.	**PLEASERS** They can be so focused on appearing a certain way to others that they could be overlooking what matters to them. Over time, they tend to make choices that aren't in service of their own success and fulfillment.

Fig. 14.2 **The Four Self-Awareness Archetypes.** These archetypes map internal self-awareness (how well you know yourself) against external self-awareness (how well you understand how others see you). (Reprinted by permission from Eurich T. What self-awareness really is [and how to cultivate it]. *Harvard Business Rev.* 2018;January 4. Copyright ©2018 by Harvard Business Publishing; all rights reserved.)

Adjusting Phase: Continuous Performance Improvement

During the adjusting phase, the learner applies any necessary changes to her skills and practice while determining the need to adapt different skills. In other words, she incorporates what she learned into regular practice. In every situation, she should be prepared to adapt her leadership style based on the context of the situation and the people she is leading. She may need to incorporate new leadership skills. Adapting leadership styles to fit the situation is smart and strategic.

At this point, the learner should challenge herself to keep pushing to hone her desired leadership skills. The learner should self-assess if her efforts are working and ask for peer feedback on progress. Using peers, coaches, or mentors to comment on leadership style and progress with skill development is a valuable technique.

Now that we have reviewed how the MAL model can be used for the development of leadership skills, we explore how leadership skills and attributes can themselves be important catalysts for medical student development into master adaptive learners.

THE INTERSECTION OF LEADERSHIP DEVELOPMENT WITH MASTER ADAPTIVE LEARNER DEVELOPMENT

At every phase of the MAL model, leadership skills and attributes can iteratively help a learner navigate the process and develop into a master adaptive learner. In ideal leaders and ideal master adaptive learners, it can and should be difficult to disentangle where the leader ends and the learner begins. Leaders can be defined by how well they learn. The best learners demonstrate the determination and purposefulness of leaders. We now highlight skills that leaders have that may accelerate their development into master adaptive learners at each phase of the process.

In the planning and learning phases, a leader with a high level of emotional intelligence can demonstrate the self-awareness and motivation needed to identify a gap, select an opportunity for learning, and capitalize on resources for learning. As a result of his prior knowledge of reflection and goal setting, initiation of the MAL process can be jumpstarted. Compared to the beginning learner, a leader is readily able to reflect to a deeper level on his gaps, design more specific learning goals, and recalibrate when ineffective learning strategies arise due to his prior experience and skill set.

During the assessing and adjusting phases, the most important leadership qualities the learner needs are teamwork, good communication, and systems literacy. Whereas beginning learners may be hesitant to share personal areas of improvement, leaders take initiative to clearly articulate their learning goals to their teams and humbly seek diverse feedback on their performance and behaviors. An effective leader would have also built trust within the team, ensuring that teammates are honest with their feedback. Once obtaining that feedback, leaders again leverage their emotional intelligence and self-awareness to incorporate learnings into everyday practice. Finally, beginning learners may have difficulty taking a high-level view of the system; conversely, leaders capitalize on their systems knowledge to apply their personal insights and new behaviors to improving the larger system.

Foundational leadership skills have the potential to drive and hasten MAL development. Medical educators can leverage this knowledge to identify learners with inherent leadership qualities and challenge them to apply these qualities to different learning domains. Ultimately, learning and leading weave together, resulting in development of well-prepared trainees who become change agents and transform the health care system.

CONCLUSION

Leadership development for physicians is important for their roles in complex and continually changing health care systems. This should start as early as possible in medical school so that medical students learn, apply, and improve upon necessary skills early and as they progress through their careers. Because these skills can vary over time depending on the situation, and honing them requires continuous deep learning, using the MAL model can be an effective framework for the development of these skills. In addition, many of the skills and attributes needed to be an effective leader are similar to those needed to be a master adaptive learner. Therefore the development of leadership skills in learners early on also contributes to their development into master adaptive learners.

Leaders like JFK, Lincoln, the Roosevelts, and LBJ planned, learned, assessed, and adjusted their leadership skills over time. They used continuous deep learning to hone the way they understood and served others, communicated critical information, and inspired positive change. As physicians are increasingly called upon to serve as leaders, they can utilize this same process. Physicians can use the MAL model to support their own leadership development, practicing adaptive expertise in an area beyond clinical knowledge to facilitate their development into well-rounded, master adaptive learners.

TAKE-HOME POINTS

1. Interpersonal literacy (an understanding of personal relationships) and systems literacy (an understanding of the health care system) are two key leadership competencies that are critical to develop in future physicians. Leadership skills that enhance interpersonal literacy include emotional intelligence, teamwork, and communication. Leaders use their systems knowledge to create change.

2. The Master Adaptive Learner model can be used to develop leadership skills. In the planning phase, learners identify a gap in their leadership skills and set goals to improve that skill. In the learning phase, they engage with leadership literature to learn about theories and frameworks. In the assessing phase, learners practice that leadership skill in different environments. In the adjusting phase, they adjust their skill and leadership behaviors based on feedback.

3. Just as the Master Adaptive Learner model can be used to develop leadership skills, leadership skills can help trainees become master adaptive learners. For example, a high level of emotional intelligence can help learners better identify gaps and self-assess progress toward goals.

4. In ideal leaders and ideal master adaptive learners, it can be difficult to disentangle where the leader ends and the learner begins. Leaders can be defined by how well they learn. The best learners demonstrate the determination and purposefulness of leaders.

QUESTIONS FOR FURTHER THOUGHT

1. What is the ideal composition of a support system that might help a trainee develop his leadership skills and master adaptive learner abilities concurrently?

2. How can leadership and master adaptive learner development be integrated into curricula to help learners prioritize these skill sets alongside basic science knowledge and clinical skills?

3. How might a learner define and measure success in reaching her leadership and master adaptive learner goals?

ANNOTATED BIBLIOGRAPHY

1. Rotenstein LS, Sadun R, Jena AB. Why doctors need leadership training. *Harvard Business Rev*. October 17, 2018. Available at: https://hbr.org/2018/10/why-doctors-need-leadership-training. Accessed January 8, 2019.
   The authors describe two key competencies of physician leaders: interpersonal literacy and systems literacy.

2. Goleman D, Boyatzis RE. Emotional intelligence has 12 elements. Which do you need to work on? *Harvard Business Rev*. December 5, 2017. Available at: https://hbr.org/2017/02/emotional-intelligence-has-12-elements-which-do-you-need-to-work-on. Accessed January 8, 2019.
   This paper defines emotional intelligence and divides the skill into leadership domains and competencies. Various examples of how emotional intelligence skills can be identified and developed are provided.

3. Giles S. The most important leadership competencies, according to leaders around the world. *Harvard Business Rev*. March 15, 2016. Available at: https://hbr.org/2016/03/the-most-important-leadership-competencies-according-to-leaders-around-the-world. Accessed January 8, 2019.
   The author reports the most important leadership competencies as discovered from a survey of 195 leaders across 30 global organizations.

REFERENCES

1. Kennedy JF. *Remarks Prepared for Delivery at the Trade Mart*. Dallas, TX: John F. Kennedy Presidential Library and Museum; November 22, 1963 [Undelivered]. Available at: https://www.jfklibrary.org/archives/other-resources/john-f-kennedy-speeches/dallas-tx-trade-mart-undelivered-19631122. Accessed January 8, 2019.

2. Goodwin DK. *Leadership: In Turbulent Times*. New York, NY: Simon & Schuster; 2018.

3. NEJM Catalyst Insights Council. *The Critical Role of Clinical Leaders: Transforming Care Today and Tomorrow*. Available at: https://www.aemh.org/images/AEMH_documents/2018/22_The-Critical-Role-of-Clinical-Leaders—Transforming-Care-Today-and-Tomorrow.pdf. 2018.

4. Rotenstein LS, Sadun R, Jena AB. Why doctors need leadership training. *Harvard Business Rev*. October 17, 2018. Available at: https://hbr.org/2018/10/why-doctors-need-leadership-training. Published. Accessed January 8, 2019.

5. Neeley SM, Clyne B, Resnick-Ault D. The state of leadership education in US medical schools: results of a national survey. *Med Educ Online*. 2017;22(1):1301697. doi:10.1080/10872981.2017.1301697.

6. Rogelberg SG, Taja U, Naseer S. Servant Leadership Chapter in the *SAGE Encyclopedia of Industrial and Organizational Psychology*.

2nd ed. 2017. Accessed March 8, 2019. doi:10.4135/9781483386874.n486.

7. Salovey P, Mayer JD. Emotional intelligence. *Imagin Cogn Pers*. 1990;9(3):185-211.

8. Goleman D, Boyatzis RE. Emotional intelligence has 12 elements. Which do you need to work on? *Harvard Business Rev*. December 5, 2017. Available at: https://hbr.org/2017/02/emotional-intelligence-has-12-elements-which-do-you-need-to-work-on. Accessed January 8, 2019.

9. Leung C, Lucas A, Brindley P, et al. Followership: a review of the literature in healthcare and beyond. *J Crit Care*. 2018;46:99-104. doi:10.1016/j.jcrc.2018.05.001.

10. Giles S. The most important leadership competencies, according to leaders around the world. *Harvard Business Rev*. March 15, 2016. Available at: https://hbr.org/2016/03/the-most-important-leadership-competencies-according-to-leaders-around-the-world. Accessed January 8, 2019.

11. Folkman J. 5 ways to build a high-performance team. *Forbes*. April 13, 2016. Available at: https://www.forbes.com/sites/joefolkman/2016/04/13/are-you-on-the-team-from-hell-5-ways-to-create-a-high-performance-team. Accessed January 8, 2019.

12. Lee TH. Turning doctors into leaders. *Harvard Business Rev*. September 7, 2017. Available at: https://hbr.org/2010/04/turning-doctors-into-leaders.

13. Lerman C, Jameson JL. Leadership development in medicine. *N Engl J Med*. 2018;378(20):1862-1863.

14. Rowland D. Why leadership development isn't developing leaders. *Harvard Business Rev*. October 14, 2016. Available at: https://hbr.org/2016/10/why-leadership-development-isnt-developing-leaders. Published. Accessed March 8, 2019.

15. Stoller JK. Developing physician-leaders: a call to action. *J Gen Intern Med*. 2009;24(7):876-878.

16. Frich JC, Brewster AL, Cherlin EJ, Bradley EH. Leadership development programs for physicians: a systematic review. *J Gen Intern Med*. 2015;30(5):656-674.

17. Eurich T. What self-awareness really is and how to cultivate it. *Harvard Business Rev*. January 4, 2018. Available at: https://hbr.org/2018/01/what-self-awareness-really-is-and-how-to-cultivate-it.

18. Epstein A. Build self-awareness with help from your team. *Harvard Business Rev*. August 13, 2018. Available at: https://hbr.org/2018/08/build-self-awareness-with-help-from-your-team.

19. Tjan AK. 5 ways to become more self-aware. *Harvard Business Rev*. February 11, 2015. Available at: https://hbr.org/2015/02/5-ways-to-become-more-self-aware.

How Can the Master Adaptive Learner Model and Health Systems Science Collaborate to Improve Health Care?

Stephanie R. Starr, MD; Michael Dekhtyar, MEd; and Jed D. Gonzalo, MD, MSc

LEARNING OBJECTIVES

1. Summarize the need to incorporate health systems science (HSS) education into the Master Adaptive Learner (MAL) model for current and future practice.
2. Define systems thinking and its relationship to the MAL model and to HSS education.
3. Describe how HSS concepts can be used to advance adaptive expertise at each phase of the MAL process.
4. Summarize the potential benefit of early HSS education with the introduction of the MAL model with regard to learner professional identity formation.
5. Identify potential outcomes of the impact of adaptive learners on the health care system.

CHAPTER OUTLINE

CHAPTER SUMMARY

Physician education must include basic science, clinical science, and health systems science (HSS) to meet societal health needs now and in the future. HSS is broad and includes health system improvement, high-value care, social determinants of health, health economics, population health, informatics, leadership, and team science. Systems thinking enables learners to see the parts and the relationship between the parts of the health care system, similar to the way the Master Adaptive Learner (MAL) model enables learners to see and make explicit the development of adaptive expertise over time. Utilizing the MAL process when addressing HSS-related clinical challenges can help trainees successfully provide clinical care. We describe HSS-related educational experiences (emphasizing systems thinking, social determinants of health, high-value care, and health system improvement), incorporating each of the four MAL model steps, and highlight the similarities between the MAL model and the Plan-Do-Study-Act cycle steps used in health system improvement. Early professional identity formation aligned with HSS and the MAL model may help learners optimize their clinical experiences and prepare for complex clinical challenges requiring adaptive expertise. Adaptive learners can add value to the health care system by applying HSS concepts and skills in authentic practice settings to improve the care of patients and by applying the MAL process to the work of their interprofessional clinical teams.

INTRODUCTION

The Master Adaptive Learner (MAL) model espouses the need to be able to adapt, using both routine and innovative expertise as necessary, to ensure physicians can solve new problems in unfamiliar contexts to maintain and improve individual patient and population (societal) health.[1] Systematically using the planning, learning, assessing, and adjusting phases of the MAL process can help ensure physician trainees are prepared to flex between routine and innovative expertise in the rapidly changing US health care system. Necessary changes to facilitate this process include updates to traditional physician areas of expertise (basic and clinical science) as well as additional integrated expertise in additional concepts (e.g., health economics, health care improvement, social determinants of health, population health, team science).[2,3] Some have termed these additional competencies or "third science" as health systems science (HSS).[4,5]

Systems thinking takes a broad approach to understanding a system's parts and the relationship of these parts.[6,7] Incorporating systems thinking takes a holistic, cohesive approach to understanding and solving challenges and facilitates the learner's ability to visualize the seen as well as unseen drivers, connections, and consequences of interactions that occur in a given context.[8,9] Integrating this approach within medical education contexts requires a reconceptualization of medical education to acknowledge the integrated components of HSS with the basic and clinical sciences.

How can faculty facilitate learners' incorporation of HSS concepts and systems thinking into their approach to patient care and, in the process, advance adaptive expertise? How does systems thinking relate to the MAL process as well as HSS education? While HSS education and the MAL process are early in their development and application, with more to learn regarding optimal integration of both, what impact might be expected on patients and the health care system due to such interventions? This chapter seeks to answer these questions based on our current

understanding, which will evolve as collaborations of medical educators continue to work toward ensuring clinicians are prepared to improve the overall health and health care of patients and populations within a complex and changing health care system.

HEALTH SYSTEMS SCIENCE AND SYSTEMS THINKING

The HSS curricular framework (Table 15.1) for undergraduate medical education (UME) was developed by

TABLE 15.1   Health Systems Science Curricular Framework

Health Systems Science

Patient experience and context
- Patient experience and values
- Patient behaviors and motivations

Health care delivery
- Structures of delivery
- Processes of delivery

Health care policy and economics
- Policy
- Economics and payment

Population, public, and social determinants of health
- Social determinants of health
- Public health
- Population health and improvement

Clinical informatics and health technology
- Informatics/data analytics
- Decision support/evidence-based medicine
- Technology and tools

High-value care
- Quality principles and dimensions
- Cost and waste
- Evaluation/metrics

Health system improvement
- Improvement principles, processes, and tools
- Data and measurement
- Innovation and scholarship

Systems thinking

Change management and advocacy

Ethics and law

Leadership

Teamwork

faculty from the American Medical Association's Accelerating Change in Medical Education Consortium based on existing or planned curricula across 11 schools. Other national HSS UME efforts include the creation of formal HSS curricula,[10-12] a textbook,[13] curricular innovations in experiential learning,[14,15] and formal faculty development programs to advance HSS expertise.[16,17] Educators have developed strategies to assess HSS-related student outcomes, including HSS milestones[18] and a national HSS subject examination.[19]

Systems thinking exists at the core of HSS. It is a philosophy, a mindset, and a set of skills and understanding that allow physicians to conceptualize the complex health care system as a series of interdependent and multidirectional parts that are linked together to make the whole. Physicians must, for example, think broadly, consider problems from multiple perspectives, and avoid premature conclusions to adequately think about and address patients' health concerns as well as to optimally operate in and improve the system. These ways of thinking are reflected in the Waters Foundation's 14 habits of a systems thinker, which have been used in many education settings[20] and are being applied by some in medical education.

A critical part of systems thinking is the ability for physicians and trainees to "see" the levels of the health care system. Students typically enter professional school conceptualizing their clinical role as providing one-to-one care of individual patients (e.g., in an outpatient setting). They may anticipate their future role as members of frontline clinical teams (or a clinical microsystem) in a hospital setting but may not always see the depth and breadth of similar teams in the outpatient setting. Trainees must have a common nomenclature to describe levels of the health care system (such as microsystems, mesosystems, and macrosystems, depicted and described in Fig. 15.1).[21] They must understand their role in clinical microsystem teams to improve the team-based care they provide via quality improvement (QI) and patient safety strategies, which can occur at any level of the health care system.

Traditionally physicians have been trained to see the parts and the relationship between the parts with which they are directly involved (such as their role during an individual patient visit or in their interprofessional team work in a clinic or hospital unit), but not other systems factors that are less apparent. For example, they may not consider their patients' experiences outside of the

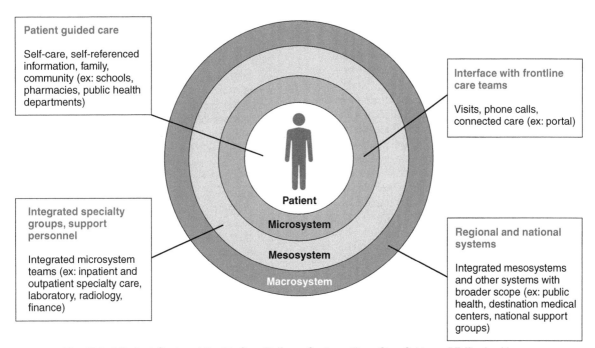

Fig. 15.1 A Patient-Centered Health Care Delivery System. (From Starr S, Nesse RE. The health care delivery system. In: Skochelak SE, Hawkins RE, et al, eds. *Health Systems Science.* Philadelphia, PA: Elsevier; 2017:24-35. Modified from Nelson EC, Godfrey MM, Batalden PB, et al. Clinical microsystems, part 1. The building blocks of health systems. *Jt Comm J Qual Patient Saf.* 2008;34[7]:367-378).

examination room, such as those that limit access to care (e.g., lack of transportation for underserved patients) or unnecessarily increase the cost of their care (e.g., the influence of fee-for-service models in physician overuse of some tests). Physicians must also understand the system and its parts at a higher level beyond their own health care organization, such as understanding the impact of medication costs on their patients resulting from nontransparent drug cost negotiations between insurance companies and pharmaceutical corporations.

Systems thinking is integral to the MAL process as well, enabling learners to see the process by which they can build their learning to develop and maintain their adaptive expertise. In both HSS and MAL development, systems thinking fosters the ability to see in a new and deliberate way. Thus health professional learners would ideally employ systems thinking within and across all levels of the health care system, beginning with a reflection of their own learning (i.e., via the MAL model).

Current and future practice requires physicians to begin their learning with a patient-centered health approach, including the knowledge that clinical practice is estimated to account for less than 20% of health outcomes, with social determinants and health behaviors having the largest impact.[22,23] Therefore physicians must first address social determinants of health and promote effective health behaviors, requiring knowledge and skills not traditionally taught in medical education. Second, physicians must embrace their responsibility to improve the system to improve health and health care for patients. This requires physicians to be systems thinkers who seek to understand and optimize each level of the system in which they learn and work. They must help solve problems for individual patients as well as for populations of patients that reflect larger societal problems, such as the cost of health care, unnecessary variation in the quality of care, lack of access to care, and medical errors.[3]

Patients perceive and contextualize their health care experiences based on aspects of care that impact them before and after their physician interactions, as well as the care they receive in those visits. Therefore, in addition to physicians' application of basic and clinical sciences based on results of their history and physical examination, an understanding of their patient's health care system experience will translate to more effective patient-centered care. In this context, systems thinking also includes the physician's ability to incorporate HSS principles as part of his application of the basic and clinical sciences in providing care. This requires that the physician utilize the MAL process in determining gaps in his knowledge related to the unique systems-based experiences of each patient as well as systemic effects on populations of patients.

EXAMPLES OF HEALTH SYSTEMS SCIENCE–RELATED EDUCATIONAL EXPERIENCES THAT INCORPORATE THE MASTER ADAPTIVE LEARNER MODEL

The MAL process provides a mechanism for trainees to integrate their basic, clinical, and HSS knowledge and skills so they are able to continue to learn as they are presented with new health care challenges. Physicians must develop a systems thinking approach and secure an early understanding of HSS concepts and skills in order to see and reflect upon clinical gaps when caring for individual patients and populations of patients. Four examples—systems thinking, social determinants of health, high-value care, and health system improvement—are highlighted in this section to demonstrate how HSS and the MAL process can be applied to address gaps related to these areas.

Systems Thinking (Focus on Phase 1 of MAL: Planning)

Vignette 1

Olivia is a fourth-year medical student interviewing Mr. Evans, a man with cough and bloody sputum for 3 months. He is coming in to see his primary care physician, Dr. Gonzales, for his symptoms. He missed a previously scheduled visit 2 months ago. Olivia listens carefully to Mr. Evans as he describes the difficulties he experienced getting the missed visit rescheduled after his plans for transportation to the last visit fell through. Olivia shares with Dr. Gonzales her concern that if Mr. Evans has a serious diagnosis (such as lung cancer or pulmonary tuberculosis) to explain his symptoms, an earlier evaluation could have resulted in a better prognosis.

1. How might Olivia's ability to see multiple levels of the health care system provide a deeper understanding of Mr. Evans' challenges and identify an opportunity to improve care for other patients?
2. How might Dr. Gonzales incorporate the Master Adaptive Learner process as part of his teaching after this clinical encounter?

Phase 1 of the MAL model (planning) requires learners to identify gaps between what is and what should be. In a traditional curriculum without an emphasis on HSS, students may find it easier to label/classify gaps in the basic and clinical sciences. In Vignette 1, Olivia might focus on the next steps of making the diagnosis and not recognize the gap in the health care provided, specifically the delay in presentation to care because of transportation difficulties. Trainees are encouraged to identify systems gaps that affect their patients using an HSS lens. Further, they are encouraged to think about systems gaps for which changing the system might influence the care of multiple patients. For example, the clinic team might choose to call patients after missed visits to see if they can address barriers to keeping appointments (e.g., arranging a medical taxi paid by county funds).

The MAL process requires deliberate reflection on top of content knowledge because knowledge application without reflection in novel, complex, or ambiguous contexts, or a combination of these, is insufficient for effective clinical decision making. In Vignette 1, Dr. Gonzales can reinforce Olivia's progression as a master adaptive learner in this phase by highlighting the importance of seeing gaps such as access challenges at multiple levels of the health care system.

Social Determinants of Health (Focus on Phase 2 of MAL: Learning)

Vignette 2
Mr. Chen presents to the emergency department with chest pain and is transferred to the hospital service team. Olivia approaches Mr. Chen's care by applying the routine expertise she has developed from the basic and clinical sciences (cardiac and pulmonary anatomy and pathophysiology, pharmacology) to accurately diagnose and treat his myocardial infarction. She recognizes her own gap—uncertainty regarding how to adapt Mr. Chen's discharge planning from what she has done for other myocardial infarction patients given his homelessness and untreated mental illness—but is uncertain how to proceed.
1. How might early learning about the social determinants of health enable Olivia to progress as a master adaptive learner?
2. How might Dr. Gonzales use this clinical encounter to help Olivia move through the learning phase?

Clinical reasoning must include HSS topics such as social determinants of health to best translate the basic and clinical sciences into optimal patient care,[24] and all clinicians need the nomenclature and ability to see, categorize, and communicate these and other HSS-related gaps to effectively innovate and solve new clinical challenges using the MAL process. Students may not see gaps that cause health inequity, such as limited access to food in urban food deserts, unless they are primed to ask about food security during visits.

Phase 2 of the MAL process (learning) requires learners to seek reliable information to help them better characterize and quantify the gap they have identified and to critically appraise the evidence in order to close their gaps in understanding. In Vignette 2, Olivia does not know how best to develop a successful discharge plan for Mr. Chen. Dr. Gonzales might prompt Olivia to consider team and other local resources (such as a team social worker with deep knowledge of community resources) and critical appraisal of best practices to help develop a plan for successful discharge to the community with at least temporary housing and connections to those who can help with longer-term needs for Mr. Chen. To deepen this understanding and its applicability to multiple future patients, Dr. Gonzales might also encourage Olivia to think upstream and consider resources to help augment her ability to take a more complete social history. She might read more broadly on the social determinants of health and consider how to incorporate an expanded social history for future patients, so she and her team can more readily identify and respond to patients with health needs that impact their hospitalization or successful discharge or both.[25]

Reflection on the social determinants of health and their impact on groups of patients (e.g., newly arrived immigrants) enables learners to consider how they, their clinical teams, and the larger system can improve health outcomes within traditional health care settings (e.g., via population health strategies to meet the needs of disadvantaged populations) as well as in the community (such as with community health workers and community-based interventions to promote health literacy and share local resources).

High-Value Care (Focus on Phase 3 of MAL: Assessing)

Vignette 3
Olivia is working in the rheumatology clinic for 1 month. She has multiple opportunities to see patients with Dr. Lake to confirm their diagnosis of rheumatoid arthritis and to codevelop a treatment plan. Dr. Lake notes that Olivia frequently elicits patient-specific challenges to care that are related to social determinants of health.

The evidence suggests several alternatives for first-line treatment of rheumatoid arthritis; the options differ in terms of cost, convenience (such as oral vs. intravenous infusion), and side effects. Dr. Lake models use of a shared decision-making aid to help her patients choose a treatment. She subsequently observes Olivia facilitating similar conversations with four other patients with rheumatoid arthritis.

1. How can a patient-centered understanding of high-value care enable Olivia to progress as a master adaptive learner?
2. How might Dr. Lake use this series of clinical encounters to help Olivia move through phase 3?

High-value care in clinical practice includes a number of HSS topics and provides an excellent opportunity to incorporate the MAL process. Trainees can learn to provide high-value care for individual patients via the Alliance for Academic Internal Medicine and the American College of Physicians' five-step model (Fig. 15.2),[26] which combines evidence-based medicine (Steps 1-3) with shared decision making (Step 4) to ensure that each patient's preferences and values are incorporated within their individual contexts.[27] The unique context of each patient (including social determinants such as financial, transportation, and other resource limitations, as well as medical comorbidities) provides variation in the teaching of concepts and opportunities for learners to embrace struggle and discovery, facets important to developing adaptive expertise.[28] In Vignette 3, for each patient with a new diagnosis of rheumatoid arthritis, Dr. Lake helps Olivia apply the current evidence to create a list of medication options to consider. Olivia facilitates conversations with each patient using a decision aid[29] to solicit the patients' preferences, values, and concerns.

Phase 3 of the MAL process (assessing) requires learners to apply their new understanding to their clinical practice, using informed self-assessment skills and external feedback. In Vignette 3, Dr. Lake can ask Olivia to reflect on her conversations with patients using the decision aid and provide feedback based on direct observation to help her facilitate future similar conversations to answer questions about treatment options and enable her patients to make treatment decisions that meet their needs.

Health System Improvement (Focus on Phase 4 of MAL: Adjusting)

Vignette 4

Olivia and a small group of students decide to plan and implement a QI project with an interprofessional clinical team. With the assistance of Dr. Lake and the clinic administrator, they implement several Plan-Do-Study-Act cycles over 4 months to consistently incorporate the shared decision-making tool for patients choosing their rheumatoid arthritis treatment.

1. How can an understanding of health system improvement enable Olivia to progress as a master adaptive learner?
2. How might Olivia use this clinical experience to move through phase 4 of the MAL model?

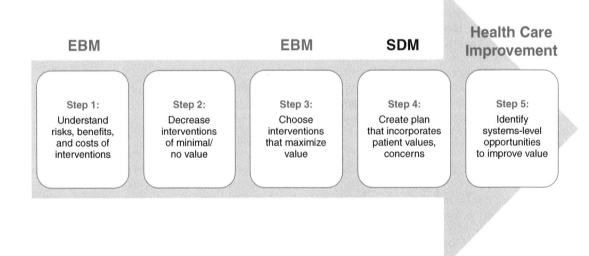

Fig. 15.2 **Five-Step Framework for Teaching High-Value Care.** *EBM,* Evidence-based medicine; *SDM,* shared decision making. (Adapted with permission from Smith CD, Alliance for Academic Internal Medicine–American College of Physicians High Value, Cost-Conscious Care Curriculum Development Committee. Teaching high-value, cost-conscious care to residents: the Alliance for Academic Internal Medicine–American College of Physicians curriculum. *Ann Intern Med.* 2012;157:285.)

Health system improvement (including QI) provides a complementary framework to the MAL process as both seek to identify and close gaps to make improvements. The relevance of the MAL process to health system improvement goes beyond the obvious similarity between the four phases of the MAL process and the Plan-Do-Study-Act (PDSA) cycle, as shown in Table 15.2.[30] QI relies on defining a gap and analyzing baseline data to develop and implement an improvement to close the gap. The QI approach complements adaptive expertise in that standardization of an estimated 80% of clinical approaches facilitates the capacity to apply adaptive expertise (innovate) for the remaining 20%,[31,32] thus balancing routine and innovative expertise.

Phase 4 of the MAL process (adjusting) requires learners to incorporate what they have learned into daily routines, to clarify how the new learning will impact daily practice, and to determine if future similar challenges will require routine or novel approaches. In Vignette 4, Olivia and her peers recognize that their QI project requires implementation at the level of their frontline clinical team. As early HSS learners, they also see that innovations developed at the microsystem level might be successfully adapted to other microsystems within the health care system to have a greater impact on patients and their families.

EARLY PROFESSIONAL IDENTITY FORMATION

Chapter 2 proposes the advantages of developing adaptive expertise early in professional development. Similarly, early professional identity of health professionals is needed to ensure that learners see their role in both doing their work and improving it.[32a] They need to apply systems thinking and problem-solving strategies that help close HSS-related gaps to meet the Institute for Healthcare Improvement's Triple Aim.[33] Some have also suggested that this may mitigate health professional burnout (i.e., achievement of the Quadruple Aim)[34] if trainees learn to see systems gaps and address inefficiencies as members of frontline clinical teams.

This evolving view of professionalism that includes HSS as part of identify formation, referred to as systems citizenship,[34,35] requires health professionals to use a systems thinking lens to understand how a patient's individual care is influenced by systemic factors and to take a proactive stance to help patient safety and prevent system errors. Despite the potential benefits of this new professionalism to improve patient care, students do not necessarily see their role as systems citizens or innovators.[36] This presents an opportunity for incorporating the MAL process within

TABLE 15.2 Comparison of the Four Phases of the Master Adaptive Learner (MAL) Model With the Plan-Do-Study-Act (PDSA) Cycle's Four Steps		
	MAL Model[1]	**PDSA Model[30]**
Goal	Optimal adaptive expertise over professional lifetime	Improve the health system and, ultimately, health and health care
Target for improvement	Learner ability to improve and maintain adaptive expertise	Health care structure, process, or outcome (with potential to also improve patient health/value, and function/wellness of clinical team)
Step 1	**Planning:** Identifying a gap, selecting an opportunity for learning, and searching for resources for learning	**Plan:** Team identifies process needing change and the target for change and (based on baseline measurement and analysis of the data) develops intervention(s)
Step 2	**Learning:** Internalizing new understandings that address an identified gap in knowledge, skill, or attitude	**Do:** Team tests the change by implementing the intervention(s)
Step 3	**Assessing:** Experimentation, informed self-assessment via external feedback	**Study:** Team studies the success or failure of the change by collecting postintervention measure and analyzing the results
Step 4	**Adjusting:** Incorporating what is learned into daily routine and identifying what is novel going forward; deciding if individual or system implementation is needed	**Act:** Team designs modifications and prepares for new cycle to retest using adapted intervention(s)

HSS education to highlight learners' responsibility and opportunity to improve their own learning and the health care system.

In the vignettes, we can observe Olivia's progression through the MAL process and describe her use of systems thinking and developing systems citizenship. In each vignette Olivia uncovers a new layer of HSS that she is able to apply to clinical care to improve both the health of patients and the functioning of the health care system. As a systems thinker, she recognizes issues of access to care and the role of varying social statuses that impact patient care, as well as the role of varying health professionals in helping her make clinical decisions. As a learner, she continues to apply her knowledge of social determinants, but also recognizes unique challenges that face each patient with regard to the cost of care. She learns about inefficiencies of the health care system through her patient interactions and focuses on her patients' needs through the use of evidence-based tools for shared decision making. Realizing the positive impact that she had on her patients through providing high-value care that takes into account their social determinants of health, she recognizes an opportunity to propagate this learning in other clinical microsystems through QI projects and implementation of PDSA cycles. In this ideal scenario, Olivia recognizes the alignment of the MAL process she has been trained to implement with the PDSA processes that she is using to improve health care system functioning and the quality of care each patient receives.

POTENTIAL IMPACTS OF MASTER ADAPTIVE LEARNERS ON THE HEALTH CARE SYSTEM

What can we expect of learners who are master adaptive learners and systems citizens? How can learners trained to continuously improve their own learning as well as the health care system positively impact care?

Adding Value to the Health Care System

Educators have already demonstrated that learners can add value to clinical practice by improving individual patient care and the health care system in which they participate.[37-41] They are able to identify novel clinical challenges because they typically have more time to do so than other team members. They can educate other team members on new technologies and care processes. They can serve as peer faculty in nonclinical learning environments for early learners in UME and can contribute to service learning of peers and improvements in systems when the learning is paired with the needs of the community served.[14,15,37]

Any QI approach reflects the MAL model in that even similar quality gaps require interventions with modifications that reflect the specific clinical context in which the improvement is being made. Learners who not only have

HSS skills, knowledge, systems thinking abilities, nomenclature, and systems citizenship identity, but also a sense of empowerment as a master adaptive learner, may be better able to see what changes they can make to fix health care system inefficiencies and reflect on how they can continue to be part of the solution. In this sense, HSS competence and experience in the MAL process is one way to create a mechanism for mitigating burnout of self and of other team members.

Advancing Teamwork Within the Health Care System

In 2011 Atul Gawande, MD, MPH, described the need to move away from the idea of physicians as independent "cowboys" and instead accelerate toward a goal of health care team "pit crews," composed of individuals with specific skill sets who need both specific expertise and, more importantly, an understanding of how to optimize the interaction of team members to ensure ideal outcomes.[42] Health care is practiced as a team, so theories of human cognition that focus on the individual mind are insufficient in medical education.

Distributed cognition is a theory of human cognition that describes how information is processed across people, teams, technologies, and culture.[43] One important focus of HSS education is the recognition that practitioners operate within a community of practice composed of interprofessional teams and learners of different levels.[44] In this context, the MAL model may be applied on a team level to address knowledge and skill gaps across a health care team. The reflexivity and systems thinking characteristics of all team members, not just the leadership, are crucial throughout this process. This provides an opportunity for the team to fully assess their challenges, understand the behaviors and systemic drivers of adverse events, and articulate the highest-leverage improvements that will increase their capacity to adapt in complex situations.

CONCLUSION

HSS education and the MAL process independently have significant potential to help health professionals achieve the Triple Aim within an evolving 21st-century health care system and meet their obligation to society. Successful learners in HSS education who utilize the MAL process are systems thinkers. Explicitly labeling clinical practice examples of HSS-related challenges can help promote adaptive learning. Educators creating programs that explicitly include both approaches in a synergistic manner can produce master adaptive learners while providing multiple opportunities to improve patient care and the systems in which they learn and practice through the development of adaptive expertise.

TAKE-HOME POINTS

1. Integrating health systems science (HSS) education with the MAL model can help health professionals better meet the needs of 21st-century society.
2. Systems thinking is central to HSS, modeled in the MAL model, and helps learners see in new ways to develop physician competence and adaptive expertise.
3. Clinical challenges that focus on HSS concepts can help advance the MAL process.
4. There may be advantages to early HSS education as well as implementation of the MAL model in learners' professional identify formation as physicians.
5. Adaptive learners can add value to current clinical practice and can help advance clinical care by interprofessional teams.

QUESTIONS FOR FURTHER THOUGHT

1. How might educators best design early clinical experiences in UME to blend the MAL model with learning both clinical science and HSS?
2. What activities might help promote both the MAL model and HSS as part of professional identity formation in these settings?
3. What are some considerations for learner assessment for programs implementing the MAL model process and HSS education?

ANNOTATED BIBLIOGRAPHY

1. Lucey CR. Medical education—part of the problem and part of the solution. *JAMA Intern Med*. 2013;173:1639-1643.
   This article is foundational in articulating the need to reform medical education and clinical learning environments to train physicians with improved knowledge and skills required for practice within an evolving health care system.
2. Gonzalo JD, Dekhtyar M, Starr SR, et al. Health systems science curricula in undergraduate medical education: identifying and defining a potential curricular framework. *Acad Med*. 2017;92:123-131.
   This research report describes the development of a health systems science framework through an inductive analysis of medical education curricula.
3. Smith CD, Alliance for Academic Internal Medicine–American College of Physicians High Value, Cost-Conscious Care Curriculum Development Committee. Teaching high-value, cost-conscious care to residents: the Alliance for Academic Internal Medicine–American College of Physicians curriculum. *Ann Intern Med*. 2012;157:284-286.
   This article describes the development and implementation of a high-value, cost-conscious care curriculum developed for residents.
4. Gonzalo JD, Dekhtyar M, Hawkins RE, Wolpaw DR. How can medical students add value? Identifying roles, barriers, and strategies to advance the value of undergraduate medical education to patient care and the health system. *Acad Med*. 2017;92:1294-1301.
   This article identifies potential stakeholders regarding the value of student work and the roles and tasks students could perform to add value to the health care system. This article also identifies key barriers and associated strategies to promote value-added roles in undergraduate medical education.
5. Gonzalo JD, Lucey C, Wolpaw T, Chang A. Value-added clinical systems learning roles for medical students that transform education and health: a guide for building partnerships between medical schools and health systems. *Acad Med*. 2017;92:602-607.
   This article discusses large-scale efforts to develop novel, required, longitudinal, and authentic health systems science curricula in classrooms and workplaces for first-year students.

REFERENCES

1. Cutrer WB, Miller B, Pusic MV, et al. Fostering the development of master adaptive learners: A conceptual model to guide skill acquisition in medical education. *Acad Med*. 2017;92:70-75.
2. Skochelak SE. A decade of reports calling for change in medical education: what do they say? *Acad Med*. 2010;85:S26-S33.
3. Lucey CR. Medical education – part of the problem and part of the solution. *JAMA Intern Med*. 2013;173:1639-1643.
4. Gonzalo JD, Haidet P, Papp KK, et al. Educating for the 21st-century health care system: An interdependent framework of basic, clinical, and systems sciences. *Acad Med*. 2017;92:35-39.
5. Gonzalo JD, Dekhtyar M, Starr SR, et al. Health systems science curricula in undergraduate medical education: Identifying and defining a potential curricular framework. *Acad Med*. 2017;92:123-131.

6. Senge PM. *The Fifth Discipline: The Art and Practice of the Learning Organization*. New York, NY: Doubleday; 2006.

7. Sweeney LB, Meadows D. *The Systems Thinking Playbook: Exercises to Stretch and Build Learning and Systems Thinking Capabilities*. White River Junction, VT: Chelsea Green Publishing; 1995.

8. Plack MM, Goldman EF, Scott AR, et al. Systems thinking and systems-based practice across the health professions: an inquiry into definitions, teaching practices, and assessment. *Teach Learn Med*. 2018;30:242-254.

9. Colbert CY, Ogden PE, Ownby AR, Bowe C. Systems-based practice in graduate medical education: systems thinking as the missing foundational construct. *Teach Learn Med*. 2011;23:179-185.

10. Gonzalo JD, Wolpaw T, Wolpaw D. Curricular transformation in health systems science: the need for global change. *Acad Med*. 2018;93:1431-1433.

11. Borkan JM, George P, Tunkel AR. Curricular transformation: the case against global change. *Acad Med*. 2018;93:1428-1430.

12. Starr SR, Agrwal N, Bryan MJ, et al. Science of health care delivery: An innovation in undergraduate medical education to meet society's needs. *Mayo Clin Proc Innov Qual Outcomes*. 2017;1:117-129.

13. Skochelak SE, Hawkins RE, Lawson LE, Starr SR, Borkan JM, Gonzalo JD, eds. *Health Systems Science*. St. Louis, MO: Elsevier; 2016.

14. Ackerman SL, Boscardin C, Karliner L, et al. The action research program: Experiential learning in systems-based practice for first-year medical students. *Teach Learn Med*. 2016;28:183-191.

15. Kaplan JA, Brinson Z, Hofer R, et al. Early learners as health coaches for older adults preparing for surgery. *J Surg Res*. 2017;209:184-190.

16. Baxley EG, Lawson L, Garrison HG, et al. The Teachers of Quality Academy: a learning community approach to preparing faculty to teach health systems science. *Acad Med*. 2016;91:1655-1660.

17. Walsh DS, Lazorick S, Lawson L, et al. The Teachers of Quality Academy: evaluation of the effectiveness and impact of a health systems science training program. *Am J Med Qual*. 2019;34:36-44.

18. Havyer RD, Norby SM, Leep Hunderfund AN, et al. Science of health care delivery milestones for undergraduate medical education. *BMC Med Educ*. 2017;17:145-150.

19. Dekhtyar M, Ross LP, D'Angelo J, et al. Validity of the health systems science examination: relationship between examinee performance and time of training. *Am J Med Qual*. 2019 Jun 10. doi: 10.1177/1062860619853349. [Epub ahead of print]

20. Benson T, Marlin S. *The Habit-Forming Guide to Becoming a Systems Thinker*. Pittsburgh, PA: Systems Thinking Group, Inc; 2017.

21. Nelson EC, Godfrey MM, Batalden PB, et al. Clinical Microsystems, Part 1. The building blocks of health systems. *Jt Comm J Qual Patient Saf*. 2008;34(7):367-378.

22. Hood CM, Gennuso KP, Swain GR, Catlin BB. County health rankings relationships between determinant factors and health outcomes. *Am J Prev Med*. 2016;50:129-135.

23. Magnan S. Social determinants of health 101 for health care: Five plus five. *NAM Perspectives*. 2017; Discussion Paper, National Academy of Medicine, Washington, DC. doi:10.31478/201710c.

24. Mylopoulos M, Woods NN. When I say … adaptive expertise. *Med Educ*. 2017;51:685-686.

25. Williams BC, Ward DA, Chick DA, Johnson EL, Ross PT. Using a six-domain framework to include biopsychosocial information in the standard medical history. *Teach Learn Med*. 2019;31(1):87-98. doi:10.1080/10401334.2018.1480958.

26. Smith CD, Alliance for Academic Internal Medicine–American College of Physicians High Value, Cost-Conscious Care Curriculum Development Committee. Teaching high-value, cost-conscious care to residents: the Alliance for Academic Internal Medicine–American College of Physicians curriculum. *Ann Intern Med*. 2012;157:284-286.

27. Hoffmann TC, Montori VM, Del Mar C. The connection between evidence-based medicine and shared decision making. *JAMA*. 2014;312:1295-1296.

28. Mylopoulos M, Kulasegaram K, Woods NN. Developing the experts we need: Fostering adaptive expertise through education. *J Eval Clin Pract*. 2018;24:674-677.

29. Rheumatoid Arthritis (RA) Choice. Mayo Clinic Shared Decision Making National Resource Center. Available at: https://shareddecisions.mayoclinic.org/rheumatoid-arthritis-ra-choice/. Accessed October 15, 2018.

30. Taylor MJ, McNicholas C, Nicolay C, Darzi A, Bell D, Reed JE. Systematic review of the application of the plan-do-study-act method to improve quality in healthcare. *BMJ Qual Saf*. 2014;23:290-298.

31. Cutrer WB, Ehrenfeld JM. Protocolization, standardization and the need for adaptive expertise in our medical systems. *J Med Syst*. 2017;41:200.

32. Pusic MV, Santen SA, Dekhtyar M, et al. Learning to balance efficiency and innovation for optimal adaptive expertise. *Med Teach*. 2018;40:820-827.

32a. Batalden PB, Davidoff F. What is "quality improvement" and how can it transform healthcare? *Qual Saf Health Care*. 2007;16:2-3.

33. Berwick DM, Nolan TW, Whittington J. The triple aim: Care, health, and cost. *Health Aff (Millwood)*. 2008;27:759-769.

34. Bodenheimer T, Sinsky C. From triple to quadruple aim: Care of the patient requires care of the provider. *Ann Fam Med*. 2014;12:573-576.

35. Hafferty FW, Levinson D. Moving beyond nostalgia and motives: Towards a complexity science view of medical professionalism. *Perspect Biol Med*. 2008;51:599-615.

36. Gonzalo JD, Singh MK. How systems citizenship is no accident in health professions education: the continued call for health systems science curricula. *AHRQ PSNet*. 2019. Available at: https://psnet.ahrq.gov/perspectives/perspective/265/Building-Systems-Citizenship-in-Health-Professions-Education-The-Continued-Call-for-Health-Systems-Science-Curricula. Accessed April 1, 2019.

37. Mylopoulos M, Regehr G. How student models of expertise and innovation impact the development of adaptive expertise in medicine. *Med Educ*. 2009;43:127-132.

38. Gonzalo JD, Dekhtyar M, Hawkins RE, Wolpaw DR. How can medical students add value? Identifying roles, barriers, and strategies to advance the value of undergraduate medical education to patient care and the health system. *Acad Med*. 2017;92:1294-1301.
39. Gonzalo JD, Lucey C, Wolpaw T, Chang A. Value-added clinical systems learning roles for medical students that transform education and health: a guide for building partnerships between medical schools and health systems. *Acad Med*. 2017;92:602-607.
40. Lin SY, Schillinger E, Irby DM. Value-added medical education: Engaging future doctors to transform health care delivery today. *J Gen Intern Med*. 2014;30:150-151.
41. Sklar D. How medical education can add value to the health care delivery system. *Acad Med*. 2016;91:445-447.
42. Gawande A. Cowboys and pit crews. *The New Yorker*. May 26, 2011. Available at: https://www.newyorker.com/news/news-desk/cowboys-and-pit-crews. Accessed January 23, 2019.
43. Hazlehurst B. When I say ... distributed cognition. *Med Educ*. 2015;49:755-756.
44. Gonzalo JD, Thompson BM, Haidet P, Mann K, Wolpaw DR. A constructive reframing of student roles and systems learning in medical education using a communities of practice lens. *Acad Med*. 2017;92:1687-1694.

16

How Does Master Adaptive Learning Ensure Optimal Pathways to Clinical Expertise?

Martin V. Pusic, MD, PhD; Kathy Boutis, MD, MSc; Sally A. Santen, MD, PhD; and William B. Cutrer MD, MEd

LEARNING OBJECTIVES

1. Review "learning how to learn," the conceptual basis of master adaptive learning.
2. Use Learning Curve Theory to describe the arc of master adaptive learning.
3. Describe the role of scientific theories in master adaptive learning.
4. Summarize the key themes of this book.

CHAPTER OUTLINE

CHAPTER SUMMARY

In this final chapter, we zoom out to take a higher perspective on master adaptive learning (MAL). We have presented a great deal of detailed evidence so as to illuminate and justify the MAL approach to learning to *be* a clinician and to learning *as* a clinician. We propose this chapter as a resting place where the interconnections can become clearer. This would not be at the atomic or detail level but at a fuzzier, less focused level where larger patterns become more apparent. At this higher level, using one selected scientific theory as an exemplar, we demonstrate how the MAL framework can serve as a recursive assembly of models and scientific theories that underpin a coherent approach to clinical learning at any stage in a physician's career.

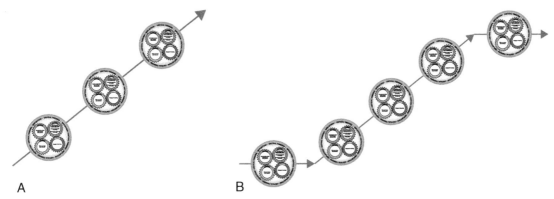

A   B

Fig. 16.1 Master Adaptive Learning in Sequential Iterations. This graphic, derived from Fig. 1.1, demonstrates the zoomed-out perspective on Master Adaptive Learning (MAL) as the learner deliberately invokes the MAL process (represented as repeated cycles) over time. (A) The aspirational trajectory with successive iterations. (B) The full nonlinear learning curve as described in the text, with the first master adaptive learner iteration emphasizing planning and organization; the next three emphasizing the engagement with learning, including desirable difficulties; and the last one representing adjusting to the developed expertise both personally and for the organization. Implicit in the processes is assessment as to where on the learning curve one is, whether the rate is enough to justify the cost, and whether the learner is on track to achieve the desired goal.

Vignette

Dr. Diana Liu, an emergency medicine physician, is the lead faculty member in her department for point-of-care ultrasound (POCUS). In this role, she is responsible for trainee and faculty development of this skill, as well as patient safety and quality improvement as impacted by the POCUS technique. Her emergency department has done well in adopting ultrasound, but there is a great deal of room for improvement. Her faculty range from ultrasound zealots to self-proclaimed Luddites who have tried to minimize their adoption of the technique.

After recently learning about the Master Adaptive Learner model, she has been trying to incorporate MAL principles within her approach to teaching POCUS. She sees learning opportunities everywhere and eagerly looks for ways of better facilitating the learning.

She feels the time is right for her to develop a very intentional curriculum built on MAL principles to facilitate learning POCUS skills and approach. She wants to change her learners and wants them to change the care provided in her emergency department.

OVERVIEW—ZOOMING OUT ON THE MASTER ADAPTIVE LEARNING PROCESS

Looked at from a higher level, successive iterations of the MAL cycle can be seen as clearly connected. Each iteration

of the MAL cycle (hopefully) leaves the learner at a new, incrementally higher, level, whether she has gained a new capacity or has become a little bit wiser after a productive failure (Fig. 16.1). This incremental improvement is itself governed by Learning Curve Theory, which posits that learning is a nonlinear but predictable phenomenon that has the property of scaling, such that the learning pattern repeats itself at multiple levels.[1] In the text that follows, we describe Learning Curve Theory in general and break it down according to the four phases of the MAL cycle, showing how the framework's activities and processes meaningfully align with an overall, generalizable learning trajectory.

LEARNING CURVE THEORY

At the outset of Chapter 2 we described an example of expertise development as a learning curve (see Fig. 2.1). The idea is that expertise develops according to a sigmoid-shaped curve that defines the relationship between effort expended in learning (typically along the horizontal axis) and the resulting improvement in functioning (represented along the vertical axis). Our argument in that chapter was to point to the nonlinear overall nature of learning from the initial more difficult (and hence flatter) initial phase necessary for a MAL approach (see Fig. 2.4), through to the active learning phase, and finally to an aspirational expert level where learning continues asymptotically, a phase that can be considered as the "learning expert."[2]

In Fig. 16.2, we show a prototypical learning curve and highlight its important features. The overall curve

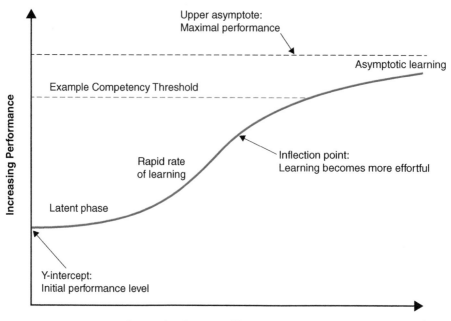

Fig. 16.2 Prototypical Learning Curve. In Learning Curve Theory, a sigmoid-shaped relationship exists between the amount of effort expended in learning and the resulting improvement in performance. Initial learning is slow and laborious. The second phase is a near-exponential increase associated with learning the easier part of the material. An inflection point signals a slowing rate of learning as it becomes more difficult (the law of diminishing returns). Finally learning enters an asymptotic phase up to a system-specific maximum. (Adapted from Pusic MV et al. Learning curves in health professions education. *Acad Med.* 2015;90[8]: 1034–1042.)

shows a nonlinear, sigmoid-shaped relationship between the amount of time and effort expended in learning and the resulting improvement in performance.[3] Different learning processes are at play in each phase of the curve. Initial learning is slow and laborious as the learner becomes oriented to the environment and the material. For example, for radiograph interpretation, the first stage involves learning how the radiographs are presented, how to access different views, what those views represent, and how they relate to the clinical situation. The second phase of the learning curve is a near-exponential increase in performance. This is associated with learning the easier part of the material—for example, obvious pathology, common presentations, or both. However, an inflection point signals the next phase where the rate of learning slows. This is also known as the law of diminishing returns, where each unit of educational effort purchases ever-smaller performance increments. Here the individual is learning rare presentations or difficult-to-perceive anomalies. Finally, learning enters an asymptotic phase in which it approaches a maximum, dictated

by the nature of the material and the context. These would be cases that are difficult for even those with expertise in the field and cases that show considerable practice variation that are resistant to routine approaches. The asymptote represents a theoretical maximum level of performance predicted by prior learning experience with the system. In Fig. 16.2, we have drawn a competency line that might represent an acceptable or aspirational level of functioning for a trainee. Suffice it to say that true expertise is hard won.[4]

This sigmoid-shaped association between learning effort and performance is remarkably reproducible whether seen in animals learning laboratory tasks, humans performing a wide range of psychomotor or cognitive tasks, or organizations learning from experience whether in building airplanes or adopting guidelines.[3,5-7] In health professions education, the association has been found at all levels of learning: from the atomic level (e.g., suture tying)[8] to cognitively complex tasks (e.g., radiograph interpretation)[3] and psychomotor skills (e.g., laparoscopy)[9] and even at organizational levels.[10]

Learning Curve Theory is thus a well-established scientific theory that describes and explains the fundamental basis for learning, with health professions education being no exception. In subsequent sections, we show how the overall iterative MAL process (see Fig. 16.1), described in considerable detail in prior chapters, aligns nicely with Learning Curve Theory. It would have been surprising were it not to align, since the process of establishing a scientific theory requires many failed attempts to falsify it.[1] In describing exactly how MAL aligns with Learning Curve Theory, we hope to provide a metacognitive perspective (yet again) for the master adaptive learners, this time on the longer arc of learning both for themselves and at the level of the organization or health care system.

PLANNING—THE LATENT PHASE OF THE LEARNING CURVE

Vignette Continued

Over the years, Dr. Liu has refined, through multiple iterations, an "Orientation to Point-Of-Care Ultrasound" curriculum given to novices, usually medical students and interns. When she first started, she presented lectures on ultrasound theory and the indications and diagnostic findings for typical applications. This gradually evolved over the years to a completely hands-on session in which pairs of learners just played with the machines, aided by a "Getting Started in POCUS: Guide to Knob-ology" visual guide to what every knob on the machine does. She used learner feedback from each session to identify gaps in her teaching approach and guide her improvement efforts as a teacher. The feedback scores improved with each change but now, as she reflects, she wonders whether her current iteration is indeed the best preparation for future learning (PFL).

She reflects deeply on her current approach to teaching and assessment, trying to understand if her approach really sets her participants up to learn by encouraging productive failure through guided discovery learning. She remembers reading in the medical education literature about letting trainees solve problems and perform tasks without direct instruction while providing some feedback. These more challenging conditions have been described as enhancing learning and equipping trainees with PFL-related behaviors.[11] At the core, she wants to provide her participants with the opportunity and feedback to help them identify gaps in their own knowledge, skills, and attitudes around the use of POCUS, and then enter

into one of the MAL cycles to deepen their expertise. She recognizes that this will likely involve constructing early activities that challenge and stretch her learners, remaining hopeful that they will persist so as to reap the benefits of their new skills.

All learning curves have a y-intercept that is, almost without exception, not zero. It is a fundamental tenet of constructivism that new learning must be grafted onto the old. A key process in master adaptive learning is having a sense of one's current level of functioning (the putative y-intercept) and recognizing the gap that exists when it is compared with another, higher aspirational level of serving patients. In prior chapters, we described the importance of informed self-assessment in initiating the MAL cycle (Chapter 6) and goal setting (Chapter 8). As we will describe here, having a metacognitive awareness of the nonlinear path of learning can serve the master adaptive learner in planning out the path to a new higher level of functioning.

The learning curve describes an initial latent phase where little improvement occurs despite effort having been invested. This initial latent phase can be divided into unproductive and productive latency divided by whether the activity advantages downstream learning. Consider a reductionist example in which a mouse repetitively learns to navigate a difficult but solvable maze in search of a target piece of cheese. Initially, the mouse would put considerable effort into random forays without much payback in terms of speed in reaching the cheese. There is a necessary period of orienting to the environment that represents learning, but not of a kind that is visible in performance. We call this unproductive (or unnecessary) latency because it could be obviated. For example, given a smarter mouse (say, Mickey or Jerry), we would hand them an orienting map such that all learning effort is now germane to the task of reaching the cheese quickly. An instructor can thus help decrease unproductive latency to a minimum.

Throughout this book, we have argued for productive latency, wherein increased initial effort results in more effective downstream learning. In Chapter 2, we made the analogy to compound interest in which learning to learn, while initially disadvantageous to direct learning of content, in the long run has a multiplicative effect of preparing for future learning. The key difference for productive latency is that we do not want to obviate it. Instead, it is the necessary price to pay for a more effective path overall. The instructor's role here is both to highlight and celebrate the investment, and to provide encouragement and faith that, in the face of no initial reward in performance, it will be worth it.[12] The instructor knows the space and the best

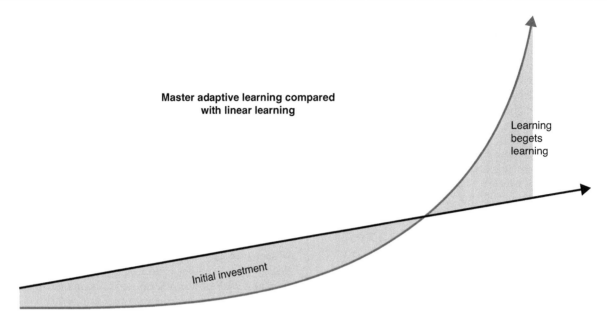

Fig. 16.3 The Latent Phase of the Learning Curve. In many respects, investment in a MAL approach represents the difference between linear *(black line)* and exponential *(blue line)* learning, as described in Chapter 2. Exponential processes are those in which the innate process feeds off itself in a manner that builds slowly initially but later explodes. It is within the nature of exponential processes that the early stages seem slower than those in linear ones.

path through it. As described in Chapter 2 and repeated here in Fig. 16.2, learning how to learn will seem to disadvantage early performance, because time must be divided between that metacognitive process and the content to be learned.

Thus we see how the planning phase of the MAL process aligns with the latent phase of the learning curve (Figure 16.3). Planning takes into account a specific learner's prior knowledge. A productive latent phase involves goal identification, organization of learning, and laying down beneficial habits of behavior and mind. The learner especially needs orientation and support during this important but often underappreciated phase of learning (Table 16.1).

LEARNING—THE RAPID PHASE OF THE LEARNING CURVE

Vignette Continued

As she considers the POCUS curriculum in totality, Dr. Liu recognizes she has a diversity of learners at many different levels of knowledge, skill, and attitude around the topic. Each group possesses its own strengths and challenges. In many respects, Dr. Liu's second-year residents are always her most joyful POCUS group. Having mastered the basics through her series of carefully considered exercises that forced them to struggle but rewarded their efforts, they are POCUS devotees, constantly looking for new opportunities and situations to apply their skills. They love bringing back ever-clearer video clips of gallbladders, fetuses, pneumonias, and Morrison pouches. Dr. Liu nurtured their quest for feedback and encouraged them to perform their own ultrasound on every willing patient they sent to ob-gyn or radiology, and to compare their read to that of the specialists. The feedback loop worked well, with each resident refining his or her technique over the course of the year, becoming more and more accurate.

Dr. Liu had systematically excluded the second years from the monthly POCUS quality improvement rounds because she felt the cases were often specialized or difficult and outside the scope of what a second-year resident should know. She wonders if she should revisit her policy and provide the enthusiastic second-year residents the opportunity to be stumped and challenged.

TABLE 16.1 Phases of the Learning Curve.		
Learning Curve Phase	**Instructor's Role**	**Master Adaptive Learner Implications**
y-Intercept	Identify and build on prior knowledge	***Planning***—Goal setting based on prior knowledge; recognize the gap; informed self-assessment
Latent Phase	Decrease nonproductive latency (orient) Highlight productive approaches Prepare for future learning Encourage and support	***Planning***—minimize unproductive latency by orienting the learner well, removing obstacles Maximize productive latency by promoting learning for learning and through the use of scripts and advance organizers
Rapid Learning	Advantage desirable difficulties approach Position in Optimal Adaptability Corridor Signal nonlinear nature of learning	***Learning***—situate learner for adaptive expertise development Assessing and monitoring with goal in mind Remediation for suboptimal trajectory
Inflection Point and Deceleration of Learning	Make explicit how inflection is different from competency Metacognitive awareness of the implications of the law of diminishing returns Judge effort-reward tradeoff	***Assessing***—need sufficient discrimination to distinguish ongoing expertise development Continuous improvement advantaging adaptive over routinized approaches
Asymptote	Theoretical maximum level of performance Identify breakthrough learning Calibrate environment to excellence Learning organization	***Adjusting***—Is the attained learning sufficient for the environment? Can we do better? Organizational change management approaches

The ascending phase of the learning curve loosely corresponds to the lay conceptualization of learning—that is to say, the nearly linear phase in which a unit increase in learning effort results in a predictable corresponding increase in performance. The learner can see himself improving at a reliable rate. The MAL instructor's or coach's role during the learning phase is to ensure that the learner structures his learning well, to support and encourage him during the learning process, and to provide feedback on his progress where necessary. Motivation is high as learners steadily march toward their learning goal. This is the sweet spot of learning.

However, a MAL approach to this progressive learning phase may differ. By taking a metacognitive perspective on the learning, a master adaptive learner will look to do even better than comfortable, linear learning and instead be open to the full range of improvement possibilities. In Chapter 2, we described the desirable difficulties learning principles espoused by the Drs. Bjork.[13,14] This is defined as an instructional strategy in which, in comparison to other possibilities, more effort is required (i.e., the learning is made more difficult than it might be) but the

increased effort engenders greater cognitive processing, which is repaid with better encoding and more durable learning.[13,14] A classic example is the difference between re-reading or highlighting text in a textbook chapter, compared with generating question-format flash cards.[15] The former is easier and feels like effective learning, but the latter difficult option has been shown to be more effective in the longer term. Other examples of desirable difficulties are delayed (not immediate) feedback to increase cognitive processing and spacing and interleaving (versus blocked practice).[16,17]

To illustrate this idea, you should read the following question and then put the book down and reflect on what you think is a potential answer:

> What is a desirable difficulty instructional strategy that is particularly appropriate for master adaptive learning? *(put book down and reflect)*

Whether you took the extra time to do the mini-exercise or just read straight through, the illustration is hopefully clear that the set-apart question, with no obvious answer, results in increased cognitive processing that reinforces both consideration of the idea of desirable difficulty as well as its relevance to the MAL model.

As you answered the question, we hope the particular desirable difficulty you proposed positioned the learner in the more difficult, more time-consuming, but potentially more rewarding Optimal Adaptability Corridor (see Chapters 2 and 3 and Fig. 3.1). This means, as in the quality improvement rounds described in the vignette, that having the master adaptive learner take extra time to consider innovation and how she might adapt and do things differently, even as she develops her skills, is important. Take for a separate example a surgical resident who is developing her skills in the management of hernia patients. She may feel an imperative to polish her routines, with fluidity or speed being perceived as a key self-assessment metric. This resident's learning could be improved by taking part in quality improvement initiatives developed at a departmental level, keeping her at the innovation interface. She could also play a role in a root cause analysis of a herniorrhaphy gone wrong. This would have her examining her core assumptions in a manner consistent with the MAL metacognitive lens.[18,19]

ASSESSING—THE INFLECTION POINT OF THE LEARNING CURVE AND PRODUCTIVE FAILURE

Vignette Continued

"Why don't EM faculty use POCUS for appendicitis?" asked one of Dr. Liu's junior residents.

"Let me tell you about how I wasted a year of my life," responded Dr. Liu. She went on to describe how, as a junior emergency medicine attending, she embarked on a quality improvement project to have the local emergency medicine physicians learn how to diagnose appendicitis by ultrasound. There were myriad problems, many out of Dr. Liu's control.

"How did it turn out?" asked the resident.

"Eventually my director sat me down and, based on our data, we abandoned the project. But I followed the literature closely. It took almost a decade for the eventual practice pattern to become established. We didn't know it then, but appendicitis ultrasound only really works in pediatrics. In retrospect, I think I would have just kept working and working at it, without my director's outside perspective. We made the right call to shut it down, but it hurt."

As he engages in the learning phase, the master adaptive learner continually assesses how his learning is progressing and whether the degree of difficulty is indeed at the right level of desirability. This metacognitive monitoring is helpful for regulating the learning but also for steering through the potential pitfalls that are inherent to gaining expertise at the highest levels. The MAL framework explicitly acknowledges that the highest levels of health professions expertise are difficult to achieve (hence the necessarily long and rigorous training). The learning at more advanced levels is complicated by the fact that assessing is more difficult. There are fewer explicit assessment instruments, and feedback is harder to come by or less clear in the face of practice variation. Thus, at advanced levels, the impact of learning may be less predictable such that learning can involve a tremendous amount of learning effort, only to finally conclude that the newly developed skill will not have the intended impact. There may be a productive failure.

Thus the assessing phase of the MAL model may properly lead to complete abandonment of the learning project, in favor of a different approach. For example, the early pioneers in laparoscopic surgery worked with initial pilot methods, some that worked and some that did not, on the way to eventual success.[20] A certain number of failures are a necessary part of learning, and learning that is guaranteed of success is a lower-ambition type of learning. Productive failure is rightly celebrated in the research world and the innovation world.[21] In medicine this is additionally challenging because failure can have significant patient consequences. With master adaptive learning we are proposing that openness to failure will sometimes be a necessary part of learning, especially at the highest levels of clinical care.

The practical implication is that master adaptive learning, done right, is not always successful. The assessing phase implies a continual comparison of learning progress against available resources (usually time) and the distance to the target state. Asking the question, "Is this the best learning project for me and/or my system, right now?" is an important component of the assessing process for any individual MAL cycle. Learning Curve Theory can provide metacognitive direction that allows the master adaptive learner to make informed, effective decisions, with the important point being, yet again, that learning is not linear. We have made this point in terms of the planning phase (see Fig. 16.2), but in assessing whether to continue a learning project, two other features of the sigmoid-shaped (or S-shaped) learning curve come into play: the inflection point and asymptotic learning.

Assessment and the Inflection Point—A False Milestone

Vignette Continued

"Why aren't the senior residents coming to our POCUS quality improvement rounds?" asked Dr. Liu of her chief residents.

"I think it's because this program does such a great job of teaching POCUS that, recognizing we obviously need to keep learning, the seniors feel they're pretty good at POCUS," replied one of the chiefs, diplomatically. "I guess they don't feel that they are learning a lot from those discussions." Slightly frustrated with the answer that they don't think there is more to learn or the chance to further deepen their expertise, Dr. Liu wonders how she might create unexpected challenges or failures to help prompt her senior learners to relook for gaps in their practice.

Looking again at the prototypical learning curve in Fig. 16.2, after the period of rapid learning, the learning slows down at an inflection point. This is because, at base, learning is an autocatalytic process in the same way that many enzymatic processes are.[1,22] Early in the process there is a lot of substrate for improvement. The learner gains facility with common, frequent, and generally typical examples. She starts with the easy-to-learn material in the domain. Learning is easy to organize and easy to accomplish. Learning is rapid and efficient. A good example would be the tremendous growth seen during the intern year of a residency program. However, as learning progresses, the next-thing-to-be-learned is necessarily less common, less accessible, and less tractable. There is less substrate for the autocatalytic process. The acceleration slows and in fact inflects to a decelerating trajectory.

The inflection point feels to the learner like a significant signpost in her personal development: "Yesterday I was gaining knowledge/skill at a tremendous rate. Today that rate has slowed a great deal. Am I done?" This deceleration can be erroneously interpreted as a competency milestone. However, for the highest levels of expertise the desired level of performance is usually well beyond what has been achieved at the inflection point (see Fig. 16.2). Ongoing, informed self-assessment in relationship to a well-described competency or excellence goal can give the master adaptive learner a more realistic view of the nonlinear path to true expertise. Reforms promoting competency-based advancement promise to reorient the learner to a more realistic assessment (see Chapter 6).[23]

Assessment and Asymptotic Learning—The Law of Diminishing Returns

As previously mentioned, the seminal work of Anders Ericsson has shown that the highest levels of expertise are hard won.[4,24,25] In the decelerating phase of learning, the so-called law of diminishing returns kicks in. The intermediate learner who feels that the learning deceleration signals achievement of expertise actually still has a long road ahead of him. In the decelerating phase, it takes more and more learning effort to accomplish the same incremental improvement in performance. In this phase, learning resources that can improve performance are no longer plentiful. There are fewer and fewer expert teachers. There is less consensus and more practice variation clouding feedback. Truly impactful cases are rare and less available for learning, and, at this stage of a professional trajectory, the time available for learning is ever more precious.

The deceleration phase makes clear the asymptotic nature of expertise development, in which the development can be judged either with respect to a community-specified competency line (as in competency-based advancement) or with regard to an asymptote that represents the best that can be done given the current state of the learning system. This last point is important in two respects. While the science of breakthroughs is beyond the scope of this chapter, the asymptote really represents the current potential of a learning system and, therefore, a target for achievement. Consider the implications of a MAL planning process in which the aspiration is to achieve an asymptotic level of performance as opposed to an intermediate competency level. Changing our expertise development systems from a competency achievement orientation to one that stresses advancing the potential of the entire learning system would have the welcome benefit of increasing the profile of excellence.[26] Also, in this chapter we have, for the purposes of illustration, been reductionist in describing expertise development as a smooth learning curve. The conceptual advance is to suggest that there are regularities underlying what can appear to be a random process. However, there is tremendous variability in learning at the individual level.[3] How an individual progresses relative to the group and relative to a system-level asymptote is an area of ongoing research.[27]

ADJUSTING—INDIVIDUAL AND ORGANIZATIONAL LEARNING

Vignette Continued

During an emergency medicine faculty meeting, Dr. Liu is caught off guard by growing resentment of the faculty around POCUS, following a recent departmental announcement. "Why do we have to get new machines? I was just getting used to the ones we have now!" The emergency medicine attending who made the comment is generally considered to be a lovable grouch who had to learn POCUS late in his career. Many of the other faculty are nodding their heads in support. Dr. Liu sinks into her chair, wishing she'd skipped this meeting.

She replies, "They're the same but better. The residents love them." Her comment is met with the rolling of eyes around the room.

Her spirits lift when one of the most senior attendings blurts out, "Oh well then, bring it on! Nothing will rival how hard it was to use my first ultrasound machine. This will be a piece of cake by comparison." She is silently thankful for his comment, but she wonders if there might have been a more effective way to roll out the new machines within the department.

In the adjusting phase, the master adaptive learner is to take her newly acquired skill or knowledge and decide whether to implement it into routine practice. This requires considering the tension between routinization and innovation as well as the interplay between the individual and the health system. To this point, we have presented a zoomed-out view of the MAL process as it can promote individual development. In many respects, the adjusting phase of the MAL model is an explicit encouragement to the learner to take just such a higher-level perspective on the implications for practice of her just-accomplished learning. In particular, this requires consideration of how learning at the individual level relates to the system level.

Routine Balanced With Innovation

"Is my newly developed skill an incremental refinement of something that is already well routinized? Or is it an innovation that will require creative destruction in order to rework practice?" In a number of places, we have made the point that adjusting one's practice can require different processes depending on whether the improvement in question is the incremental refinement of a routine practice or involves implementing a significant innovation. Refining a routine practice is in many ways easier. There already exists a shared understanding of the clinical action. The new skill may simply extend current practices. An example might be the updating of a clinical guideline wherein the goals of therapy remain the same, but the thresholds for therapy have been refined or the medication/dosages have changed. Another example might be an ultrasound machine that undergoes an iterative refinement. In essence, the learner and the system continue on the mature part of the learning curve, doing the incremental work that ensures ongoing improvement.

A significant innovation, on the other hand, is more difficult to digest even if it has the potential to improve the system as a whole. Here, existing routines need to be disrupted to accommodate the new learning or technology. Well-studied examples are the introduction of laparoscopic techniques to general surgery or, as in the vignette, the initial adoption of POCUS in emergency medicine.[28] Learning to use augmented intelligence systems will require a new normal for all clinicians in the coming years.[29] However, these large disruptions can be considered as extreme examples for a continuous spectrum ranging from learning that completely redefines a field of clinical practice to well-honed, encapsulated clinical processes that are stable and foundational.[19] In between is the space described in Fig. 2.2 that encompasses all sorts of intermediate everyday improvements that affect individuals, teams, and systems. Negotiating this space requires adaptive expertise (see Chapter 2).

Individuals vary in their propensity to adjust in this way, as has been described by Rogers, including his canonical Innovation Curve (Fig. 16.4).[30] This is a key principle underlying the adjusting phase of the MAL process, with the master adaptive learner expected to be more disposed to the innovator/early adopter end of the spectrum. However, this is not a blind expectation, given that a well-informed, reflective late majority or laggard master adaptive learner who is well versed in critical appraisal could be the most valuable member of a diverse team that seeks to rationally implement costly learning across a complex clinical environment (see Chapter 11). Nonetheless, in many respects the disruptive innovation is the greatest challenge to the master adaptive learner. To learn, in mid-career, an entirely new method or process like POCUS calls for all the intangibles that drive master adaptive learning: resilience, motivation, a growth mindset, and curiosity. It may seem unusual to consider an organizational learning conceptualization, like the Rogers Innovation Curve, in a book on individual learning. However, no learning happens in isolation, as was stressed in our consideration of the learning environment (see Chapter 11). Master adaptive learning occurs best when the individual-system interaction is explicitly taken into account.

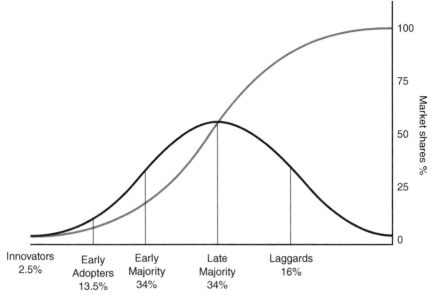

Fig. 16.4 Rogers Innovation Curve. The Rogers Innovation Curve is a first derivative of the learning curve. As a new technology or idea is taken up by a community, individuals vary in their propensity to adjust their practice to the new method in a fashion that is approximately normally distributed *(black curve)*. This adoption/adjustment process is a key driver of organizational learning *(blue curve)*. (From Rogers E, 2012; public domain. based on Rogers E. *Diffusion of Innovations*. New York: Free Press; 1962. Available at: https://commons. wikimedia.org/w/index.php?curid=18525407.)

Individual Balanced With Organizational Imperatives

In the adjusting phase, the other zoomed-out perspective that can be helpful to the master adaptive learner is that of the system-level implications of his new learning:

- Does my health care system have a learning curve?
- Where am I with respect to it?
- Can I influence it?

We have touched on this in describing the Rogers Theory of Innovation adoption, but there are many additional factors to consider in the interaction between a master adaptive learner and his system. Some of these have been described in Chapter 15. Here we reiterate that learning theories can guide the master adaptive learner in his efforts. Well-developed theories of organizational change, essentially learning theories, can predict the road ahead even in complex learning environments.[31,32] An example of an organizational change management theory was put forth by Elisabeth Kubler-Ross after her seminal work on the stages of grieving. The same stages (Denial-Anger-Bargaining-Depression-Acceptance) that apply to grieving have dismaying applicability to organizational change

management.[33,34] Taking a metacognitive approach, knowing that the stages are coming and in what order, can help the master adaptive learner in adjusting his own learning and in adjusting his organization. In Fig. 16.5, we show how these mitigations are meant to help an organization digest a disruptive innovation, one that results in an initial performance hit in service of an eventual rise to a new, higher level of functioning.[35]

A more proactive conceptualization, Kotter's change management theory outlines an eight-step process that describes a systematic approach to influencing a complex learning environment, as the adjusting phase of master adaptive learning would advocate. The Kotter model includes modulating the level of urgency in the organization, building a team with a consensus vision of the desired change, and then breaking down the change into manageable chunks that are implemented with clear communication and commitment.[36,37] The idea is to set a goal of lasting culture change and to commit up front to providing the necessary organizational energy and resources—a kind of organizational "desirable difficulty." The point is that the same qualities of openness to

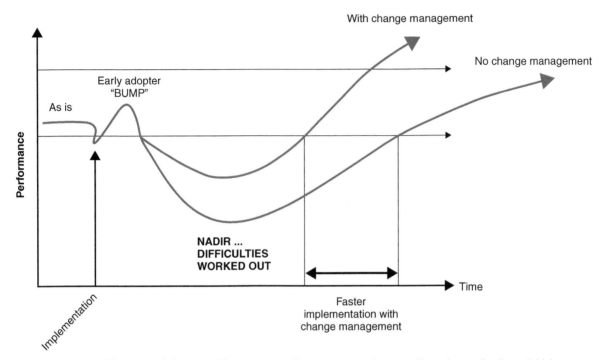

Fig. 16.5 Theories of Change Management. As a system adopts a disruptive technology, initial performance can suffer until the full adjustment has been made. Change management can mitigate this predictable process. (Adapted from Mulholland B. 8 Critical change management models to evolve and survive. *Process Street.* 2017;July 24. https://www.process.st/change-management-models/. Accessed April 10, 2019.)

innovation that make a master adaptive learner a valuable addition to clinical care can roll up to the institutional level, where they can similarly have a positive impact within an organizational learning framework.

SCIENTIFIC THEORIES AND THE MASTER ADAPTIVE LEARNING FRAMEWORK

Throughout this book, we have stressed the solid theoretical underpinnings of the MAL process and the traits we would inculcate in a master adaptive learner. Indeed, a key aspiration of master adaptive learning is to integrate a number of evidence- and theory-based pedagogical principles into a shared language, a shared attitude to the enterprise of learning in clinical care. The model adds value insofar as it can guide the everyday judgments of a learner in a 21st-century clinical learning environment.

In this chapter, we have used one exemplar theory, that of learning curves, to demonstrate the foundation on which the MAL framework is built. We could have chosen

any of several others. For example, the connections between master adaptive learning and the precepts of self-regulated learning are considerable.[38] Besides being an important consideration during the learning phase, we could highlight the need for self-direction in the planning, assessing, and adjusting phases.

In Table 16.2, we have listed some of the component theories that underpin the MAL model. The intent is to highlight its robustness. These component parts, dissected and described in detail in the chapters leading to this one, are the well-established, empirically tested foundations of our field. What could have been a disparate collection of theories and methods instead knits together nicely into a four-phase cycle so that, in the words of Cutrer and colleagues from the original paper, "this shared conceptual model will facilitate conversation between teachers and learners that allows for the analysis and diagnosis of learning struggles, as well as motivate individuals to be more effective and impactful in learning that improves the delivery of high-quality health care."[39]

TABLE 16.2   Education Science Theories Relevant to the Master Adaptive Learner Framework.

Learning Theory	Main Tenets	Key Investigators[a]	Relevance to MAL Framework	Chapters
Overall				
Preparation for Future Learning	Downstream learning can be advantaged by learning designs that emphasize deep mechanistic and meta-cognitive understanding.	Schwartz & Bransford; Woods, Brooks, & Norman	Master adaptive learning considers learning in the moment both for the good it does now and for how it will advantage learning in the future.	2, 9
Self-Determination Theory (SDT)	SDT is an approach to human motivation and personality that highlights the importance of evolved inner resources for personality development and behavioral self-regulation.	Deci & Ryan	Developing MAL traits and habits requires self-direction and self-regulation on the part of the learner.	1, 13
Situated Cognition	Learning is a social co-constructed process between people as opposed to being entirely in one's head. Early participation advantages learning.	Lave & Wenger	During both the learning and the adjusting phases, the learning between and among people is an important part of adaptive expertise and its place in health systems.	11
Living Systems Theory	The general behavior of living systems is determined among seven levels ranging from cells through to supranational interactions.	J. G. Miller	The master adaptive learner exists in a complex learning environment that interacts with levels below and above it. The master adaptive learner can positively influence each interlocking system.	11
Learning Curve Theory	Learning consistently follows a sigmoid-shaped pattern relating effort with learning.	L. L. Thurstone	MAL process cycles lead to iterative development of adaptive expertise along a predictable but nonlinear path.	16
Planning				
Cognitive Dissonance	Mental discomfort is experienced when a person holds two or more contra-dictory beliefs or ideas.	L. Festinger	The feeling of cognitive dissonance can stimulate the master adaptive learner to enter the learning process.	1, 3
Informed Self-Assessment	Self-assessment is difficult, with success depending on pursuing outside information.	J. Sargeant	Appropriate calibration and adjustment of clinician functioning depends on feedback data, both internal and external.	1, 6

Continued

TABLE 16.2 Education Science Theories Relevant to the Master Adaptive Learner Framework—cont'd.

Learning Theory	Main Tenets	Key Investigators[a]	Relevance to MAL Framework	Chapters
Scientific Management Theory (SMT)	SMT uses the scientific method to analyze and optimize workflows. The planning of an activity can be separated from the doing.	F. W. Taylor	SMT can come into the MAL process, in terms of both planning and managing a learning workflow, but also for MAL questions that engender new, better clinical methods, whether routine or innovative (adjusting).	2, 14
Learning				
Encapsulation of Knowledge	Biomedical knowledge becomes encapsulated with clinical experiences and clinical learning to form illness scripts.	H. Schmidt	Master adaptive learning is advantaged by particular attention to the encapsulation process and the ability to metacognitively examine an illness script and its limits.	3
Zone of Proximal Development (ZPD)	The ZPD is an optimal learning zone between what a learner cannot do unaided and what he can already do unaided.	L. Vygotsky	Each learner has a different ZPD. The MAL process works best when customized for each learner.	2, 5
Cognitive Load Theory	Human cognitive architecture includes specific bottle-necks that can be mitigated by instructional design.	J. Sweller; R. Mayer	Clinical information can be deliberately apportioned to the master adaptive learner, allowing increased cognitive resources to be brought to bear on key concepts.	13
Desirable Difficulties	Deep learning approaches can be disadvantageous in the short term but result in more durable learning over the longer term.	Bjork & Bjork	Master adaptive learning is often advantaged by choosing the path that is more difficult in the short term. The Optimal Adaptability Corridor is a master adaptive learner–specific example.	2, 13, 16
Dual-Process Theory of Clinical Decision Making	Two distinct cognitive systems influence clinical decision making: one fast and intuitive, the other slow and analytic.	P. Croskerry; Kahneman & Tversky	MAL learning is best supported by an understanding of human cognitive architecture.	5

TABLE 16.2   Education Science Theories Relevant to the Master Adaptive Learner Framework—cont'd.

Learning Theory	Main Tenets	Key Investigators[a]	Relevance to MAL Framework	Chapters
Habit Formation	The process of routinizing new behaviors into stereotyped routines starts with the early stages of learning according to a cycle in which a triggering cue invokes the routine that is then reinforced with a specific reward.	C. Duhigg	MAL behaviors can be most effective when they become a deliberately cultivated habit.	5
Assessing				
Cognitive Biases in Self-Assessment	Self-assessment is difficult, with success depending on metacognitive awareness.	Kruger & Dunning	Early in the learning cycle, the master adaptive learner knows not to rely on unguided self-assessment; at high levels of expertise, the master adaptive learner carries a beneficial bias to underestimating her level of performance.	6
Reflective Practice	Learning occurs best when organized according to a metacognitive framework that includes specific opportunities for reflection.	D. Schön	MAL debriefing and learning strategies that invoke self-monitoring, reflection, or both are more effective.	12
Adjusting				
Adaptive Expertise	Higher levels of expertise include a balance between innovation and routinization.	Hatano; Bransford & Schwartz; Mylopoulos & Scardamalia	Master adaptive learning occurs best in the Optimal Adaptability Corridor where the learner can deliberately practice balancing routine and innovative approaches.	2, 10
Systems Thinking	Systems thinking is a theory of systems that emphasizes the interrelationships between elements favoring holistic, organic approaches.	Von Bertalanffy & Senge	In the adjusting phase, the MAL approach emphasizes interaction with the health care system and adapting to the complexity of a clinical micro- or macrosystem.	11, 15
Innovation Adoption	Rogers' Innovation Adoption curve makes clear that the propensity to adopt a new technology follows a normal distribution ranging from early to late adopters.	Rogers	Implementation of learning is variable across learners. Master adaptive learners may have a positive disposition to new innovations, informed by critical appraisal.	16

Continued

TABLE 16.2   Education Science Theories Relevant to the Master Adaptive Learner Framework—cont'd.

Learning Theory	Main Tenets	Key Investigators[a]	Relevance to MAL Framework	Chapters
Batteries (Capacity)				
Curiosity	Intellectual curiosity is the individual preference for engaging in mentally challenging tasks and the purposeful pursuit of knowledge. Both trait and state curiosity are positively predictive of classroom and workplace learning and performance.	Berlyne; Fitzgerald	Curiosity drives learners to identify gaps and unknowns for learning and can sustain each of the phases of the MAL process even when learning is difficult.	1, 4
Motivation	Self-Determination Theory describes the continuum from amotivation to external to intrinsic motivation. Positive learner feelings of autonomy, competence, and relatedness drive the move toward intrinsic motivation.	Deci & Ryan	Intrinsic motivation provides the critical drive for all four phases of the MAL process, especially when the learner experiences setbacks.	1, 4
Mindset	Mindsets, or implicit theories of self, are core assumptions individuals hold about the malleability of their personal traits, such as their intelligence or ability to learn.	C. S. Dweck	Adopting a growth mindset impacts each phase of the MAL process by ensuring the learner believes that he can and will improve with effort.	1, 4
Resilience	Resilience allows learners to adapt well in the face of adversity, trauma, tragedy, threats, or even significant sources of threat. It is vital to addressing increasing burnout in the medical field.	Newman (APA); Dyrbye & Shanafelt; Duckworth	Learners will face trials and setbacks during each MAL phase of their learning, in both the classroom and the workplace.	1, 4

[a]**References:**
Berlyne DE. Curiosity and exploration. *Science.* 1966;153(3731):25-33.
Bjork EL, Bjork RA. Making things hard on yourself, but in a good way: creating desirable difficulties to enhance learning. In: Gernsbacher MA, Pew RW, Hough LM, Pomerantz JR, eds. *Psychology and the Real World: Essays Illustrating Fundamental Contributions to Society.* New York: Worth Publishers; 2011:56-64.
Croskerry P. Clinical cognition and diagnostic error: applications of a dual process model of reasoning. *Adv Health Sci Educ.* 2009;14(1):27-35.
Deci EL, Ryan RM, eds. *Handbook of Self-Determination Research.* Rochester, NY: University of Rochester Press; 2004.
Duckworth AL, Peterson C, Matthews MD, Kelly DR. Grit: perseverance and passion for long-term goals. *J Pers Soc Psychol.* 2007;92:1087-1101.
Duhigg C. *The Power of Habit: Why We Do What We Do in Life and Business.* New York: Random House; 2012.
Dweck CS. *Mindset: The New Psychology of Success.* New York: Random House Digital, Inc.; 2008.
Festinger L. *A Theory of Cognitive Dissonance.* Stanford, CA: Stanford University Press; 1957.

Fitzgerald FT. Curiosity. *Ann Intern Med.* 1999;130(1):70-72.

Hatano G, Inagaki K. Two courses of expertise. *Research and Clinical Center for Child Development Annual Report.* Sapporo, Hokkaido, Japan: Hokkaido University; 1984;6:27-36.

Kahneman D, Egan P. *Thinking, Fast and Slow.* New York: Farrar, Straus and Giroux; 2011.

Kruger J, Dunning D. Unskilled and unaware of it: how difficulties in recognizing one's own incompetence lead to inflated self-assessments. *J Pers Soc Psychol.* 1999;77(6):1121.

Lave J, Wenger E. *Situated Learning: Legitimate Peripheral Participation.* Cambridge, UK: Cambridge University Press; 1991.

Mayer RE, Moreno R. Nine ways to reduce cognitive load in multimedia learning. *Educ Psychol.* 2003;38(1):43-52.

Miller JG. *Living Systems.* New York: McGraw-Hill; 1973.

Mylopoulos M, Brydges R, Woods NN, Manzone J, Schwartz DL. Preparation for future learning: a missing competency in health professions education? *Med Educ.* 2016;50(1):115-123.

Mylopoulos M, Scardamalia M. Doctors' perspectives on their innovations in daily practice: implications for knowledge building in health care. *Med Educ.* 2008;42(10):975-981.

Newman R. APA's resilience initiative. *Prof Psychol Res Pract.* 2005;36(3):227.

Rogers EM. *Diffusion of Innovations.* New York: Simon and Schuster; 2010.

Ryan RM, Deci EL. Self-determination theory and the facilitation of intrinsic motivation, social development, and well-being. *Am Psychol.* 2000;55(1):68.

Sargeant J, Armson H, Chesluk B, et al. The processes and dimensions of informed self-assessment: a conceptual model. *Acad Med.* 2010;85(7):1212-1220.

Schmidt HG, Rikers RM. How expertise develops in medicine: knowledge encapsulation and illness script formation. *Med Educ.* 2007;41(12):1133-1139.

Schön DA. *Educating the Reflective Practitioner: Toward a New Design for Teaching and Learning in the Professions.* Jossey-Bass Higher Education Series. 1st ed. San Franscisco: Jossey Bass; 1987.

Schwartz DL, Bransford JD, Sears D. Efficiency and innovation in transfer. In: Mestre JP, ed. *Transfer of Learning From a Modern Multidisciplinary Perspective.* Greenwich, CT: Information Age Publishing; 2005:1-51.

Shanafelt TD, Boone S, Tan L, et al. Burnout and satisfaction with work-life balance among US physicians relative to the general US population. *Arch Intern Med.* 2012;172(18):1377-1385.

Sweller J. Cognitive load theory. *Psychol Learn Motivat.* 2011;55:37-76. (See also Mayer RE. *Learning and Instruction.* Upper Saddle River, NJ: Merrill; 2003.)

Taylor FW. *Scientific Management.* New York: Routledge; 2004.

Thurstone LL. The learning curve equation. *Psychol Monogr.* 1919;26(3).

Von Bertalanffy L. *General System Theory.* New York: Braziller; 1968:40.

Vygotsky—see, for example: Mayer RE. *Learning and Instruction.* Upper Saddle River, NJ: Merrill; 2003.

Woods NN, Brooks LR, Norman GR. The value of basic science in clinical diagnosis: creating coherence among signs and symptoms. *Med Educ.* 2005;39(1):107-112.

CONCLUSION

Master adaptive learning is an evidence-based, rich response to the imperatives of modern health care. It acknowledges the increasingly dynamic and complex nature of the clinical care but also celebrates the progress that health professions education has made in advancing and contextualizing learning science. An overview of the book's chapters provides a summary of the potential of master adaptive learning. In the first three chapters, we described a new kind of clinical learning, arguing that the clinician of the future will be, to an even greater extent, constantly learning and adapting. While the superb learners who enter the health professions have already demonstrated considerable learning ability, we have made the claim that a new focus on the exact nature of "learning for clinical learning" will be repaid with a higher level of expertise. In particular, we pointed to the important balance between

routinization and innovation that needs to be practiced during training so the clinician can exercise adaptive expertise as she innovates in the moment and as she seeks to influence and adapt to her changing environment.

In subsequent chapters, we presented different perspectives on learning how to become a master adaptive learner. From its intersection with clinical reasoning (Chapters 3 and 5) to consideration of what personal characteristics are necessary (Chapter 4), a metacognitive perspective allows the master adaptive learner to explicitly consider his development as a learner and as an expert. Mapping out the path, as stressed in this chapter, can lead to more intentional, effective, and efficient personal development that includes a capacity for self-direction. We have stressed the importance of well-designed assessment the locus of control of which can be with the master adaptive learner but that is tempered by a metacognitive awareness of the limits of unguided self-assessment (Chapters 6 and 7). This is not to say that master adaptive learning falls entirely on the learner. Good instructional design is as important as ever but needs to be reoriented. In Chapter 8 we discussed where and how teaching to the MAL principles can be most effective, with additional chapters on the most important learning contexts, the classroom and the bedside (Chapters 9 and 10). With the locus of learning control taken on by an empowered master adaptive learner, the shift from direct transmission of instruction to supportive individualized coaching is a natural progression, as outlined in Chapter 12 and reinforced as it relates to the struggling learner in Chapter 13. However, perhaps the richest picture of the MAL conceptualization occurs when the modern clinical learning environment, with all its dynamic complexity, is considered as it interacts with a learner tuned to both its difficulties and its affordances (Chapter 11). The emphasis on adaptive expertise is an explicit nod to the dynamic nature of this interaction and the increasingly dynamic nature of the interaction between the learner and the clinical context. Here the welcome development is increased recognition of the third pillar of medical education, health systems science.[40] As its educational importance for clinicians is characterized in the coming years, the integral role of adaptive expertise will undoubtedly be made more explicit, as Chapter 15 begins to describe, with an important component being the leadership skills (Chapter 14) that help master adaptive learners effect change within those systems. Finally, in this chapter we have tried to make the point that MAL process cycles accumulate to affect change in individuals and can influence the learning trajectories of microsystems and, ultimately, organizations, all according to predictable trajectories.

The MAL conceptualization emerged from the decades-long work of Don Moore,[41] building on the work of H. B. Slotnick,[42] that of Fox, Mazmanian, and Putnam,[43] and the many others who invested significant time and energy into better understanding how practicing physicians learn. Dr. Moore masterfully gathered and aligned the work to create a unified understanding about the learning stages of practicing physicians. Combining his work with the self-regulated learning work of Zimmerman[44] (general education), White, Gruppen, and Fantone[45] (medical education), and Schumacher, Englander, and Carraccio[46] (master learner) allowed the group to more explicitly consider the learning process–focused knowledge, skills, and attitudes necessary for development in physicians-in-training. Finally, the focus on using preparation for future learning and setting the target on adaptive expertise development of Mylopoulos and colleagues[11] provided significant alignment and motivation for the American Medical Association's (AMA's) MAL interest group's efforts.

The AMA's MAL interest group hopes that, in picking up the baton, we have done justice to this rich conceptualization. The best testament would be that the model continues to evolve in the way that it promotes clinical learning.

TAKE-HOME POINTS

1. Learning takes a nonlinear path in most instances, with the master adaptive learning process being no exception. Knowing the elements of the sigmoid-shaped learning curve can allow the master adaptive learner to map a more intentional path to her learning goals.
2. Regularities in learning trajectories are seen not only in individuals but also at progressively higher levels of learning such as at the clinical microsystem or the organization. Metacognitive awareness of these regularities can help the master adaptive learner, especially during the adjusting phase as he considers the potential impact of his learning on the health system.
3. Perhaps the greatest test of a master adaptive learner will come when a disruptive innovation requires complete reformulation of an aspect of her clinical practice. The metacognitive perspective promoted in the MAL model will facilitate such a transition.

QUESTIONS FOR FURTHER THOUGHT

1. Name a skill that you are developing in the service of improved care. Where are you on your learning curve? How will you know when you have achieved expertise? What does the path ahead look like? What nonlinearities await?
2. What are your organization's mechanisms for promoting organizational learning? Does the organization engage in preparation for future learning (PFL)? How does the organization promote PFL? What are the barriers?
3. Name a time when you stopped your own learning curve. What went into the decision? Was it an intentional decision? Or did you just peter out? What could help you the next time in making a more effective or efficient decision?

ANNOTATED BIBLIOGRAPHY

1. Rogers EM. *Diffusion of Innovations.* New York, NY: Free Press; 2003. https://books.google.com/books?id=9U1K5LjUOwEC. Accessed April 4, 2019.

   This seminal conceptualization allows for understanding of how innovation and learning diffuse among individuals at differential rates. Early adopters and late adopters can have different but equally valuable roles in the healthy consideration of innovations within an organization.

2. Pusic MV, Boutis K, McGaghie WC. Role of scientific theory in simulation education research. *Simul Healthc.* 2018;13 (3S suppl 1):S7-S14.

   This article on scientific theories as a basis for educational practice is similar in structure to this chapter but with a deeper consideration of what goes into a scientific theory. It includes consideration of the roles of falsification, scalability, and explanatory power.

3. Barrow JM, Toney-Butler TJ. *Change Management.* Treasure Island, FL: StatPearls Publishing; 2019. Available at: http://www.ncbi.nlm.nih.gov/pubmed/29083813. Accessed April 7, 2019.

   Organizational learning models abound. In this chapter we have discussed only a few. A broad survey, starting with this article, allows the reader to consider the intersection of a master adaptive learner with these organizational conceptualizations of learning.

4. Firestein S. *Failure: Why Science Is So Successful.* 1st ed. New York, NY: Oxford University Press; 2016.

   Health professions education has a laudable orientation toward success. However, as noted by Firestein, an eminent scientist who wrote this very accessible book, some of the best learning occurs from failure. In fact, learning from failure may be the key ingredient for developing wisdom.

REFERENCES

1. Pusic MV, Boutis K, McGaghie WC. Role of scientific theory in simulation education research. *Simul Healthc.* 2018;13 (3S suppl 1):S7-S14.
2. Kalet A, Pusic M. Defining and assessing competence. In: Kalet A, Chou C, eds. *Remediation in Medical Education.* 1st ed. Boston, MA: Springer; 2014:3-15.
3. Pusic MV, Boutis K, Hatala R, Cook DA. Learning curves in health professions education. *Acad Med.* 2015;90(8):1034-1042.
4. Ericsson KA, Lehmann AC. Expert and exceptional performance: evidence of maximal adaptation to task constraints. *Annu Rev Psychol.* 1996;47:273-305.
5. Wright TP. Factors affecting the cost of airplanes. *J Aeronaut Sci.* 1936;3(4):122-128.
6. Flavio S, Fogliatto FS, Anazanello MJ. Learning curves: the state of the art and research directions. In: Jaber MY, ed. *Learning Curves: Theory, Models, and Applications.* Boca Raton, FL: CRC Press; 2011:3-22.
7. Boston Consulting Group. *Perspectives on Corporate Strategy.* Boston, MA: Boston Consulting Group; 1968. Available at:
   http://www.worldcat.org/title/perspectives-on-corporate-strategy/oclc/643223488?referer=di&ht=edition. Accessed March 13, 2012.
8. Gas BL, Buckarma EH, Cook DA, Farley DR, Pusic MV. Is speed a desirable difficulty for learning procedures? An initial exploration of the effects of chronometric pressure. *Acad Med.* 2018;93(6):920-928.
9. Ramsay CR, Grant AM, Wallace SA, Garthwaite PH, Monk AF, Russell IT. Statistical assessment of the learning curves of health technologies. *Health Technol Assess.* 2001;5(12):1-79.
10. Warm EJ, Held JD, Hellmann M, et al. Entrusting observable practice activities and milestones over the 36 months of an internal medicine residency. *Acad Med.* 2016;91(10):1398-1405.
11. Mylopoulos M, Brydges R, Woods NN, Manzone J, Schwartz DL. Preparation for future learning: a missing competency in health professions education? *Med Educ.* 2016;50(1):115-123.
12. Sung SY, Choi JN. Do organizations spend wisely on employees? Effects of training and development investments on learning and innovation in organizations. *J Organ Behav.* 2014;35(3):393-412.
13. Schmidt RA, Bjork RA. New conceptualizations of practice: common principles in three paradigms suggest new concepts for training. *Psychol Sci.* 1992;3(4):207-217.
14. Bjork EL, Bjork RA. Making things hard on yourself, but in a good way: creating desirable difficulties to enhance learning. In: Gernsbacher MA, Pew RW, Hough LM, Pomerantz JR, eds. *Psychology and the Real World: Essays Illustrating Fundamental Contributions to Society.* New York, NY: Worth Publisher; 2011:56-64.
15. Larsen DP, Butler AC, Roediger HL. Test-enhanced learning in medical education. *Med Educ.* 2008;42(10):959-966.
16. Kerfoot BP, DeWolf WC, Masser BA, Church PA, Federman DD. Spaced education improves the retention of clinical knowledge by medical students: a randomised controlled trial. *Med Educ.* 2007;41(1):23-31.
17. Rohrer D, Pashler H. Recent research on human learning challenges conventional instructional strategies. *Educ Res.* 2010;39(5):406-412.
18. Schwartz D, Bransford J. Rethinking transfer: a simple proposal with multiple implications. *Rev Res Educ.* 2008;24:61-100.
19. Pusic MV, Santen SA, Dekhtyar M, et al. Learning to balance efficiency and innovation for optimal adaptive expertise. *Med Teach.* 2018;40(8):820-827.
20. Blum CA, Adams DB. Who did the first laparoscopic cholecystectomy? *J Minim Access Surg.* 2011;7(3):165-168.
21. Firestein S. *Failure: Why Science is so Successful.* 1st ed. New York, NY: Oxford University Press; 2016.
22. Singer JD, Willett JB. *Applied Longitudinal Data Analysis: Modeling Change and Event Occurrence.* Oxford, UK: Oxford University Press; 2003.
23. Frank JR, Snell LS, Cate OT, et al. Competency-based medical education: theory to practice. *Med Teach.* 2010;32(8): 638-645.
24. Ericsson KA. Acquisition and maintenance of medical expertise: a perspective from the expert-performance approach with deliberate practice. *Acad Med.* 2015;90(11): 1471-1486.

25. Ericsson KA. Deliberate practice and acquisition of expert performance: a general overview. *Acad Emerg Med.* 2008;15(11):988-994.
26. Gallagher AG. Metric-based simulation training to proficiency in medical education:- what it is and how to do it. *Ulster Med J.* 2012;81(3):107-113.
27. Pusic MV, Boutis K, Pecaric MR, Savenkov O, Beckstead JW, Jaber MY. A primer on the statistical modelling of learning curves in health professions education. *Adv Health Sci Educ Theory Pract.* 2017;22(3):741-759.
28. Ramsay CR, Grant AM, Wallace SA, Garthwaite PH, Monk AF, Russell IT. Assessment of the learning curve in health technologies. A systematic review. *Int J Technol Assess Health Care.* 2000;16(4):1095-1108.
29. Quer G, Muse ED, Nikzad N, Topol EJ, Steinhubl SR. Augmenting diagnostic vision with AI. *Lancet.* 2017;390(10091):221.
30. Rogers EM. *Diffusion of Innovations.* New York, NY: Free Press; 2003.
31. Barrow JM, Toney-Butler TJ. *Change Management.* Treasure Island, FL: StatPearls Publishing; 2019.
32. Warm EJ, Kinnear B, Kelleher M, Sall D, Holmboe E. Transforming resident assessment: an analysis using Deming's system of profound knowledge. *Acad Med.* 2018;94(2):195-201.
33. *Major Approaches & Models of Change Management.* Cleverism. 2019. Available at: https://www.cleverism.com/major-approaches-models-of-change-management/. Accessed April 4, 2019.
34. McAlearney AS, Hefner JL, Sieck CJ, Huerta TR. The journey through grief: insights from a qualitative study of electronic health record implementation. *Health Serv Res.* 2015;50(2):462-488.
35. Sayles C. Transformational change—based on the model of Virginia Satir. *Contemp Fam Ther.* 2002;24(1):93-109.
36. Appelbaum SH, Habashy S, Malo J, Shafiq H. Back to the future: revisiting Kotter's 1996 change model. *J Manag Dev.* 2012;31(8):764-782.
37. Kotter JP. *Leading Change.* Boston, MA; Harvard Business Press; 2012.
38. Zimmerman BJ. Investigating self-regulation and motivation: historical background, methodological developments, and future prospects. *Am Educ Res J.* 2008;45(1):166-183.
39. Cutrer WB, Miller B, Pusic MV, et al. Fostering the development of master adaptive learners: a conceptual model to guide skill acquisition in medical education. *Acad Med.* 2017;92(1):70-75.
40. Skochelak SE, Hawkins RE, Lawson LE, Starr S, Borkan J, Gonzalo J. *Health Systems Science.* Philadelphia, PA: Elsevier; 2017.
41. Moore Jr DE. How physicians learn and how to design learning experiences for them: an approach based on an interpretive review of evidence. In: Hager M, Russell S, Fletcher SW, eds. *Continuing Education in the Health Professions: Improving Healthcare Through Lifelong Learning.* New York: Josiah Macy, Jr. Foundation; 2008;30.
42. Slotnick HB. How doctors learn: physicians' self-directed learning episodes. *Acad Med.* 1999;74(10):1106-1117.
43. Fox RD, Mazmanian PE, Putnam RW, eds. *Changing and Learning in the Lives of Physicians.* New York, NY: Praeger; 1989.
44. Zimmerman BJ. Self-regulated learning and academic achievement: an overview. *Educ Psychol.* 1990;25(1):3-17.
45. White CB, Gruppen LD, Fantone JC. Self-regulated learning in medical education. In: Swanwick T, ed. *Understanding Medical Education: Evidence, Theory and Practice.* 2nd ed. Chichester, West Sussex, UK: John Wiley & Sons; 2014;201-211.
46. Schumacher DJ, Englander R, Carraccio C. Developing the master learner: applying learning theory to the learner, the teacher, and the learning environment. *Acad Med.* 2013;88(11):1635-1645.

MASTER ADAPTIVE LEARNER GLOSSARY

ABC analysis   A prioritization strategy. Learners group tasks into categories. Category A includes tasks that are urgent and important. Category B includes tasks that are important yet not urgent, and category C includes tasks that are unimportant but can be urgent or not urgent.

Academic Resilience Scale   A 30-item instrument that focuses on the process of resilience rather than attitudes about resilience. The instrument provides a measure of academic resilience based on learners' specific adaptive cognitive-affective and behavioral responses to academic adversity.

adaptive expertise   The combination of routine and innovative problem solving. An individual demonstrating adaptive expertise recognizes when a "routine" approach will not work, and subsequently reframes the problem in a way that allows her to explore new concepts (learning) and to invent new solutions (innovation).

adjusting phase   Part of the Master Adaptive Learner framework. Involves a physician incorporating what she has learned into daily work routines, at the individual, microsystem, and/or organizational level.

advising   Provides the learner with expert answers to his questions. Not to be confused with coaching or mentoring.

appreciative inquiry   Uses a strengths-based approach to engage a learner in identifying her strengths and postulating how those strengths can be used to achieve a desired outcome.

assessing phase   Part of the Master Adaptive Learner framework. Involves physicians seeking feedback and examining practice patterns.

change management   At the organizational level, change is difficult but can be managed by a thoughtful approach that acknowledges the predictable aspects of change and common problems that arise.

coaching   A coach evaluates the performance of learners via review of objective assessments, assisting the trainee to identify needs and create a plan to achieve them. A coach helps the learner to be accountable, to improve his own self-monitoring, and to realize his full potential. Not to be confused with advising or mentoring.

cognitive apprenticeship   Theory that accounts for the problem that, when they are teaching novices, masters of a skill often fail to take into account the implicit processes involved in carrying out complex skills. Cognitive apprenticeships are designed to bring these tacit processes into the open, where learners can observe, enact, and practice them with help from the teacher.

conceptual knowledge   One of the three categories of knowledge (along with content and procedural knowledge). A deeper understanding using schemas and mental models.

conceptual model   Conceptual knowledge about a particular system that is codified to reliably explain or predict the way it works, or both.

content knowledge   One of the three categories of knowledge (along with conceptual and procedural knowledge). Facts and information stored in memory.

critical thinking   The ability to apply higher-order cognitive skills (conceptualization, analysis, evaluation) and the disposition to be deliberate about thinking (being open-minded or intellectually honest) that lead to action that is logical and appropriate.

curiosity   One of the four internal characteristics that drive the Master Adaptive Learning process. It is the internal desire of the learner to know and understand more. It drives the learner to enter the learning cycle rather than leave questions unanswered. The other three characteristics are motivation, growth mindset, and resilience.

deliberate practice   Purposeful, systematic practice in service of attaining a defined learning goal; contrast with unguided repetitive practice. Tailored feedback/coaching is a key component.

desirable difficulty   An instructional design wherein a more difficult path is chosen in service of more durable, effective learning for the long term or for optimal transfer to where it will be applied.

disruptive innovation   In the business world, a disruptive innovation is one that creates a new market, eventually disrupting and potentially replacing the old one. In health care, disruption can occur in work processes that may have been well established.

Eisenhower decision matrix   A model to help the learner prioritize tasks. Using the Eisenhower model, the coach should help the learner decipher between urgent versus not urgent and important versus not important goals (also see ABC analysis).

extrinsic motivation   One of two basic types of motivation. Drives a person to seek a reward or avoid a punishment.

Gibbs model of reflection   Breaks down the act of reflection into six steps: description, feelings, evaluation, analysis, conclusions, and action plan.

growth mindset   One of the four internal characteristics that drive the Master Adaptive Learning process. It is a positive belief pattern held about one's own intelligence and capacity for learning being open to ongoing improvement. The other three characteristics are motivation, curiosity, and resilience.

health systems science   The study of how health systems deliver care to patients, how patients receive and access that care, and how care can be improved.

informed self-assessment   Use of external information to inform and generate a more accurate concept of the individual's knowledge, skills, and attitudes.

innovation expertise   In contrast to routinized expertise, innovation expertise requires a bespoke, individualized solution developed in the moment for a particular context or problem. Typically associated with more complex problems.

instructional design   A systematic approach to the creation, implementation, and monitoring of instruction. For example, choosing a desirable difficulty over a superficial approach can be an advantageous instructional design decision.

intrinsic motivation   One of two basic types of motivation. Drives an individual to pursue an activity because of a personal interest.

ISMART   Acronym that prompts the learner to articulate a goal that is Important, Specific, and Measurable, offers Accountability, is Realistic, and contains a Timeline.

L

learning curve theory   Posits that learning is a nonlinear but predictable phenomenon that has the property of scaling, such that the learning pattern repeats itself at multiple levels.

learning environment   The contexts, cultures, and diverse physical locations in which individuals learn, which is all the more complex in health care.

learning phase   Part of the Master Adaptive Learner framework. Period of intense focus when a physician develops and internalizes new understandings that address identified gaps in knowledge, skills, or attitudes.

M

master adaptive learner   A learner who uses a metacognitive approach to self-regulated learning that leads to the development and demonstration of adaptive expertise.

mastery orientation   Defines success in terms of how well the knowledge, skills, and abilities have been demonstrated.

Melbourne Curiosity Inventory   A self-reported measure that employs distinct trait and state subscales. Forty items (20 per subscale) assess thoughts and feelings about learning, exploring, problem solving, and questioning.

mentoring   Mentors often have in-depth, personal knowledge of their learners. Assumes a more intimate relationship. The mentor feels personal responsibility and, in turn, fulfillment when the protégé succeeds. Not to be confused with coaching or advising.

metacognition   Awareness and understanding of one's own thought processes.

metacognitive monitoring   More commonly known as reflection. A careful analysis of the evidence to generate an approach to the situation using a form of critical thinking.

Miller framework   A way of ranking clinical competence in educational settings and in the workplace. Distinguishes between knowledge at the lower levels and action in the higher levels.

motivation   The psychological energy that drives and directs us to accomplish defined goals. One of the four internal characteristics that drive the Master Adaptive Learning process. The other three are curiosity, growth mindset, and resilience.

motivational interviewing   A counseling method that helps people resolve ambivalent feelings and insecurities to find the internal motivation they need to change their behavior.

O

optimal adaptability corridor   A learning situation, or desirable difficulty, in which the individual's learning is situated to ensure that she balances innovation and routinization imperatives as she learns.

P

performance orientation   Emphasizes success in terms of markers of success outside the individual (grades, promotion, etc.)

Plan-Do-Study-Act   A health care system quality improvement strategy that can be incorporated into improvement strategies for individual physicians.

planning phase   Part of the Master Adaptive Learner framework. Incorporates three stages: identifying a gap, selecting an opportunity for learning, and searching for resources for learning.

preparation for future learning   Education theory that states downstream learning can be advantaged by learning designs that emphasize deep mechanistic and metacognitive understanding.

problem-based learning   The classroom method that most closely aligns with the priorities of the Master Adaptive Learner model. Small teams of learners identify learning objectives that will help them understand a clinical case. Following self-study, teams reassemble and discuss their learning.

procedural knowledge   One of the three categories of knowledge (along with conceptual and content knowledge). Knowledge applied to a given problem or task so as to affect a desired outcome.

R

reflective practice   The ability to reflect on one's actions so as to engage in a process of continuous learning.

resilience   One of the four internal characteristics that drive the Master Adaptive Learning process. Resilient learners cultivate specific skills, habits, and attitudes that enhance their capacity to have a healthy response to stress and achieve goals. The other three characteristics are motivation, growth mindset, and curiosity.

Rogers Innovation Curve   An organizational learning conceptualization acknowledging that organizations learn in a progressive fashion across individuals, among whom some are early adopters, some are late adopters, and the majority are somewhere in between.

routine expertise   Mastering a process to such an extent that a learner becomes highly efficient and accurate, even appearing to perform the process automatically. Contrast with innovation expertise and adaptive expertise.

S

scaffolding   Just enough, just-in-time, and just for the individual support from the group, instructors, and self-selected resources.

schemas   Cognitive structures that learners build over time to represent what they know about something.

scientific theory   Allied to the idea of a conceptual model but with a much higher standard of proof through the scientific method.

self-determination theory   Postulates that motivation is a continuum, ranging from amotivation (lack of motivation) to intrinsic motivation (pursuit of an activity for one's personal interest) self-generated by the individual.

self-directed learning   Learning that is metacognitively guided, is at least partly intrinsically motivated, and follows a strategic plan. Very similar to self-regulated learning, but self-directed learning places greater emphasis on the learner's independent definition of goals and evaluation of learning resources. It stems from adult education.

self-efficacy   The beliefs a learner holds about how successful he can be under adverse circumstances.

self-regulated learning Learning that is metacognitively guided, is at least partly intrinsically motivated, and follows a strategic plan. Very similar to self-directed learning but is somewhat more narrowly focused in school environments. It stems from childhood education.

systems thinking Enables learners to see the parts and the relationship between the parts of a system.

T

team-based learning Learners work on the same problem, thereby precluding individualized learning plans but maximizing opportunities for diverse group learning.

transfer of learning The process of applying learned knowledge or skill in a time and context remote from where it was developed. Implies the variable nature of such transfer and that instructional design can mitigate losses during the transfer.

U

unguided self-assessment Process wherein a trainee makes a judgment on her performance without examining external information about that performance.

W

WOOP A tool that can be used for goal creation. Stands for Wish-Outcome-Obstacle-Plan. The learner is prompted to focus on visualization (the Outcome) and anticipate and plan for a way of overcoming the obstacle(s) to his vision.

Z

zone of proximal development Learning that is hard enough to be worth doing, but not so hard that success is impossible, though success may follow a failure or two.

INDEX

Page numbers followed by *f* indicate figures; *b*, boxes; *t*, tables.